THIRD ED...

D1031504

THE DOCTOR OF NURSING PRACTICE ESSENTIALS

A New Model for Advanced Practice Nursing

Edited by

Mary E. Zaccagnini, DNP, APRN, ACNS-BC

Assistant Professor Ad Honorem
University of Minnesota
Minneapolis, Minnesota

Kathryn Waud White, DNP, APRN, CRNA

Associate Professor
University of Minnesota
Minneapolis, Minnesota

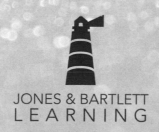

JONES & BARTLETT
LEARNING

World Headquarters
Jones & Bartlett Learning
5 Wall Street
Burlington, MA 01803
978-443-5000
info@jblearning.com
www.jblearning.com

Jones & Bartlett Learning books and products are available through most bookstores and online booksellers. To contact Jones & Bartlett Learning directly, call 800-832-0034, fax 978-443-8000, or visit our website, www.jblearning.com.

Substantial discounts on bulk quantities of Jones & Bartlett Learning publications are available to corporations, professional associations, and other qualified organizations. For details and specific discount information, contact the special sales department at Jones & Bartlett Learning via the above contact information or send an email to specialsales@jblearning.com.

The content, statements, views, and opinions herein are the sole expression of the respective authors and not that of Jones & Bartlett Learning, LLC. Reference herein to any specific commercial product, process, or service by trade name, trademark, manufacturer, or otherwise does not constitute or imply its endorsement or recommendation by Jones & Bartlett Learning, LLC and such reference shall not be used for advertising or product endorsement purposes. All trademarks displayed are the trademarks of the parties noted herein. *The Doctor of Nursing Practice Essentials: A New Model for Advanced Practice Nursing, Third Edition* is an independent publication and has not been authorized, sponsored, or otherwise approved by the owners of the trademarks or service marks referenced in this product.

There may be images in this book that feature models; these models do not necessarily endorse, represent, or participate in the activities represented in the images. Any screenshots in this product are for educational and instructive purposes only. Any individuals and scenarios featured in the case studies throughout this product may be real or fictitious, but are used for instructional purposes only.

The authors, editor, and publisher have made every effort to provide accurate information. However, they are not responsible for errors, omissions, or for any outcomes related to the use of the contents of this book and take no responsibility for the use of the products and procedures described. Treatments and side effects described in this book may not be applicable to all people; likewise, some people may require a dose or experience a side effect that is not described herein. Drugs and medical devices are discussed that may have limited availability controlled by the Food and Drug Administration (FDA) for use only in a research study or clinical trial. Research, clinical practice, and government regulations often change the accepted standard in this field. When consideration is being given to use of any drug in the clinical setting, the health care provider or reader is responsible for determining FDA status of the drug, reading the package insert, and reviewing prescribing information for the most up-to-date recommendations on dose, precautions, and contraindications, and determining the appropriate usage for the product. This is especially important in the case of drugs that are new or seldom used.

Production Credits

VP, Executive Publisher: David D. Cella
Executive Editor: Amanda Martin
Associate Acquisitions Editor: Rebecca Myrick
Editorial Assistant: Lauren Vaughn
Senior Production Editor: Amanda Clerkin
Senior Marketing Manager: Jennifer Scherzay
VP, Manufacturing and Inventory Control: Therese Connell

Composition: S4Carlisle Publishing Services
Cover Design: Kristin E. Parker
Rights & Media Specialist: Wes DeShano
Media Development Editor: Troy Liston
Cover Image: © tatko aparatko/Shutterstock
Printing and Binding: Edwards Brothers Malloy
Cover Printing: Edwards Brothers Malloy

Library of Congress Cataloging-in-Publication Data
The doctor of nursing practice essentials : a new model for advanced practice nursing/edited by Mary E. Zaccagnini, Kathryn Waud White. — Third edition.
    p. ; cm.
Includes bibliographical references and index.
ISBN 978-1-284-07970-8 (pbk.)
I. Zaccagnini, Mary E., editor. II. White, Kathryn Waud, editor.
[DNLM: 1. Education, Nursing, Graduate—United States. 2. Nurse Clinicians—education—United States. 3. Nurse Practitioners—education—United States. WY 18.5]
RT75
610.73092—dc23
                                  2015028480

6048

Printed in the United States of America
19 18 17 16 15   10 9 8 7 6 5 4 3 2 1

Dedication

This book is dedicated to all of our current and future DNP colleagues, especially those who so graciously gave of their time and volunteered to author this book.

Kathy & Mary

This book is also dedicated to my sister Karen, who passed away suddenly during the writing of the first edition of our book.

Mary

Contents

Preface

The Affordable Care Act, which has dramatically transformed every aspect of American health care, was signed into law on March 23, 2010 (Ray & Norbeck, 2014). More changes are undoubtedly coming. The societal forces driving the transformation of health care have been dissected, researched, and exhaustively discussed, debated, and documented. The primary question continues to be how to implement these changes in health care. Advanced practice nurses are now and will continue to be the nexus of that change. With the development of the doctor of nursing practice (DNP) program of study and the American Association of Colleges of Nursing's (AACN's) *Essentials of Doctoral Education for Advanced Nursing Practice*, we have the opportunity to place these ideas into action, to bring them into nursing practice in a way never before done. This text provides a nursing framework for transforming health care and the tools to make those changes.

The pace of change in advanced nursing education is rapid as well, and thus we are bringing the third edition of *The Doctor of Nursing Practice Essentials* to DNP students, graduates, and educators. In this edition, we have attempted to update all chapters and ideas, keeping in mind the changes in health care already brought about by legislative and economic forces. This edition includes a great depth of educator resources and expanded information about the DNP project. It continues to be unique in outlining a step-by-step template for the development of the DNP scholarly project.

It is important to mention that this text is unique in that it is authored by nurses who practice at an advanced level and who have achieved the DNP degree. Some fulfill traditional advanced practice roles and some have expanded roles as administrators, educators, and entrepreneurs. We are grateful for each of these nurses who took hours out of his or her busy practice to author these materials.

Purpose of the Text

This is intended to serve as a core text for DNP students and faculty to use to achieve mastery of the AACN Essentials as well as a "shelf reference" for practicing DNPs. The DNP Essentials are all covered herein; each essential is covered in adequate detail to frame the foundation of the DNP educational program. This text provides the infrastructure for students, faculty, and practicing DNPs to achieve and sustain the highest level of practice. Students who are exploring advanced practice nursing have Chapters 8 and 9 to refer to when investigating and imagining their new roles.

This text gives students the foundation necessary to enter into the highest level of advanced practice nursing and develop that practice to the highest level possible for the benefit of their patients and the health of the country and the world. For faculty, this text provides a framework that they can partner with their creativity to make their own unique programs, different from each other but all coming to the same endpoint: graduates who practice at the clinical doctorate level. For doctorally prepared advanced practice nurses, this book serves as a reference to reinforce their knowledge and skills as they take on leadership roles in health care. This text will help nurses prepared with clinical doctorates engage in advocacy, lead large and small organizations, integrate the skills of collaboration, and use informatics to demonstrate the value of nursing interventions, document quality clinical competencies, and improve the health of the nation.

Reference

Ray, W., & Norbeck, T. (2014). A look at how the president was able to sign Obamacare into law four years ago. *Forbes*, March 26, 2014.

Contributors

Laurel Ash, DNP, RN, FNP-BC
Essential Health Proctor
Proctor, Minnesota

Susan F. Burkart-Jayez, DNP, RN, FNP-BC
Occupational Health, Program Manager
Department of Veterans Affairs
VA Healthcare Network
Upstate New York at Albany
Albany, New York

Sandra R. Edwardson, PhD, RN, FAAN
Professor and Dean Emerita
School of Nursing
University of Minnesota
Minneapolis, Minnesota

Carole R. Eldridge, DNP, RN, CNE, NEA-BC
Vice President, Post-Licensure Programs
Chamberlain College of Nursing
Arlington, Virginia

Joy Elwell, DNP, FNP-BC, FAANP
Faculty
Frontier Nursing University
Hyden, Kentucky
Owner
Joy Elwell–FNP, LLC
Scarsdale, New York

Carol Flaten, DNP, RN
Clinical Assistant Professor
University of Minnesota
School of Nursing
Minneapolis, Minnesota

Timothy F. Gardner, DNP, FNP-BC
CEO/Family Primary Care Provider
Count to Ten Holistic Health Center
Gary, Indiana

Heather Jelnik, DNP, APRN, CNM
Riverside Clinic
Fairview Health System

Dan Lovinaria, BSN, MBA, DNP, APRN, CRNA
Assistant Clinical Professor
School of Nursing
University of Minnesota
Minneapolis, Minnesota

Sandra L. McPherson, DNP, RN-BC, CPHIMS
Director of Clinical Informatics
Lawrence and Memorial Hospital
New London, Connecticut

Catherine Miller, DNP, RN, CNP
Essential Health Spooner
Spooner, Wisconsin

Angela Mund, DNP, CRNA
Assistant Professor, Program
  Director
Anesthesia for Nurses
Medical University of South
  Carolina
Charleston, South Carolina

**Garrett J. Peterson, DNP, RN,
  CRNA**
Staff Nurse Anesthetist
Minneapolis Veterans Affairs Health
  Care System
Minneapolis, Minnesota

**Jeanne Pfeiffer, DNP, MPH,
  RN, CIC**
Clinical Associate Professor
School of Nursing
University of Minnesota
Minneapolis, Minnesota

**Sandra Wiggins Petersen, DNP,
  APRN, FNP-BC, GNP-BC,
  PMHNP**
Associate Professor
Family Nurse Practitioner Program
College of Nursing and Health
  Sciences
University of Texas
Tyler, Texas

**Deborah Ringdahl, DNP, RN,
  CNM**
Clinical Associate Professor
School of Nursing
University of Minnesota
Minneapolis, Minnesota

Melissa Saftner, PhD, APRN, CNM
Clinical Associate Professor
School of Nursing
University of Minnesota
Minneapolis, Minnesota

**Diane Schadewald, DNP, RN,
  CNP, WHNP, FNP**
Clinical Associate Professor
University of Wisconsin
Milwaukee, Wisconsin

**Gwendolyn Short, DNP, MSN,
  MPH**
Faculty
Frontier Nursing University
Hyden, Kentucky

**Catherine Tymkow, DNP, MS,
  APN, WHNP-BC**
CNE Associate Professor of Nursing
  and DNP Program Coordinator
Department of Nursing
College of Health and Human
  Services
Governors State University
University Park, Illinois

**Mary Jean Vickers, DNP, RN,
  ACNS-BC**
Program Manager, Clinical
  Development
University of Minnesota Medical
  Center, Fairview
Minneapolis, Minnesota

**Kathryn Waud White, DNP,
  RN, CRNA**
Clinical Associate Professor
School of Nursing
University of Minnesota
Minneapolis, Minnesota

**Mary E. Zaccagnini, DNP, RN,
  ACNS-BC**
Clinical Assistant Professor Ad
  Honorem
School of Nursing
University of Minnesota
Minneapolis, Minnesota

Imagining the DNP Role

Sandra R. Edwardson

Doctoral preparation in nursing has had a long development. From programs designed to prepare nursing faculty to the doctor of nursing practice (DNP), the profession has experienced several forms of doctoral education. Before describing the development of the DNP concept, its roots in doctoral education in nursing will be summarized.

Beginning in the mid-1950s with the first pre- and postdoctoral research grants and the research fellowship program of the Division of Nursing Resources (precursor of the Division of Nursing within the U.S. Public Health Service), nursing leaders have gradually won recognition at both the federal and university levels. Although the first emphasis was on preparing faculty and developing research programs, the call for clinical or professional programs was ever present.

Stevenson and Woods (1986) identified four generations of nurses with doctorates:

- 1900–1940: EdD or other functional degree offered through colleges of education to prepare nursing faculty
- 1940–1960: PhD in basic or social science with no nursing content
- 1960–1970: PhD in basic science with minor in nursing through nurse scientist programs offered in conjunction with basic science programs
- 1970–present: PhD in nursing or DNS
- 2000 and beyond: programs projected "greater specificity within nursing" and "formalized postdoctoral programs" (p. 8)

To this chronology we can now add the practice doctorate. Since formally approved by the American Association of Colleges of Nursing (AACN) in October 2004, a special study commissioned by AACN reported that, by April 2014, there were programs offered by more than 250 schools. Although many of the programs are offered by schools that also offer research doctorates, many are the only doctoral program in the school (AACN, 2011). Clearly the degree has made it possible for many schools unable or unwilling to offer research degrees to move into doctoral education. The Commission on Collegiate Nursing Education (CCNE) reported at least 177 accredited programs as of fall 2014 (CCNE, 2015).

From the beginning, the primary reason for wanting doctoral preparation in nursing was to develop the knowledge necessary for practice and to gain credibility within the academy. Some of the early programs were DNS[1] (doctor of nursing science) programs. In their earliest incarnations, the DNS programs were established as substitutes for the PhD (Meleis, 1988). This was because some states only allow the PhD to be offered through the main campus of the system or because the school was a baccalaureate-granting institution (Downs, 1989). In other cases, university officials believed that there was insufficient research and scholarship in nursing to justify a PhD degree. Therefore, some of the early schools seeking permission to establish PhD programs lacked a mechanism for doing so and chose the DNS as an option.

Early thinkers recommended PhD preparation for generation of new knowledge, and DNS programs to prepare individuals to apply that knowledge (Cleland, 1976; Peplau, 1966). This was in keeping with the statements of the Association of Graduate Schools and the Council of Graduate Schools, which distinguished the PhD from professional degrees: "The professional Doctor's degree should be the highest university award given in a particular field in recognition of completion of academic *preparation for professional practice*, whereas the Doctor of Philosophy should be given in recognition of *preparation for research* whether the particular field of learning is pure or applied" (Council of Graduate Schools in the United States, 1966, p. 3).

Over time, the purpose of DNS programs tended to move toward research preparation. Noting the number of articles describing the differences and similarity in types of nursing doctoral programs, Starck, Duffy, and Vogler (1993) proposed that the DNS prepares individuals "in a specialized area of practice for the purpose of testing and validating application of" knowledge that extends and generates nursing practice protocols (p. 214). They advocated for content, including healthcare practices; biologic, psychosocial, economic, legal, and ethical knowledge; and research methods for investigating clinical problems.

---

[1]DNS is used as a shorthand for Doctor of Nursing Science (DNS or DNSc), Doctor of Science in Nursing (DSN).

An analysis of the curricula of PhD and DNS programs showed that there was more clinical emphasis in the latter, but the differences between the programs as they were implemented were very subtle (Edwardson, 2004). Florence Downs (1989), the long-term editor of *Nursing Research*, conducted an informal review of topics by PhD and DNS authors in the journal. It revealed essentially the same number of manuscripts on clinical topics by each. Her bottom line was that she was less concerned about the structure and content of the programs than with their quality and excellence.

Practice Doctorates

There are subtle though uncertain distinctions between professional degrees such as the DNS and practice degrees such as the DNP. The Council of Graduate Schools appointed a task force to examine the growth of professional programs, but it too has been grappling with defining exactly what they are (Council of Graduate Schools, 2007). European and Australian universities have also attempted to make meaningful distinctions between professional and research degrees. In those countries, professional doctorates have been attempts to make the doctorate more focused on the application of knowledge to the solution of societal problems (Maxwell, Shanahan, & Green, 2001).

In the United States, professional doctorates have existed for many years in fields such as education (EdD). Although subtle, the major distinction between a professional and a practice degree seems to be in the goals. In the view of Starck et al. (1993), the DNS has as its purpose the testing and validation of knowledge to extend and generate nursing practice protocols. In other words, the purpose is to extend the knowledge generated by research doctorates by testing it in practice. The practice doctorate, on the other hand, is the highest level preparation for the actual practice of the discipline. Holders of practice doctorates are in the business of applying knowledge as they provide direct service to clients. In so doing, they may also do systematic inquiry similar to that of the holders of professional or research degrees, but the primary purpose of the degree is to prepare practitioners.

The first nursing doctoral degree dedicated solely to practice was the doctor of nursing (ND) established at Case Western Reserve University in 1979 (Case Western Reserve University, n.d.). It began as an entry-level nursing degree but evolved into a program offering preparation for advanced practice. Few other schools embraced the ND degree, and by the late 1990s, only one program (University of Colorado) offered an entry-level program.

There are many examples of practice-focused degrees in other disciplines, including entry-level degrees such as the doctor of medicine (MD) and juris doctor (JD), and advanced practice degrees such as the doctor of psychology (PsyD). In the early part of the 21st century, existing practice-focused degrees in nursing were mainly advanced practice doctoral degrees. They included the ND at Case Western Reserve University, Rush University, and the University of South Carolina; a DNSc at the University of Tennessee, Memphis; the doctor of nursing practice (DNP) at the University of Kentucky; and the DrNP at Columbia University.

The DrNP (now DNP) offered by Columbia provides greater depth and breadth of knowledge and practice than existing master's programs in clinical science, informatics, and research methods. It is also designed to prepare students to admit and co-manage patients as well as discharge patients from hospitals. They are expected to be able to provide care from the outpatient to the inpatient setting and vice versa (Mundinger, 2005).

The AACN Role in Creating the DNP

This brief review of our history brings us to 1999. In that year, the board of the AACN appointed a task force to revise quality indicators for doctoral education and to address the differences among three types of nursing doctorates: PhD, DNSc/DNS/DSN, and ND degrees. The task force was able to prepare a revised version of the *Indicators of Quality in Research-Focused Doctoral Programs in Nursing* (2001) but found that, for all its attempts to make distinctions between research degrees (PhD) and professional degrees (DNS, DNSc, DSN), the faculty of programs that offer the DNS/DSN degrees saw the need for a common set of quality indicators for both. The task force members concluded that there may be differences in the roles for which the graduates are prepared and in the curricular content of the programs, but the basic requirements for quality programs were viewed as the same for research and professional degrees.

Based on its analysis, the quality indicators task force constructed **Figure 1** to describe what was happening in the field. Although it was able to address the research half of the model, there was insufficient time and clarity to deal with the practice-focused half of the model. There seemed to be only one true entry-level doctorate (ND) left at the time, although the discussion suggested that a number of AACN member deans thought that the idea ought to be resurrected. Other programs, such as those at the University of Kentucky, Columbia University, and the

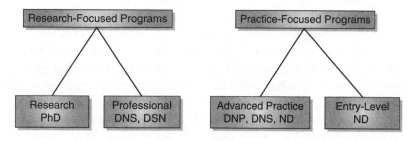

Figure 1 Proposed Classification of Nursing Doctorates
Reprinted from *Journal of Professional Nursing, 20*(1), Edwardson, S. R., Matching standards and needs in doctoral education in nursing, Pages 40–46, Copyright 2004, with permission from Elsevier.

University of Tennessee–Memphis had emerged to give nurses advanced practice preparation at the doctoral level, but they too differed in goals and structure.

Because of the lack of clarity concerning the right half of the model, the quality indicators task force recommended appointment of a second group to study it, and the Task Force on the Clinical Doctorate in Nursing (later renamed the Task Force on the Practice Doctorate in Nursing) was established to focus on that issue alone (AACN, 2004). There were several resources available for the group's work, but the task force also found it necessary to gather some information on its own.

Marion and colleagues noted discernible differences between practice-focused and research-focused programs. Practice-focused programs place less emphasis on theory, meta-theory, and research methods than do research-focused programs. Capstone projects are designed to solve practice problems or inform practice with an emphasis on scholarly practice and outcome evaluation. Clinical practica or residencies are required (Marion et al., 2003).

After considering published definitions and consulting with leaders in health care and nursing education, the task force defined *practice* as follows:

> *The term practice, specifically nursing practice, as conceptualized in this document, refers to any form of nursing intervention that influences health care outcomes for individuals or populations, including the direct care of individual patients, management of care for individuals and populations, administration of nursing and health care organizations, and the development and implementation of health policy. Preparation at the practice doctorate level includes advanced preparation in nursing, based on nursing. (AACN, 2004)*

There was controversy about including in the definition roles other than nurse practitioner, clinical nurse specialist, nurse-midwife, or nurse anesthetist. But the task force concluded that caring for populations and seeing to the arrangements under which nursing is practiced were equally important as direct clinical care for advancing the health of the public. Omitted from the definition was preparation for nursing education. This omission is consistent with PhD and practice education in other disciplines in which preparation concentrates on the specific specialty or subspecialty, and preparation for faculty roles is something that is added as a separate discipline. In short, the task force concluded that nursing faculty need substantive expertise in the subject matter of the discipline and not just pedagogical theory and practice.

Another topic of considerable discussion was the title. Whereas many in the task force might have preferred the simple doctor of nursing or DN label, a search of titles revealed that DN was reserved for the doctor of naprapathy (NaturalHealers, 2015). Similarly, the ND degree title was in use by doctors of naturopathy (American Association of Naturopathic Physicians, n.d.) in some states and not available to us. It was finally concluded that there should be only one title and that it should be doctor of nursing practice. It was thought to be the most descriptive title despite the assumption of some that it referred only to nurse practitioners. The task force recommended that the ND be phased out.

A transitional plan was also proposed. Knowing that most of the graduates of the programs would want or need specialty certification, it was clear that the education sector could establish the educational preparation for the role but had no control over the certification process. Therefore, the recommendation was that the many bodies that certify nurses set the year 2015 as the time when initial certification would require the DNP degree.

A final discussion focused on quality control. Whereas the quality of PhD programs is the responsibility of graduate schools, professional and practice degrees are typically awarded by professional schools without the built-in quality control mechanisms provided by graduate schools. For this reason, the task force recommended that an accreditation process similar to that for master's and baccalaureate programs be established to assure quality in DNP programs. The CCNE took up the challenge immediately, developed the criteria, and began reviewing DNP programs in the fall of 2008. The CCNE has since accredited at least 177 programs (CCNE, 2015). As of July 2014, 243 programs were enrolling students across the nation, with another 70 under development (AACN, 2014).

Factors Propelling the Practice Doctorate

From the outset, the DNP had significant opposition. Several nationally recognized leaders in nursing objected based on the fears that the degree would detract from the hard-fought growth and recognition of research in nursing and of nursing in the academy. Meleis and Dracup (2005) argued that the MS and PhD degrees are widely understood and accepted and that a new doctoral degree would amount to second-class citizenship. They believe that the nursing doctorate should be dedicated to advancing and translating knowledge and that separating the practice and research foci could thwart knowledge development and interfere with establishing evidence for quality and safety in health care. Having been among those who fought most vigorously for the acceptance of nursing as a bona fide academic discipline, they feared the DNP would lead to remarginalization within the academy. Others see the two degrees as complementary to one another (Edwardson, 2010).

Many factors led to the perceived need for the DNP. First was the growing complexity of the healthcare environment, coupled with the rapid expansion of knowledge required for practice. Groups such as the Institute of Medicine, the Robert Wood Johnson Foundation, and others urged health profession educators to meet this growing complexity with educational programs that acknowledge the high levels of scientific knowledge and practice expertise required to ensure high-quality patient outcomes. The Institute of Medicine, for example, emphasized the need for all health professions programs to prepare students able to deliver patient-centered care as members of interdisciplinary teams that emphasize evidence-based practice, quality improvement, and informatics (Institute of Medicine, 2003a).

Another Institute of Medicine report observed how management decisions in healthcare organizations had expanded the responsibilities of chief nursing executives, increased the scope of responsibilities for all nursing managers, and led to the loss of mid-level nurse managers (Institute of Medicine, 2003b). The result has been that nurses at all levels need increased knowledge and administrative skills to provide the needed leadership. The Institute of Medicine recommended preparation of nursing leaders for all levels of management and encouraged nursing managers to participate in executive decisions (Institute of Medicine, 2003b).

Another factor propelling the DNP was the movement to doctoral entry levels in related health professions such as pharmacy and physical therapy. These professions had recognized the need for advanced preparation to realize fully their potential contribution to health care. Lest it appear that this was a keeping-up-with-the-Joneses rationale, there were others who saw the need for doctoral preparation of practitioners. For example, a landmark study by the National Research Council of the National Academies (2005) noted the following: "The need for doctorally prepared practitioners and clinical faculty would be met if nursing could develop a new non-research clinical doctorate, similar to the M.D. and Pharm.D. in medicine and pharmacy, respectively" (p. 74). But the DNP, which is designed for nurses who are already licensed practitioners, is unlike the doctoral degrees in other health disciplines that are required for entry into the professions.

Leaders of national nursing, medical, and healthcare organizations with whom the Task Force on the Practice Doctorate met confirmed the need for nurses able to deal with the increasing complexity and sophistication of health care. In response to concerns that the DNP might amount to degree creep, they were sympathetic to the need for additional preparation and expressed confidence that such preparation would add value (AACN, 2004).

As noted earlier, eight clinically focused programs were in existence when the Task Force on the Practice Doctorate began its work. The task force survey of these programs showed considerable variation among the programs in design but also revealed some commonalities. The commonalities included content related to advanced clinical practice (including both patient and practice management), organizations, systems, and leadership skills, research methods, and basic scientific underpinnings for practice (AACN, 2004).

Yet another issue propelling the development of the DNP was the way master's programs had responded to the inexorable growth in scientific knowledge and technological sophistication. To fulfill their obligation to provide adequate preparation and to meet the requirements of specialty certification bodies, nursing schools had gradually expanded their master's curricula. In many schools, programs required upward of 50% more credits than typical for master's programs, increasing the cost and time for completing the program. At one school, for example, the minimum credits required from high school graduation to program completion for a family nurse practitioner degree and a PharmD degree were equal. This suggested that it was time to recognize the preparation with an appropriate degree.

Of course, curriculum length should not be the only criterion for a new degree. Despite the expanded credit requirements of master's programs, practicing nurse practitioners continued to ask for additional preparation in health policy, management, informatics, evaluation of evidence, and advanced diagnosis and care management (Lenz, Mundinger, Hopkins, Clark, & Lin, 2002). Therefore, the Task Force on the Practice Doctorate and its successor, Task Force on the Essentials of the DNP, both recommended curricula that would not only meet the requirements of existing master's programs but would also respond to the Institute of

Medicine's call for greater facility with evidence-based practice, quality improvement, and informatics (Institute of Medicine, 2003a). This is in keeping with the position of the National Organization of Nurse Practitioner Faculties, which called for additional preparation in business practices, information management, health literacy, end-of-life care, genetics, mental health concepts, caring for older adults, and managed care (Bellack, Graber, O'Neil, Musham, & Lancaster, 1999).

Some have objected to the DNP based on the assumption that it was preparation to replace physicians. This was especially troublesome to the American Medical Association (AMA), which saw the emergence of the degree as an attempt to educate nursing students with skills equivalent to primary care physicians. Its House of Delegates in June 2008 passed Resolution 214, which stated "that our AMA adopt a policy that those nurses who are Doctors of Nursing Practice must only be able to practice under the supervision of a physician and as part of a medical team with the final authority and responsibility for the patient under the supervision of a licensed physician" (AMA, 2008a). Resolution 232 from the same meeting declared that "the title 'Doctor,' in a medical setting, apply only to physicians licensed to practice medicine in all its branches, dentists and podiatrists" and that the organization should serve to protect, through legislation, the titles "Doctor," "Resident," and "Residency" (AMA, 2008b).

Some nurses, too, feared that the growing role of advanced practice nurses in primary care could lead to abandoning the unique role and contribution of nurses. Yet there is growing evidence that advanced practice nurses can and do provide services that allow for the full expression of the nurse's role while also filling gaps for needed services in the system (Brooten, Youngblut, Deatrick, Naylor, & York, 2003; Brooten et al., 1986; Lenz, Mundinger, Kane, Hopkins, & Lin, 2004; Naylor & McCauley, 1999). Nurses are proving to have important roles in filling the need for primary and chronic care for all population groups, but especially the growing number of elderly and those living longer with chronic illnesses.

Finally, the shortage of doctorally prepared nursing faculty has been a growing concern within the discipline as schools find themselves turning away qualified applicants partly because of a shortage of faculty. Although the number of PhD programs grew substantially throughout the 1990s, most schools graduated fewer than four or five new PhDs per year (Edwardson, 2004). Schools, including those with PhD programs, had employed master's-prepared practitioners to fill the need for faculty prepared to supervise beginning and advanced nursing students. Although the DNP was specifically designed as advanced preparation for the *practice* of the discipline, many saw DNPs as one way to fill the void for faculty with advanced practice expertise. They could complement and supplement PhD-prepared faculty whose time is increasingly consumed with the scholarship so necessary for the growth and contribution of the discipline (Sebastian & Delaney, 2013). As O'Sullivan, Carter, Marion, Pohl, and Werner (2005) argued, the myth that a practice doctorate would have an adverse impact on the PhD degree was countered by the reality that it will help "to preserve the integrity of the PhD as a true research degree" (p. 7).

The Future

Although educators, practitioners, and administrators agree that the added content found in the DNP education brings value to health care, the master's of science in nursing (MSN) continues to be the primary route for entry into advanced practice nursing, with limited impetus to replace the MSN with the direct path to the DNP from the BSN degree. Several barriers to the growth of the BSN-to-DNP, as entry into practice, have been elucidated by the RAND study completed in 2014. Those barriers include lack of faculty resources, budgetary concerns, lack of administrative support, and lack of differentiation between MSN- and DNP-prepared nurses on the part of employers (Auerbach et al., 2014).

The nursing profession has followed a long and varied path for preparing its practitioners. DNP graduates hold promise for investigating and solving some of the vexing problems facing our healthcare system and delivering the highest level of nursing practice. As knowledge workers, nurses can no longer rely on tradition and task orientation as their substantive base. Rather, they need facility with obtaining and maintaining the most current and evidence-based knowledge to inform their practice. The DNP has been designed to give its practitioners the tools for navigating complex systems and mining the latest available knowledge. Early indications are that DNP-prepared nurses are up to the task.

References

American Association of Colleges of Nursing. (2001). *Indicators of quality in research-focused doctoral programs in nursing.* Washington, DC: Author.

American Association of Colleges of Nursing. (2004). *AACN position statement on practice doctorates in nursing.* Washington, DC: Author.

American Association of Colleges of Nursing. (2011). *The doctor of nursing practice.* Washington, DC: Author. Retrieved from http://www.aacn.nche.edu/media-relations/fact-sheets/dnp

American Association of Colleges of Nursing. (2014). *DNP talking points.* Retrieved from http://www.aacn.nche.edu/dnp/about/talking-points

American Association of Naturopathic Physicians. (n.d.). *What is naturopathic medicine?* Retrieved from http://www.naturopathic.org

American Medical Association. (2008a, June). House of Delegates Resolution 214.

American Medical Association. (2008b, June). House of Delegates Resolution 232.

Auerbach, D. I., Martsolf, G., Pearson, M. L., Taylor, E. A., Zaydman, M., Muchow, A., . . . Dower, C. (2014). *The DNP by 2015: A study of the institutional, political, and professional issues that facilitate or impede establishing a post-baccalaureate doctor of nursing practice program.* Santa Monica, CA: The RAND Corporation.

Bellack, J. P., Graber, D. R., O'Neil, E. H., Musham, C., & Lancaster, C. (1999). Curriculum trends in nurse practitioner programs: Current and ideal. *Journal of Professional Nursing, 15*(1), 15–27.

Brooten, D., Kumar, S., Brown, L. P., Butts, P., Finkler, S. A., Bakewell-Sachs, S., . . . Delivoria-Papadopoulos, M. (1986). A randomized clinical trial of early discharge and home follow-up of very low birth weight infants. *New England Journal of Medicine, 315*(15), 934–939.

Brooten, D., Youngblut, J. M., Deatrick, J., Naylor, M., & York, R. (2003). Patient problems, advanced practice nurse interventions, time and contacts among five patient groups. *Journal of Nursing Scholarship, 35*(1), 73–79.

Case Western Reserve University. (n.d.). *DNP: The future of advanced nursing practice.* Retrieved from http://fpb.case.edu/DNP

Cleland, V. (1976). Develop a doctoral program. *Nursing Outlook, 2*(6), 631–635.

Commission on Collegiate Nursing Education. (2015). *Accredited doctor of nursing practice (DNP) programs.* Washington, DC: Author. Retrieved from http://directory.ccnecommunity.org/reports/rptAccreditedPrograms_New.asp?sort=institution&sProgramType=3

Council of Graduate Schools in the United States. (1966). *The doctor's degree in professional fields. A statement by the Association of Graduate Schools and the Council of Graduate Schools in the United States.* Washington, DC: Author.

Council of Graduate Schools. (2007). *Task Force Report on the Professional Doctorate* (p. 1). Council of Graduate Schools, Washington, DC.

Downs, F. S. (1989). Differences between the professional doctorate and the academic/research doctorate. *Journal of Professional Nursing, 5*(5), 261–265.

Edwardson, S. R. (2004). Matching standards and needs in doctoral education in nursing. *Journal of Professional Nursing, 20*(1), 40–46.

Edwardson, S. R. (2010). Doctor of philosophy and doctor of nursing practice as complementary degrees. *Journal of Professional Nursing, 26*(3), 137–140.

Institute of Medicine. (2003a). *Health professions education: A bridge to quality.* Washington, DC: National Academies Press.

Institute of Medicine. (2003b). *Keeping patients safe: Transforming the work environment of nurses.* Washington, DC: National Academies Press.

Lenz, E. R., Mundinger, M. O., Hopkins, S., Clark, J., & Lin, S. (2002, September). *Patterns of nurse practitioner practice: Results from a national survey.* Presented at State of the Science Conference, Washington, DC.

Lenz, E. R., Mundinger, M. O., Kane, R. L., Hopkins, S. C., & Lin, S. X. (2004). Primary care outcomes in patients treated by nurse practitioners or physicians: Two-year follow-up. *Medical Care Research and Review, 61*(3), 332–351.

Marion, L., Viens, D., O'Sullivan, A., Crabtree, C., Fontana, S., & Price, M. (2003). The practice doctorate in nursing: Future or fringe? *Medscape.* Retrieved from http://www.medscape.com

Maxwell, T. W., Shanahan, P., & Green, B. (2001). Introduction: New opportunities in doctoral education and professional practice. In B. Green, T. W. Maxwell, & P. Shanahan (Eds.), *Doctoral education and professional practice: The next generation?* (pp. 1–13). Armidale, New South Wales, Australia: Kardoorair.

Meleis, A. I. (1988). Doctoral education in nursing: Its present and its future. *Journal of Professional Nursing, 4*(6), 436–446.

Meleis, A., & Dracup, K. (2005, September 30). The case against the DNP: History, timing, substance, and marginalization. *Online Journal of Issues in Nursing, 10*(3). Manuscript 2. Retrieved from http://www.nursingworld.org/MainMenuCategories/ANAMarketplace/ANAPeriodicals/OJIN

Mundinger, M. O. (2005). Who's who in nursing: Bringing clarity to the doctor of nursing practice. *Nursing Outlook, 53,* 173–176.

National Research Council of the National Academies (2005). *Advancing the nation's health needs: NIH research training programs.* Washington. DC: National Academies Press.

NaturalHealers. (2015). *Naprapathic medicine training and careers.* Retrieved from http://www.naturalhealers.com/naprapathy/

Naylor, M. D., & McCauley, K. M. (1999). The effects of a discharge planning and home follow-up intervention on elders hospitalized with common medical and surgical cardiac conditions. *Journal of Cardiovascular Nursing, 14*(1), 44–54.

O'Sullivan, A., Carter, M., Marion, L., Pohl, J., & Werner, K. (2005, September 30). Moving forward together: The practice doctorate in nursing. *Online Journal of Issues in Nursing, 10*(3), Manuscript 4. Retrieved from http://www.nursingworld.org/MainMenuCategories/ANAMarketplace/ANAPeriodicals/OJIN/TableofContents/Volume102005/No3Sept05/tpc28_416028.aspx

Peplau, H. E. (1966). Nursing's two routes to doctoral degrees. *Nursing Forum, 5*(2), 57–67.

Sebastian, J. G., & Delaney, C. W. (2013). Doctor of nursing practice programs: Opportunities for faculty development. *Journal of Nursing Education, 52*(8), 453–461.

Starck, P. L., Duffy, M. E., & Vogler, R. (1993). Developing a nursing doctorate for the 21st century. *Journal of Professional Nursing, 9*(4), 212–219.

Stevenson, J. S., & Woods, N. F. (1986). Nursing science and contemporary science: Emerging paradigms. In G. E. Sorensen (Ed.), *Setting the agenda for the year 2000: Knowledge development in nursing* (pp. 6–20). Kansas City, MO: American Academy of Nursing.

Part I

Essentials for Practice

Chapter 1

Nursing Science and Theory: Scientific Underpinnings for Practice

Carole R. Eldridge

> *All truth passes through three stages. First, it is ridiculed. Second, it is violently opposed. Third, it is accepted as being self-evident.*
>
> —Arthur Schopenhauer

> *Nursing requires knowledge.*
>
> —Mark Risjord

Advanced practice nurses tend to be pragmatic in their view of nursing, focusing on whether something "works" in their practice and with their clients. We look for actions and their consequences, believing that every effect has a discernible and, it is hoped, treatable cause. We understand that science is essential to clinical practice. We can apply scientific knowledge to real-life problems. However, clinical practitioners are often inclined to discard theory as too abstract for practical purposes and too broad to have meaningful application to daily nursing practice.

This view, which seems to eschew the value of philosophical thought, is actually a philosophical stance of its own. Whether we appreciate it or not, every nurse operates from a philosophical and theoretical base. The mature doctor of nursing practice (DNP) acknowledges this and seeks to understand the values, beliefs, and ideas that inform his or her daily practice. Practicing at the doctoral level is a highly complex, rich, multileveled experience that demands deeper insights if we are to effectively help our clients and represent our profession. Nursing knowledge is built on relevant science and theory, and understanding that foundation is central to effective advanced nursing practice.

As we explore the meaning of our practice as doctorally prepared advanced practice nurses, there are several questions to consider. What are the scientific and theoretical concepts that should underpin DNP practice? Where do we find this knowledge? How does the DNP-prepared advanced practice nurse close the gap between theory and practice to use scientific concepts at the bedside? How might the DNP graduate manipulate theoretical and scientific concepts differently than other healthcare providers? What philosophies and values guide the decisions and actions of the DNP in the clinical setting?

DNP-prepared advanced practice nurses bring specific expertise to their work, based on a very particular grounding in the scholarship of application and translational science. This chapter examines some of the scientific and theoretical concepts that undergird the DNP.

Nursing Science

What Is Nursing Science?

Before defining the specific domain of nursing science, we should examine science itself. Science is variously defined as the study of something, the knowledge gained by that study, or the methodological activity required to gain the knowledge. Burns and Grove (2001) defined science as a body of knowledge—as the research findings and theories that have been developed, tested, and accepted by a specific discipline. They agreed with numerous others who have said that science is both a product (knowledge) and a process of methodical study. Barrett (2002) postulated that science is our ongoing effort to discover truth. As such, it is always evolving and being revised.

The scientific underpinnings of DNP practice are not confined to nursing science and theory. Nursing has always drawn its knowledge from a wide array of other domains, including biology, physiology, zoology, medicine, psychology, sociology, physics, mathematics, chemistry, communication, philosophy, and theology. Risjord (2010) argued that when the nursing profession attempts to differentiate nursing science within a specific nursing metaparadigm, the effort "isolates nursing inquiry from other domains, and . . . has contributed to the theory-practice gap" (p. 219). An integrated view of science as a multifaceted body of knowledge from which nursing science draws and to which it contributes serves the profession better, particularly as we develop interdisciplinary approaches to patient care.

That said, we should seek to understand the specific contributions of nursing science to scientific knowledge, starting with the definition of nursing. Nursing has been defined in multiple ways, depending on the particular philosophical or professional paradigm of those doing the defining. The view of nursing as a function is captured in Fawcett's (2000) definition of nursing as actions taken by nurses and the outcomes achieved by those actions. Parse (1997) offered a different focus when she wrote that nursing is a discipline organized around nursing knowledge and that the practice of nursing is a performing art. Rogers (1994) wrote that it is not the practice of nursing that defines nursing; rather, it is the use of nursing knowledge to improve the human condition. King (1990) spoke of nursing as a process of interactions within and between systems. Reed (1997) proposed that, just as archeology is the study of ancient things and biology the study of living things, nursing is the study of promoting well-being.

Actions and outcomes, a discipline, special knowledge, an art, a process, a study of processes, and interacting systems represent just some of the varied definitions of nursing. Four metaparadigm concepts of nursing have gathered general, although not exclusive or universal, acceptance in the nursing body of knowledge: person, environment, nursing, and health. *The Essentials of Doctoral Education for Advanced Nursing Practice* by the American Association of Colleges of Nursing (AACN) reflects nursing's conceptual heritage with this statement describing the focus of the discipline of nursing:

- The principles and laws that govern the life-process, well-being, and optimal function of human beings, sick or well;
- The patterning of human behavior in interaction with the environment in normal life events and critical life situations;
- The nursing actions or processes by which positive changes in health status are effected; and
- The wholeness or health of human beings recognizing that they are in continuous interaction with their environments. (Donaldson & Crowley, 1978; Fawcett, 2005; and Gortner, 1980, as cited in AACN, 2006, p. 9)

These foundational concepts address nursing in its many facets—as a discipline with special knowledge of human beings, human behavior, health, and human interaction with the environment, as well as the actions and processes that affect health.

The attempt to define nursing science is complicated by the debate over whether nursing is a pure or fundamental science, also called basic science, or an applied science. Pure science focuses on building knowledge without the concern shown by applied science for the practical applications of theories and concepts. A number of influential nurse authors have promoted the idea that nursing is a basic science with its own body of knowledge focused on the human environment (or universe) health process (Parse, 1999). The DNP-prepared nurse is generally taught to use existing evidence to create practice change, which promotes practical application. Translational science is a multidisciplinary approach that translates laboratory science to the bedside or the community. Translational science and the scholarship of practice can close the theory–practice gap while adding to the scientific body of knowledge.

The way scientific knowledge is obtained in a given field varies. Observation and measurement of the phenomena being studied, followed by description and explanation of the findings, is the most familiar form of scientific research. Experiments or interventions may be performed on the phenomena and the impact recorded. Replication of scientific studies, with similar results each time, is required before the information gained can be included in the body of accepted knowledge. Research is the process we use to create science. Theories are often developed from research findings, and more research may be conducted to test the theories. Scientific theories form the framework that holds research together and builds scientific knowledge (Barrett, 2002; Burns & Grove, 2001).

In nursing, certain research methodologies and theoretical frameworks have been, and continue to be, developed that are unique to the discipline. Many nurse researchers believe that the progress of nursing as a discipline, science, and practice depends on developing distinctive, nursing-specific theories and research methods. Other factors and methods besides replicable laboratory studies can contribute to scientific knowledge; indeed, such things as abstract thought, intuition, judgment, and experience are essential to scientific advancement (Phillips, 1996).

Instead of emphasizing the uniqueness of nursing science, Meleis (1992) proposed that a mature nursing science will be part of an integrated approach to healthcare science, with some of the theories developed and tested by nurses and some of the theories contributed by other domains of knowledge. This view attempts to close the theory–practice gap by placing nursing theory and science in the midst of other disciplines that are adding to, and sharing, the knowledge of human health.

Risjord (2010) proposed a new view of nursing science built on these principles: (1) practice problems should guide nursing research, (2) theory and practice are in a dynamic relationship, (3) theory-based research should build the knowledge needed for nursing interventions, and (4) nursing research and theories are strengthened when integrated with, and confirmed by, the research and theories of other disciplines.

In *The Essentials of Doctoral Education for Advanced Nursing Practice* (2006), the AACN adopted a definition of nursing science as an entity in itself, with a growing body of scientific knowledge, while acknowledging the value of incorporating knowledge from other sciences. Nursing science is unique, with a particular concern for the factors that affect human wellness, but it draws from any and all of the broader realms of theoretical and scientific thought that can contribute to the nursing body of knowledge. The document states,

> *Preparation to address current and future practice issues*
> *requires a strong scientific foundation for practice. The*
> *scientific foundation of nursing practice has expanded and*
> *includes a focus on both the natural and social sciences. . . .*
> *In addition, philosophical, ethical, and historical issues*
> *inherent in the development of science create a context for*
> *the application of the natural and social sciences. Nursing*
> *science also has created a significant body of knowledge*
> *to guide nursing practice and has expanded the scientific*
> *underpinnings of the discipline. (p. 9)*

Phillips (1996) emphasized that nursing science is not made up solely of facts. Instead, nursing science is a pattern, a particular way of obtaining, understanding, and using scientific knowledge. This pattern brings unity to the body of nursing knowledge. Silva (1999) questioned the necessity of requiring linear reasoning and logic in nursing science, believing that nursing science should encompass other ways of knowing besides mechanistic data-in, knowledge-out empirical processes. Some have argued for the dynamic coexistence of multiple paradigms or ways of knowing. Monti and Tingen (1999) proposed that multiple paradigms in nursing science are indicative of a flourishing science in which creativity, debate, diversity, and open inquiry serve to strengthen the exchange of multiple points of view and the growth of knowledge.

The definition of nursing science offered by Stevenson and Woods (1986) provides a useful point of view by emphasizing practical knowledge about the health problems DNP graduates encounter in practice: "Nursing science is the domain of knowledge concerned with the adaptation of individuals and groups to actual or potential health problems, the environments that influence health in humans and the therapeutic interventions that promote health and affect the consequences of illness" (p. 6).

How Nursing Science Differs from Medical Science

Much of the controversy about nursing science centers on the distinctiveness of nursing's body of knowledge, particularly its differentiation from medical science. The study and practice of medicine focuses on the diagnosis and treatment of disease. Nursing focuses on the human response to illness and its treatment. Yet, medicine and nursing overlap at many points, and seemingly even more so in advanced practice nursing. Do medicine and nursing truly differ in anything besides mere scope of practice?

As a general rule, people enter the healthcare system because they have a problem. A sick person wants to know what is causing his or her symptoms and wants the healthcare provider to make the symptoms go away. Medical providers seek to solve the diagnostic riddle and apply a treatment to cure the disease or, at the least, calm the symptoms. This approach is mechanistic and could imply that humans are machines that can be fixed by identifying the problem and intervening at the point of the breakdown. In this context, nurses usually operate as assistants to physicians or as providers operating under the approval and guidance of a physician (Parse, 1999). This paradigm confines nurses to the boxes drawn and controlled by medical thought and perspectives. If we follow the medical model, nursing science is an applied science that is concerned primarily with using things learned in other disciplines.

If, however, we view nursing science as a basic science, we open new ways of thinking and acting as advanced practice nurses. Holistic theories and approaches address broad concepts of health, wholeness, caring, and healing of entire systems instead of being limited to the medical concept of curing a disease. Taking this broader, patient-centered, holistic view presents significant challenges in a healthcare system based on the medical model. The current healthcare system, however, is infamously dysfunctional, and the time has arrived for a reexamination of the ways we conceptualize and implement nursing.

When we start from the premise that nursing science is a unique body of knowledge containing theories and evidence intuited, observed, and tested by nurses involved in the processes of human health, we can follow where the evidence leads (Parse, 1999). This is the difference that advanced practice nurses can make, the contribution the DNP graduate should provide to nursing science. The advanced practice nurse begins with the human being, not with the disease, and with the individual human's unique values and goals. The person and the nurse embark on an experiential journey together, with the nurse's knowledge informing and guiding the person along a path that belongs only to the person within his or her special environment.

Every advanced practice nurse should be a nurse scientist, gathering evidence at the patient's side, making observations, having experiences, responding to the patient's experiences, and thinking about reasons, theories, or concepts that might organize the evidence. DNP graduates should examine their own thinking and that of others, testing the concepts and gathering new evidence as an essential part of the nursing process. Throughout the nursing–human interaction, the advanced practice nurse views the individual holistically, as a complex person with unique values and goals, and never treating the patient as an object that can be passively acted on by a benevolent, all-knowing medical and nursing force.

Nursing is commonly accepted as a human science that focuses on human experiences, and nursing's holistic framework is widely acknowledged, but this framework is not always thought to include medicine and the biomedical model. Nursing should incorporate, but not be limited to, biomedical science as part of its holistic approach to healing and health. Rather than merely performing delegated medical tasks, professional nurses incorporate medical treatments and cures within their broader approach to health and wellness, treating the whole person with nursing interventions that do not spring solely from a limited biomedical approach (Bunkers, 2002; Engebretson, 1997).

Fawcett (1999) painted a vision of nursing scholarship and advanced nursing practice that placed nurses squarely and constantly at the patient's side. In her vision, research and practice occur at the bedside by the nurse using nursing concepts, methodologies, and theories. Each interaction between the nurse and the patient is a research case that tests the nursing model guiding the encounter. Clinical data are examined to support, refute, or revise nursing theories. Every nurse and every patient contributes continuously to the ongoing development of nursing knowledge and nursing science. This vision can and should inform advanced nursing practice as we move into the future. It is nursing science that can and should distinguish the DNP from other midlevel healthcare providers and from physicians, and it is nursing knowledge and care that can and should foster health and wholeness in our patients.

Scientific Foundations of Nursing Practice

Philosophical Foundation

The philosophical underpinning of any scientific body of knowledge provides the bones on which the body is built. Our philosophy is the over-arching way we explain the world, the enduring beliefs we hold (Parker, 2006). The values we adhere to, whatever they are, frame the approach we take to science, theory, and research. Nurse scientists vary in their philosophical positions, but themes common to the profession include the concepts of holism, quality of life, and the relativity of truth based on each individual's perceptions (Burns & Grove, 2001). Advanced practice nurses have a responsibility to define and refine the philosophies and values informing our theories, our research, and our application of research.

Two major philosophical orientations have guided nursing's knowledge development: positivism or empiricism, which is the foundation for research in the hard or natural sciences, and antipositivism, which embraces the soft or interpretive human sciences (Kim, 1997). Contemporary empiricism, also known as postpositivism, recognizes that knowledge is developed within specific social and historical contexts. Postpositivism acknowledges the value of observable reality as well as the complex nature of human phenomena (Fawcett, 1997b; Schumacher & Gortner, 1992).

The discipline of nursing benefits from the philosophical body of knowledge available to all scientists, but we build our own philosophical positions based on individual and collective perceptions and experiences. These positions heavily influence the research we conduct and the way we frame that research (Burns & Grove, 2001). For example, one belief commonly held by advanced practice nurses is that the practical application of knowledge is the only worthwhile goal of scientific inquiry. With this in mind, doctorally prepared advanced nurse practitioners generally frame their research within middle-range theoretical concepts that are focused enough to be useful in clinical settings. Nursing metaparadigms provide insights that can guide practice approaches, but the middle-range nursing theories provide a bridge from grand theory to nursing practice, firmly within the realm of clinicians with practice-based value systems (Parker, 2006).

Ethical Knowledge

Ethical issues in health care are complex and varied, and ethical decisions can have significant impact on our patients' lives. Most nurses face ethical dilemmas from time to time in individual practice, but doctorally prepared advanced practice nurses should be prepared to actively address ethical decisions on an ongoing basis and from a broad professional and organizational perspective (Hamric & Reigle, 2005). DNP graduates understand the dominant ethical theories and are cognizant of their practical applications.

The American Nurses Association's Code for Nurses is grounded in the principle-based model of ethical decision making, which appeals to principles such as respect for persons and autonomy. Ethical reasoning using the principled approach begins with general rules and moves to specific instances. A contrasting ethical theory is the casuistic model, wherein ethical dilemmas are examined in context and compared with similar cases. The ethics of care, or care-based theory, is another ethical decision-making model relevant to nursing. Care-based theory focuses on responsibilities, not rights, and encourages ethical responses based on relationships and needs. Although all the different ethical theories have inherent limitations, possessing an understanding of ethical reasoning will help the DNP guide patients and organizations through the process of moral decision making. At the core of most contemporary nursing theories that guide advanced practice is wide agreement that the old medical ethics of paternalism are replaced in nursing by respect for the individual's autonomy (Hamric & Reigle, 2005).

The ethical conduct of both research and clinical practice is of great concern to many scientific disciplines and endeavors, including nursing. Although research on human subjects is essential to building knowledge about human response to health and illness, human research must not harm the subjects. Additionally, researchers need to report results with scrupulous honesty and full disclosure if their findings are to add useful information to the discipline's body of knowledge. Ethics regulations have been developed to protect human rights, guard intellectual property, and promote integrity in reporting (Burns & Grove, 2001).

Federal regulations require that research involving human subjects be subjected to an institutional review process. The review of such research is conducted by a research review board (RRB) or institutional review board (IRB), a committee responsible for ensuring that human rights and safety are protected and that research is carried out ethically and in compliance with federal guidelines. Although the composition and processes of specific IRBs vary, federal law requires that members have adequate expertise to review research. Members must not have conflicts of interest pertaining to the research they review (Burns & Grove, 2001).

An IRB can decide that research submitted to the committee is either exempt from review, appropriate for expedited review, or required to undergo a complete review. The decision about the level of review is based on the risk to human subjects inherent in the proposed research. A proposed nursing study that posed nothing more than a small cost of time or inconvenience to subjects, such as a survey about working conditions, would probably be considered exempt from review. That decision cannot be made by the researcher, however. The researcher must submit information about the proposed study to the IRB. Usually the chair of the IRB will decide whether the research proposal is exempt or should be presented to the full committee for review. No nurse researcher should conduct even the smallest human study in any institution without first obtaining approval from the IRB (Burns & Grove, 2001).

Doctorally prepared nurse practitioners are obligated to learn and follow the ethical codes that apply to scientific research. Many apparently benign clinical practices have turned out eventually to have adverse consequences, and a clinical researcher can never assume that an intervention will not have a negative impact where human subjects are concerned.

The World Medical Association developed the Declaration of Helsinki: Ethical Principles for Medical Research Involving Human Subjects. Originally based on the Nuremberg Code, a response to the Nazi medical experiments, the Declaration of Helsinki was adopted in Finland in 1964 and amended numerous times, most recently in 2008. Although targeted primarily to physicians, the declaration encourages adoption by anyone conducting medical research on human subjects. The *Code of Ethics for Nurses with Interpretive Statements* (American Nurses Association, 2001) stipulates that nurses have an ethical obligation to protect human rights. When conducting nursing research, nurses must protect subjects' rights to privacy, self-determination, confidentiality, fair treatment, and protect them from harm (Burns & Grove, 2001). DNP graduates should familiarize themselves with these principles before undertaking clinical research.

Historical Knowledge

Knowledge of how the discipline of nursing achieved its current state is essential for understanding its philosophical, theoretical, ethical, and scientific foundations. History gives context to data; facts interpreted outside their context usually result in misinformation and erroneous conclusions.

Biophysical and Psychosocial Knowledge

As a human science, nursing benefits from knowledge accumulated in many other disciplines, including such important areas as biology, physiology, psychology, and sociology. Nurses are generally well educated regarding biophysical and psychosocial sciences in their nursing preparation, but the rapid changes and discoveries occurring in these fields necessitate constant updating of the advanced nurse practitioner's knowledge. Graduation with a DNP degree should be only one stage of an ongoing, lifelong quest for knowledge and growth. Providing safe, high-quality care is an imperative that requires current information, up-to-date clinical and technical skills, and familiarity with the latest research in the biological and human sciences. Professional development should never end; it should be supported by lifelong learning that brings fresh insights from science and newly discovered evidence to the practice environment.

Analytical Knowledge

Analytical reasoning provides an important underpinning for scientific knowledge in any discipline. When we analyze an issue, we make judgments about it based on the evidence in our possession, using thought processes to make connections and derive meaning.

Organizational Knowledge

Organizational science brings an essential dimension to advanced nursing practice. Organizations, whether simple or complex, can only be fully understood as whole systems in motion, with intricate relationships among multiple parts. Small particles of organizations cannot be properly understood in isolation from one another. Organizational scientists look for patterns of behavior and interactions. Systems thinking is a framework for seeing wholes. Human beings, and organizations containing humans, are open systems that change in response to even very small occurrences (Senge, 1994; Wheatley, 2006).

Organizational structure is much more important to nursing practice than many nurses realize. Some DNPs choose organizational leadership as their area of clinical practice because they have learned that patient care at the bedside is intricately interwoven with the systems of management and administration that support, and sometimes hinder, health care. It is the business of doctorally prepared clinical nurse leaders to work within complex systems to secure and implement the resources and education needed to provide safe, high-quality patient care. We know, for example, that the majority of medication errors are not caused by any single person or event. Instead, these errors are caused by problems inherent within the system of medication administration used by the organization. DNPs who want to protect their patients need to understand the organizational system, help to uncover the causes of inefficiencies and errors, and collaborate with others to improve and strengthen the system in order to support both providers and patients.

Knowledge of organizational structure and science is critical for understanding and affecting nursing effectiveness and outcomes. The advanced nurse practitioner who has a grasp on how complex systems affect nursing satisfaction and patient safety will be able to operate within the system to effect change. Organizational theories that DNP graduates should be familiar with include scientific management, bureaucratic management, administrative theory, the neoclassical approach, participative management, systems theory, the sociotechnical approach, and contingency or situational theory. Shared governance of nursing practice by the professional nurses who work in an organization is based on some of these theories and approaches.

Nursing Theory

Nursing Theory–Guided Practice

Nursing theory–guided practice is the recognition and use of models, concepts, and theories from nursing and other disciplines in our work with clients. Theories provide the base from which we seek to understand patients and their health problems and from which we plan interventions to help them. Nursing theory improves our care by giving it structure and unity, by providing more efficient continuity of care, by achieving congruence between process and product, by defining the boundaries and goals of nursing actions, and by giving us a framework through which to examine the effectiveness of our interventions. When advanced practice nurses use theory to guide care, they achieve higher quality in their care while simultaneously elevating nursing's professional standards, accountability, and autonomy. Considering the often fragmented, inefficient, and disorganized care typical of the current healthcare system, we need nursing theory–guided practice to provide a coherent antidote (Kenney, 2006; Meleis, 1997; Smith, 1994).

Scientific research and practice require a framework. Whether the framework is explicitly described or merely implied does not change the fact that the framework exists. There are many theories and conceptual models to consider in advanced nursing practice, and the DNP's responsibility is to become knowledgeable about a broad range of theoretical frameworks in order to intelligently use them in clinical practice. Kenney

(2006) believed that nurses should choose the appropriate model or theory of care for a particular client's situation as part of the initial assessment.

Burns and Grove (2001) offered a framework that links nursing research to the rest of nursing, proposing a continuum between the concrete world of nursing practice and the abstract realms of philosophy and theory. Because nurses traditionally have been expected to perform tasks, nursing thought has tended to be concrete and action oriented. Skillful, concrete thought is essential for planning and carrying out necessary interventions. Although abstract thought seems to have less application to nursing's everyday work, in reality, it is required if we are to recognize the patterns and implications that underlie events, symptoms, and behaviors exhibited by our patients. In clinical practice, the advanced practice nurse must probe beneath the symptoms to find causes and relationships. Theory and research depend on abstract thought, and nursing theory and research are essential for developing the scientific knowledge that nurses need to provide evidence-based health care.

What makes a theory a nursing theory? Nurses use knowledge from many disciplines to frame nursing research, and the knowledge gained, although shared with others, is important to nursing and is used by nursing in distinctive ways. A theory that organizes nursing knowledge and offers a systematic way to explain or describe nursing practice is a nursing theory. Nursing theories clarify what we do and help establish the parameters of our profession (McEwen & Wills, 2006). The DNP graduate knows how to "integrate nursing science with knowledge from ethics, the biophysical, psychosocial, analytical, and organizational sciences as the basis for the highest level of nursing practice" (AACN, 2006).

Developing Middle-Range Theories and Concepts to Guide Practice

Theories are variously classified according to philosophy, perspective, and scope or scale. In nursing, grand theories have the widest scope and are the most abstract, aiming to explain or describe broad issues. Middle-range theories are specific descriptions, explanations, or predictions about a phenomenon of interest, more explicitly focused and concrete than grand theories. A middle-range theory has a limited number of concepts, and these concepts can be defined in operational terms for generating testable hypotheses. Because middle-range theories can be tested, they are the theories most amenable to clinical nursing research, putting them within the exploratory domain of the advanced practice nurse scientist (McEwen & Wills, 2006; Parker, 2006).

Nursing Theories

The many nursing theories that have been developed cannot be described here in detail, but we will examine some of the work of nurse theorists as it applies to advanced nursing practice. Before doing so, it is useful to consider how the DNP should select and implement theories in nursing practice.

Fawcett (1997a) wrote that nurses must first make a conscious decision to use theories in practice. The DNP should understand that nursing theory is what differentiates us from physicians and the medical model of practice. In the traditional medical model, humans are reduced to decontextualized pieces of data. In contrast, nursing practice occurs in the interactions between nurse and person. This process is human based and can only be properly guided by values and principles, theories, and philosophical orientation, not by discrete bits of data (Mitchell, Schmidt Bunkers, & Bournes, 2006). Many nurse researchers and theorists believe that professional nursing is uniquely distinguished from other healthcare professions only by its use of nursing models and theories to guide practice (Kenney, 2006).

For example, when patients come to the DNP with problems caused by lifestyle choices, we unavoidably interact with the patients based on our values. If we follow the traditional medical model, we instruct the patient to change the behavior that is causing the illness and advise him or her to use available medications or treatments. We define the goals of therapy and the state of health we want for the patient, and we expect the individual to follow our advice. If, on the other hand, we apply a nursing model, our interaction with the patient is entirely different. The nursing values of autonomy and nonjudgmental acceptance of the patient's choices will direct us to follow different processes of assessment and intervention. Depending on the theory we apply to the situation, we join our patients' struggles to define and create a state of health that is unique to them (Mitchell, 1999).

Using nursing theories means that we must change the way we think and act in our work with clients. One of the decisions we must make as DNPs is whether we should use only one nursing model throughout our clinical practice. Using only one nursing theory to guide our care of every patient could limit our assessment and narrow our vision, so that we see only the things we need to see to fit the client into our chosen model. To create individualized care for each patient, we can benefit from knowing and using a variety of theories, selecting the conceptual models that are most suitable for particular situations. In doing so, however, we need to maintain congruence with the philosophical underpinnings, principles, and propositions that form the different theories (Kenney, 2006).

Kenney (2006) provided five steps that nurses should follow once the decision has been made to use theory-based nursing practice:

1. Consider your personal values and beliefs about nursing, clients, health, and environment.
2. Examine the underlying assumptions, values, and beliefs of various nursing models, and how the major concepts are defined.
3. Identify several models that are congruent with your own values and beliefs about nursing, clients, and health.
4. Identify the similarities and differences in client focus, nursing actions, and client outcomes of these models.
5. Practice applying the models and theories to clients with different health concerns to determine which ones best "fit" specific situations and guide nursing actions that will achieve desired client outcomes. (pp. 306–307)

It is worth noting that the majority of nurse theorists developed their theories in an effort to improve the care that nurses provide to clients. Nurse theorists were and are experienced practitioners whose theories grew out of their clinical experiences and their attempts to do a better job in the delivery of care. By reflecting on their practice and observations, nurse theorists recognize patterns and gain insights into concepts that lead to theoretical formation (Sitzman & Eichelberger, 2003). This is the same process the DNP student should follow in practice and research, forming middle-range theories that are testable at the bedside.

When studying and selecting a theoretical basis for nursing practice, the DNP should study the theory of interest in its entirety. The brief summaries provided here should serve only to pique the DNP student's interest in studying an appealing theory more thoroughly. The purpose of these summaries, which are presented in chronological order, is to consider how various theories can inform the DNP's practice. The majority of the theories will be familiar to the nurse involved in graduate studies but should be viewed by the DNP student with a fresh focus on applying nursing theory in practice and developing middle-range theories from within a grand theoretical perspective.

Florence Nightingale's Philosophy

Although Florence Nightingale is not generally considered a theorist in the formal sense, her vision of nursing and her philosophy of care resonate with many modern nurses and often inform the work of advanced practice nurses. Nightingale, who wrote *Notes on Nursing* in 1859, put the patient at the center of her model and taught that the goal of nursing is to meet the patient's needs and manipulate the patient's environment so that he or she can attain a healthy state. The work of nursing was not, in Nightingale's view, something delegated to nurses by physicians; rather, nursing was a management role, separate and distinct from medicine, with the job of managing the environment, observing the patient and the patient's interactions with the environment, and assisting the patient toward health. Nightingale perceived patients holistically and considered the impact of environmental conditions on the person's physical, intellectual, psychological, and spiritual components. Nurses were defined as those who had responsibility for another person's health, and in this role, nurses make health possible by arranging for clean, warm, properly lit, quiet surroundings and a correct diet (Dunphy, 2006; Lobo, 1995).

Peplau's Interpersonal Model

Like Nightingale, Hildegard Peplau believed that nursing concepts should come from making observations in nursing situations. Her book, *Interpersonal Relations in Nursing*, published in 1952 and again in 1988, presented her ideas about nursing's roles, the interpersonal process, and how to study nursing as an interpersonal process. Peplau taught a system of theoretical development that combined inductive reasoning, based on observation, with deductive reasoning, based on known concepts. Peplau used qualitative methods to examine something of interest and then used quantitative methods to test an intervention targeted at the problem (Belcher & Fish, 1995; Peden, 2006).

Peplau's interpersonal model pictures nursing as an interpersonal process between the nurse and patient, who are working toward mutually agreed-on goals. The sequential steps taken to reach the goals are: (1) orientation, in which the patient's problems are defined; (2) identification, in which the nurse and patient clarify expectations and figure out how to work together; (3) exploitation, in which the patient uses the services offered by the nurse that the patient finds useful; and (4) resolution, in which the patient's needs have been met and the patient moves toward independence. Even when conflict arises or things do not proceed smoothly, these therapeutic interactions can and should cause growth in both the nurse and the patient (Belcher & Fish, 1995).

Virginia Henderson's Definition of Nursing

Henderson, who developed and published her theory of nursing from 1955 to 1966, sought to differentiate nursing from other healthcare work by defining it as the performance of health-enhancing activities that patients cannot do without help. She described 14 components of nursing care: breathe normally; eat and drink adequately; eliminate body wastes; move and maintain posture; sleep and rest; select suitable clothing; maintain body temperature; keep body clean and well-groomed; avoid dangers in the environment; communicate; worship according to one's faith; work to achieve a sense of accomplishment; participate in recreation; and learn, discover, or satisfy curiosity. By assisting the patient with these basic components of care, the nurse works to help the patient become independent again (Furukawa & Howe, 1995; Gesse, Dombro, Gordon, & Rittman, 2006).

Hall's Care, Core, and Cure Model

Lydia Hall conceptualized the patient as a person, a body, and a disease, which she placed into overlapping, dynamic, and interactive circles of core (the person), care (the body), and cure (the disease). Her theory was honed over a period covering the latter half of the 1950s and the early 1960s. Nursing is concerned with all of these circles, with different parts of the model becoming the predominant nursing focus at different times. Practically speaking, Hall believed that nursing is most crucial after the patient's acute crisis has stabilized, when nurses should nurture and educate the patient and assist him or her in making changes that will prevent a repeat of the original crisis (George, 1995; Touhy & Birnbach, 2006).

A central tenet of the care, core, and cure model is that intimate personal care such as bathing belongs exclusively to nursing and that nursing is needed when an individual cannot take care of these bodily requirements unassisted. The professional nurse is able to perform personal care in such a way that it provides comfort but also engenders learning, growth, and healing. The nurse in this caring role is a nurturer, using these intimate interactions to take the client beyond cleanliness and comfort to health (George, 1995; Touhy & Birnbach, 2006).

Orem's Self-Care Deficit Theory of Nursing

First published in an early form in 1959, three interrelated theories compose Dorothea Orem's self-care deficit theory of nursing: theory of self-care, self-care deficit theory, and theory of nursing systems. To understand her general theory, it is essential to grasp the six central concepts and one peripheral concept within the overarching theory:

1. Self-care is initiating and performing activities on one's own behalf to maintain life, health, and well-being.
2. Self-care agency is the individual's ability to practice self-care.
3. Therapeutic self-care demand is the set of self-care activities needed to meet self-care needs.
4. Self-care deficit is the gap between self-care agency and self-care demand, between the self-care activities the individual can do and the self-care activities that are needed.
5. Nursing agency is the nurse's ability to meet the therapeutic self-care demands of others.
6. The nursing system is the package of nursing responsibilities, roles, relationships, and actions that is organized to meet the client's therapeutic self-care demand. (Foster & Bennett, 1995; Orem, 2006)

The self-care deficit nursing theory has been used extensively in nursing practice. As a general theory, it is relevant for guiding practice in any care setting or specialty area. Backscheider (1974) used Orem's theory to organize nursing care in a diabetic nurse management clinic, structuring the nursing system based on the nature of the clients' self-care deficits. Nursing agency overcomes the self-care deficits caused by, in this case, diabetes. Crews (1972) applied Orem's theory to nurse-managed cardiac clinics. The theory has been used to guide inpatient, outpatient, and community settings; across a variety of age groups and disease states; in the care of families and communities; to inform administration and management of nursing care; and as a basis for nursing research and education.

Orem believed that nursing is a practical science with both theoretical and practical knowledge. She taught that nursing is different from other disciplines and services because of its focus on human beings. The broad applicability of her theory to a variety of situations and its focus on designing nursing care to meet clients' needs make the self-care deficit theory a useful theoretical base for the DNP's practice and research (Isenberg, 2006).

Johnson's Behavioral Systems Model

Dorothy Johnson was influenced by Florence Nightingale in her early publications, including her 1959 proposal that nursing should draw on the basic and applied sciences in developing the science of nursing. In "The Significance of Nursing Care," Johnson (1961) reflected Nightingale again by writing that nursing care should support the patient's maintenance of equilibrium in the face of stressful, destabilizing stimuli. Based on systems thinking and developmental theories, Dorothy Johnson's 1968 behavioral systems model conceptualizes humans as open systems with interdependent subsystems. The person is a behavioral system existing within an environment (both internal and external) of multiple components, and the human/system interacts with the environment in various ways. Johnson drew analogies between five core general systems principles and concepts of human development: wholeness and order form the basis for human identity and continuity; stabilization or balance is the basis of development; reorganization correlates with change and growth; hierarchic interaction is analogous to discontinuity; and dialectical contradiction provides the basis for motivation (Holaday, 2006).

The behavioral system (person) in Johnson's model is composed of subsystems that perform specialized functions to meet a specific goal. The activities that a person employs to meet the system's goals differ based on the individual's values, motives, gender, age, self-concept, and other variables. The system's overall goal is to maintain equilibrium in the face of internal and external environmental pressures. Each subsystem works to achieve its own equilibrium, contributing to the balance or homeostasis of the whole person. Balance is attained and maintained by accommodation to the environment, and the individual with a large bank of possible accommodating behaviors will be more adaptable to changing forces (Holaday, 2006).

Nursing action is intended to help the person arrive at a state of equilibrium when possible. Johnson stated that whereas medicine sees the patient as a biological system, nursing sees the patient as a behavioral system. And although nursing's responsibility is to assist the patient toward behavioral system balance, Johnson made it clear that individuals must make their own choices about the level of functioning and balance that they want to achieve. It is the nurse's responsibility to help the client understand the function and balance that is possible and how to achieve it, and then to guide progress toward the goals of the patient's choosing (Holaday, 2006).

When practicing with this model as a guide, the nurse assesses the client to determine the source of the problem and then uses nursing interventions to create change. In the behavioral systems model, the nurse might provide essential functions or help the patient obtain essential functions, negotiating a plan with the patient. Or, the nurse might act as a regulatory force, enacting controls to restore stability. A third possible intervention is to attempt to change the person's guiding set of concepts and choices in order to bring about actions that can repair the damage (Holaday, 2006).

Johnson's model has found useful application in studies of cancer patients, psychiatric patients, education, and administration, among others. The behavioral systems model establishes behavioral system balance as a clear goal for nursing, gives a way to identify the cause of the imbalance, and guides the nurse as an external force that helps the system achieve equilibrium.

Abdellah's Problem-Solving Approach

Faye Abdellah's theoretical stance, described in 1960, was nursing centered and focused on solving nursing problems. She developed 21 nursing problems as a way to help nurses systematically identify problems presented by clients. The problems, although written from the perspective of the nurse, bear similarities to Henderson's basic nursing care components, which were written from the patient's view. For example, instead of Henderson's "keep body clean and well-groomed," Abdellah identified the nursing problem as "to maintain good hygiene and physical comfort." In practice, the nursing problems are useful for directing the nurse's actions and for providing a structure for developing principles of care (Falco, 1995).

Roy's Adaptation Model

Sister Callista Roy's adaptation model was first presented in 1964 as part of Roy's graduate work under the mentorship of Dorothy Johnson (Galbreath, 1995). In its final form, the theory contains four essential elements: the person receiving nursing care, the environment, health, and nursing (Roy & Andrews, 1991). The person, or group, is a holistic adaptive system. People and groups use coping processes to adapt to, interact with, transform, and be transformed by their environment. Human behavior results from adaptation in various modes. Health is integration and wholeness, and adaptation is used to support the process and state of health (Roy & Zhan, 2006).

Roy's model is broadly applicable to all types of nursing practice and nursing research. In particular, the adaptation model lends itself well to guiding research and practice regarding the changes that occur in human development and aging. Life stages that require significant adjustment, such as adolescence and the older adult years, are good areas for research into appropriate interventions to support the processes of adaptation. The theory emphasizes finding ways to enhance the coping processes of the individual or group experiencing change. The DNP who bases practice on this model will seek to understand the patient's adaptation processes and work with patients to help them cope with their environment and adapt toward a state of health (Roy & Zhan, 2006).

Levine's Conservation Model

Writing in 1969, Myra Levine taught that nursing's role is to support the human process of adaptation to achieve the goal of conservation, which includes conservation of energy, structural integrity, personal integrity, and social integrity. Conservation protects the integrity and wholeness of living systems in the face of change. Levine illustrated the principle of conservation by referring to a thermostat. A thermostat does not respond until there is a change in the environment, at which time it activates the heating or cooling system until the temperature in the environment is restored to the set point. The thermostat conserves energy until it is needed to restore balance, just as a successful living system in a state of homeostasis is conserving energy until action is needed to bring the system back into balance (George, 1995).

The principles of conservation form the foundation of the model: people are always acting within a complex environment that affects behavior; people protect themselves by learning everything they can about the environment; nurses are active participants in a patient's environment; and nursing care works to restore and strengthen the patient's adaptive responses to survive within the environment, including responses that help the patient deal with disease and difficulties (Schaefer, 2006).

Levine believed that knowing and using a variety of nursing theories was essential because there could never be a theory of nursing appropriate for every situation. Her conservation model has been used widely in practice, across the life span, and in clinical settings ranging from community care to critical care. The model assumes that health is the goal and that nurses should develop interventions that focus on conservation of the system's energy and integrity to achieve wholeness. The interventions will vary widely within this theory depending on the problem, the person, and the environment (Schaefer, 2006).

Rogers's Science of Unitary Human Beings

Evolving during the decades between 1961 and 1994, the science of unitary human beings is based on five assumptions about humans, described in Martha Rogers's 1970 publication, *The Theoretical Basis of Nursing*: (1) a human is a unified whole, more than and different from the sum of its parts; (2) humans and their environment are continuously exchanging energy and matter in an open system; (3) human beings evolve in one direction and cannot go backward to a previous state; (4) life's patterns identify humans and reflect their wholeness; and (5) humans are capable of abstract thought. Theorist Rogers identified four building blocks based on the five basic assumptions: energy fields (human beings and their environment are energy fields of concern to nursing); openness and dynamic movement among energy fields; pattern, or distinguishing characteristics of an energy field; and pandimensionality, meaning without boundaries of space and time (Falco & Lobo, 1995; Malinski, 2006).

Rogers's three principles of homeodynamics are grounded on the five assumptions and four building blocks. Integrality is the first principle of homeodynamics, which is defined as the continuous interaction between humans and the environment. The second principle is resonancy, which addresses the continuous changes occurring between human and environmental fields and the identification of the fields by wave patterns. Helicy, the third principle, proposes that the changes occurring between human and environmental fields are moving in the direction of increasing diversity and complexity in unpredictable and nonrepeating ways (Falco & Lobo, 1995; Malinski, 2006).

Rogers believed that many theories could be developed from the science of unitary human beings. She devised the theory of accelerating evolution, postulating that human–environment field interactions become faster and more diverse over time. There can be no such thing as a static state of normalcy in a world of accelerating evolution. A second theory, of the emergence of paranormal phenomena, suggested that experiences we usually consider paranormal are actually glimpses of innovation in field patterns. Her third theory, manifestations of field patterning in unitary human beings, is focused on the process of evolution as a nonlinear movement forward to increasing diversity (Malinski, 2006).

In clinical practice, the science of unitary human beings leads to highly individualized nursing and healthcare services. Rogers was opposed to nursing diagnosis and care mapping schemata that try to standardize care. Instead, she taught that increasing diversity meant increasingly individualized care. She emphasized each person's right to choose his or her own path to health and believed that noninvasive methods of treatment should form the basis for nursing practice. In Rogers's view, the goal of practice is to promote well-being, and nurses do this as part of a mutual process with clients (Malinski, 2006).

Rogers considered the nursing process too static, reductionistic, and sequential to apply within her paradigm of dynamic, infinite, open energy fields integrally interacting in constant change. Other practice methodologies have been developed from the principles of the science of unitary human beings. Barrett's 1988 Rogerian practice method for health patterning is widely accepted as a Rogerian alternative to the nursing process. There are two processes in Barrett's model. The first, pattern manifestation knowing, is the process of becoming familiar with the human and environmental fields. The second process is called voluntary mutual patterning and involves the nurse in helping the client to choose ways to change as part of achieving well-being. Both processes are continuous and simultaneous, not sequential or linear. The outcomes cannot be predicted or controlled (Butcher, 2006).

Scientific advances in quantum mechanics and research based on chaos theory have lent strength to Rogers's ideas. In quantum mechanics, researchers are learning that everything has an impact on everything else, and it is impossible to predict where and how all the influences will come from or what effect they will have. Studies of the electromagnetic field of the brain are revealing how awareness correlates with synchronous firing of neurons, so that the seat of consciousness seems to reside in the patterns of the field (Wheatley, 2006). DNPs will invariably benefit from integrating nursing science with knowledge from a variety of other sciences.

Neuman's Systems Model

In Betty Neuman's model, developed in 1970 and based on systems theory, each individual or group is a client system. Each system, although unique, is composed of common characteristics within a normal range. Environmental stressors disturb a system's stability to various degrees. A system has normal defenses against stressors, but when these are inadequate, the client can be negatively or positively affected. Each client has resistance factors that stabilize and move the system toward health. Nursing interventions can affect the client's move toward health on a number of levels. The goal of nursing is to promote the system's stability by assessing the impact of stressors and helping the client adjust to the environment.

The model's three types of prevention—primary, secondary, and tertiary—are interventions that promote wellness. The purpose of primary prevention is to reduce risk factors and prevent identified or suspected stressors before the client experiences a reaction to the stressors, thereby *retaining* wellness. Health promotion is an example of a primary prevention intervention. The aim of secondary prevention is to intervene in ways that strengthen the client's internal resistance to a stressor once a reaction to the stressor has occurred, thereby *attaining* a new state of health. Tertiary prevention is used as an intervention once the client has returned to a stable state after a stressor reaction and secondary prevention have occurred. Tertiary prevention focuses on *maintaining* wellness by supporting the system's strengths and conserving its energy.

Neuman's systems model was first developed for use in nursing education, but it has found wide use in a variety of settings around the world. Nursing administration, psychiatric nursing, case management, gerontological nursing, occupational health nursing, and other specialties have benefited from applying the model in practice (Aylward, 2006).

King's Interacting Systems Framework and Middle-Range Theory of Goal Attainment

Imogene King's interacting systems framework, introduced in 1971's *Toward a Theory for Nursing*, is grounded in general system theory, a philosophy of science that emphasizes wholeness and the interaction of elements within systems. King sought to identify the essence of nursing and found that this brought her to the nature of human beings because nurses are humans who give nursing care to other humans. From this abstract conceptualization, she derived the middle-range theory of goal attainment. She used concepts of self, perception, communication, interaction, transaction, role, and decision making in her theory. She theorized that the goal of nursing is to help human beings attain, maintain, or regain health and developed a "transaction process model" that she observed in human interactions. In King's transaction model, the nurse and patient interact to set goals they mutually agree on and then can mutually achieve (King, 2006).

King linked her theory of goal attainment to the nursing process, which strengthened the theory's use and applicability in clinical practice. She considered the nursing process to be a method, and the transaction process model provided theoretical grounding for the method. A nurse uses perception, communication, and interaction to gather the data needed for assessment and the judgment needed to diagnose. When the nurse and patient decide on the goals and the means to achieve them, they are planning and implementing the plan using the transactional process. Evaluation is theoretically based on the feedback loop that often begins the transactional process again (King, 2006).

Other middle-range theories have grown from the interacting systems framework. Sieloff devised the theory of departmental power to help explain group power in organizations. Frey used King's framework to develop a theory about chronic illness, families, and children. Brooks and Thomas built a theory of perceptual awareness. The framework has shown broad applicability across the life span and across a variety of systems, including personal, interpersonal, and social. It has been used to address many different client concerns and conditions in multiple nursing specialties and work settings. Several instruments have been developed to measure and test these middle-range theories, such as King's Goal Attainment Scale; Killeen's Nursing Care Survey; the Sieloff-King assessment of group power within organizations; and Rawlins, Rawlins, and Horner's Family Needs Assessment Tool (Sieloff, Frey, & Killeen, 2006).

The interacting systems framework and the middle-range theory of goal attainment have a broad scope and have been used to generate a significant amount of nursing knowledge. Sieloff et al. (2006) noted that King's work provides a theoretical base for research that can be readily applied in nursing practice as part of the continued development of evidence-based nursing.

Watson's Theory of Human Caring

Jean Watson wrote that her theory of human caring, developed between 1975 and 1979, was an effort to explicate her view that nursing practice, knowledge, and values focus on the patient's own healing processes and personal world of experiences. While complementing the medical practitioner's work, Watson's *carative factors*, as she termed them, also contrasted sharply with medicine's *curative factors* (Watson, 2006). The theory's major concepts include the 10 carative factors, the transpersonal caring relationship, the caring moment, and the caring-healing modalities. The 10 carative factors are, in brief, the promotion of and/or assistance with the following: (1) a humanistic-altruistic value system, (2) faith-hope, (3) sensitivity to self and others, (4) helping-trusting relationship, (5) expression of feelings, (6) creative problem solving, (7) transpersonal teaching-learning, (8) a supportive environment, (9) need gratification, and (10) existential-phenomenological-spiritual forces (Talento, 1995; Watson, 1979).

The original 10 caring factors evolved over time and were transposed by Watson into "clinical caritas processes." These translated factors moved from basic abstractions to open processes, such as (1) a practice of loving kindness, (2) being authentically present, (3) cultivation of spiritual practices, (4) developing a helping-trusting relationship, (5) supporting the expression of feelings, (6) creative use of self in the caring process, (7) engaging in teaching-learning from within another's perspective, (8) creating a healing environment, (9) helping with basic needs with caring consciousness, and (10) opening to spiritual and existential dimensions; soul care for self and others (Watson, 2006).

The transpersonal caring relationship, the second major concept in Watson's theory, describes an intentional attempt to connect with another person through caring. It requires the one providing care to move beyond the self in order to access the spirit of the one being cared for. The third conceptual understanding in the theory is the caring moment, when the nurse and another person interact. Caring-healing modalities, the fourth concept, are the intentional acts, words, behaviors, and various means of communication exercised by the nurse in the process of helping the client heal (Watson, 2006).

The theory of human caring has been used effectively as a framework for studying nursing leadership and management. Anne Liners Kersbergen Brett (1992) studied the caring attributes received or needed by nurse administrators at work, finding that the interpersonal caring attributes were most needed by nurse managers. Ray (1984) examined the implications of differing definitions of caring in a healthcare organization, developing a classification system of institutional caring. Data from these studies reveal that nurses and nurse administrators greatly value interactional caring, yet perceive that they do not frequently receive the kind of social caring that they need. Ray (1989) developed a middle-range theory of bureaucratic caring for nursing practice as a result of her work within Watson's grand theory.

Nursing leaders who thought that caring was being devalued in their highly technology-oriented hospital unit used Watson's theory of human caring to inform their study of caring attributes among nurses and patients. The researchers discovered that the nurses and patients felt there was a high level of relational and contextual caring on the unit and that caring behaviors were essential to maintain energy and motivate more caring behaviors. The nurse leaders discussed these findings with the unit and identified ways to systematically support caring behaviors and promote a caring culture (Carter et al., 2008).

The effects of caring on client outcomes have been tested by research that has shown preliminary linkage between nurse caring behaviors and such outcomes as patient satisfaction, perceived health status, total length of stay, and nursing care costs (Duffy, 1992), and the economic value of caring to healthcare organizations (Issel & Kahn, 1998). Duffy and Hoskins (2003) proposed a model blending caring concepts with an evidence-based practice framework, stating that these apparently diverse paradigms used together might produce the best outcomes for clients and nurses. Nyberg's 1998 model of caring administration is grounded in Watson's theory, as is the attending nurse caring model (ANCM), which was piloted at the Children's Hospital in Denver, Colorado (Watson, 2006). The DNP scholar will find fertile soil for exploration and development of practice modalities from within the theory of human caring.

Paterson and Zderad's Humanistic Nursing Theory

Published in 1976, Josephine Paterson and Loretta Zderad's *Humanistic Nursing* laid out a multidimensional and interactive theory that seeks to bridge theory and practice. Humanistic nursing theory postulates nursing as an existential experience, a shared dialogue between nurse and patient that puts the nurse in the role of nurturing and comforting someone in need. An individual, or group of individuals, generates a call for help with a health-related need, and one or more nurses respond with assistance. Nursing is what happens in the process. The theory is a broad guide for the interactions that occur in this call-and-response model (Kleiman, 2006; Praeger, 1995).

Health, in Paterson and Zderad's theory, is not just the absence of illness. Being healthy means finding meaning in existence and becoming everything one can be within the experiences, relationships, and options of life. The theory speaks of creative relationships characterized by the nurse and patient meeting, relating to each other, and providing an open, receptive presence to each other in a lived dialogue. This process leads to community and makes it possible for people to find meaning and become healthy through sharing with others (Praeger, 1995).

Paterson and Zderad developed a method of inquiry they called *phenomenologic nursology*. Phenomenology seeks to describe phenomena without explaining or predicting them. Phenomenologic nursology follows a five-step process: (1) the nurse prepares to know something or someone by opening the mind and spirit to the unknown, (2) the nurse gains knowledge of the patient through intuitive impressions and learning about the patient's experiences, (3) the nurse gains scientific knowledge of the patient by analyzing the data, (4) the nurse synthesizes the subjective and objective information to gain perspective on the situation, and (5) the nurse arrives at a new truth, a concept that includes all the information gained, refined into a descriptive construct (Kleiman, 2006; Praeger, 1995).

Newman's Theory of Health as Expanding Consciousness

In her 1978 theory of health as expanding consciousness, Margaret Newman drew from concepts in Martha Rogers's science of unitary human
beings, particularly the view that health and illness are a unitary process—
manifestations of the greater whole—and not mutually exclusive states.
Within this paradigm, then, the nurse's job is to help people recognize and
use their own power to evolve to a higher condition. Health, as defined
by Newman, is the expansion of consciousness, and nurses go with their
patients and support them in discovering wholeness and meaning. Consciousness is the system's ever-expanding information capability, which
is continuously influenced by the forces of time, movement, and space
(George, 1995; Pharris, 2006).

Nurses who use Newman's theory in practice do not set goals, predict
outcomes, or follow a defined nursing pathway. Rather, nurses enter into
partnership with people who have arrived at a point of disruption and
uncertainty. Nursing provides a caring relationship in which patients can
explore meaning and potential and grow from disorganization to a higher
level of organization. Chaos presents an opportunity for transformation,
and the nurse joins the patient in the chaos as new patterns develop. The
focus is on being with the person who is in turmoil, not on doing things
for him or her. When practicing from this perspective, nurses must focus
on what is meaningful to the patient (George, 1995; Pharris, 2006).

Parse's Human Becoming School of Thought

Rosemarie Parse's human becoming school of thought, first presented
in 1981, is philosophically rooted in the simultaneity paradigm, which
views human beings as unitary and the human–universe process as irre-
ducible and dynamic. Health is an ever-changing state, based on the human being's choices, values, and priorities. Research and practice focus
on discerning patterns and improving quality of life. The individual's desires and opinions about his or her health are more important than anyone else's perspectives. This view contrasts with the totality paradigm,
used in the medical model, in which the person is seen in biological,
psychological, social, and spiritual parts, with health as a state of well-
being in the various pieces of the person. Societal norms define health,
and research and practice focus on preventing disease and promoting
an acceptable state of health. Nurses operating within the totality paradigm use defined goals and treatment regimens to effect change in their
patients, whereas nurses who live and work within the simultaneity

paradigm are primarily concerned with escorting patients on a journey of discovery (Parse, 2006).

Growing numbers of nurses use Parse's framework to guide practice. For example, the health action model for partnership in community was developed in the 1990s in the Department of Nursing at Augustana College in Sioux Falls, South Dakota. Based on Parse's theory, the model is the result of collaboration between academia and community nursing practice. The health action model addresses human connections and disconnections, focusing on the importance of the nurse's presence with underresourced and low-income individuals (Bunkers, Nelson, Leuning, Crane, & Josephson, 1999). Another example is a parish nursing practice model, the congregational health model, first used in the 1990s by the First Presbyterian Church in Sioux Falls, South Dakota. The congregational health model draws parallels between concepts in human becoming theory and the eight beatitudes found in Christian scripture, emphasizing life in community, nursing/human presence, and respect for the choices of others (Bunkers & Putnam, 1995). Both of these models recognize the transformative impact of the nurse interacting with the community and honor the individual's definition of quality of life (Mitchell et al., 2006).

Leininger's Theory of Culture Care Diversity and Universality

Grounded in a philosophy of caring, the theory of culture care diversity and universality draws many of its concepts from the discipline of anthropology. Madeleine Leininger established the following major principles within her theory, first published in 1985: both similarities and differences can be found within cultures, and it is the job of nursing to discover the culturally universal components of care and to discern diverse ways of caring; cultural influences of all kinds have a significant impact on healthcare outcomes; and significant differences and similarities exist between professional care and traditional or folk care, and because these can be the source of problems or benefits, they must be identified. The theory of culture care diversity and universality assumes the essentialness of care for health and growth and emphasizes that culturally congruent care is necessary for well-being (Leininger, 2006).

Anne Boykin and Savina Schoenhofer: Nursing as Caring

Boykin and Schoenhofer postulated in 1993 that need-based models such as the nursing process do not appropriately address what nurses should be doing. Their grand theory of nursing as caring is based on caring in a way that is specific to each nurse, person, and situation, requiring personal as well as empirical knowledge of each patient. All humans are caring, and each person grows in caring by participating in nurturing relationships. Nursing is a discipline, a response to the social call to help others, that requires knowing and developing nursing knowledge. Nursing is also a profession, in which nursing knowledge is used to respond to the human needs that arise from the commitment to help. Nursing is a creative process that evolves moment by moment as part of a caring relationship (Boykin & Schoenhofer, 2006; George, 1995).

Nursing as caring proposes that caring is the central value of nursing. Boykin and Schoenhofer warned that if nursing does not focus on being intentionally caring, the profession will lose its unique meaning and place in health care. The nurse who is committed to caring, knowing, and nurturing other people must intentionally express this care in the face of a healthcare environment filled with dehumanizing technology, depersonalizing routines, requirements for measurable outcomes, and an emphasis on financial profits (Boykin & Schoenhofer, 2006; George, 1995).

Conceptual Models for Transcultural Nursing

Recent trends in the population and diversity profile of the United States have brought the need for theoretical underpinnings of transcultural nursing to light. In 2007, the American Academy of Nursing (AAN) released 12 recommendations for cultural competence, including Recommendation 11: "The AAN must take the lead in promulgating support of research funding for investigation with emphasis on interventions aimed at eliminating health disparities in culturally and racially diverse groups and other vulnerable populations in an effort to improve health outcomes" (Gizar et al., 2007).

A few of the conceptual models for cultural diversity include: Dr. Madeleine Leininger's Sunrise Model; Campinha-Bacote's Model of the Process of Cultural Competence in the Delivery of Healthcare Services; Giger and Davidhizar's Transcultural Assessment Model; and Purnell and Paulanka's Model of Cultural Competence (Dayer-Berenson, 2011, p. 9). Dr. Madeleine Leininger's *Culture Care: Diversity and Universality* provides the basic foundation for cultural competency in nursing (p. 15). From that work, she developed the sunrise model, which demonstrates a utilitarian model of the relationships between cultural care, diversity, and universality in a graphic model of four intersecting areas (p. 20). Giger and Davidhizar's transcultural assessment model describes a framework for cultural assessment with six foci that they postulate shape transcultural nursing care: communication, space, social organization, time, environmental control, and biological variations (p. 21). Purnell and Paulanka's model of cultural competence is designed to be utilized by all members of the healthcare team (p. 28). This model has a framework of 12 domains that reach across all cultures: heritage, communication, family roles and organization, workforce issues, biocultural ecology, high-risk health behaviors, nutrition, pregnancy and childbearing practices, death rituals, spirituality, healthcare practices, and healthcare providers (pp. 29–30). Campinha-Bacote's model, called the process of cultural competence in the delivery of healthcare services, is built on five concepts: cultural **a**wareness, cultural **s**kill, cultural **k**nowledge, cultural **e**ncounters, and cultural **d**esire (p. 31). These constructs are arranged in the ASKED mnemonic to assist the individual nurse in his or her path to cultural competence (p. 32).

Core Themes of Nursing Theory

DNPs must bring analysis and critical thinking to bear on a variety of client problems, drawing from a broad base of knowledge in multiple scientific disciplines to synthesize the data and make creative inferences to help the client. We are guided in this complex reasoning process by nursing theories that shape and inform our reflections and provide the foundation for our clinical practice (Kenney, 2006).

Early nursing models, such as those proposed by Henderson and Abdellah, were often based on an empirical, reductionistic philosophy, following traditional cause-and-effect scientific thinking. Nursing theories from the late 20th and early 21st centuries tend to come out of the philosophical framework of systems thinking, holism, and continuous unpredictable change unfolding in dynamic, interactive processes. Modern theorists generally center their models on the human or organizational system interacting with its environment, not on the disease. In these models, nurses come alongside the patient to engage in health-promoting processes and achieve the client's goals, whatever those may be. Regardless of the model chosen for a particular situation, theory-based nursing defines the DNP and is at the heart of advanced nursing practice (Benner & Wrubel, 1989; Kenney, 2006).

Rolfe (1993) advocated for a reconceptualization of the relationship between theory and practice, saying that nursing theory should come not from abstract ideas but should be generated from practice. The relationship of theory and practice then becomes circular, as theories are derived from practice and circle around to inform and modify practice, which in turn produces new theories, which again changes practice. Viewing theory in this way eliminates the theory practice gap, because each depends fully on the other, and both theory and practice are grounded in clinical realities. Nursing praxis, the joining of theory and practice, applies theoretical knowledge in unique ways in every individual patient encounter.

When advanced nurse practitioners use knowledge, experience, and reflection with a specific patient, we become both theorists and researchers while engaging in clinical practice. It's not just what we know that matters. What matters is how we use what we know, and then how we continually improve our knowledge and understanding the more we practice.

References

American Association of Colleges of Nursing. (2006). *The essentials of doctoral education for advanced nursing practice*. Washington, DC: Author.

American Nurses Association. (2001). *Code of ethics for nurses with interpretive statements*. Washington, DC: Author.

Aylward, P. D. (2006). Betty Neuman: The Neuman systems model and global applications. In M. E. Parker (Ed.), *Nursing theories and nursing practice* (2nd ed., pp. 281–294). Philadelphia, PA: F. A. Davis.

Backscheider, J. E. (1974). Self-care requirements, self-care capabilities and nursing systems in the diabetic nurse management clinic. *American Journal of Public Health, 64*(12), 1138–1146.

Barrett, E. A. M. (2002). What is nursing science? *Nursing Science Quarterly, 15*(1), 51–60.

Belcher, J. R., & Fish, L. J. (1995). Hildegard E. Peplau. In J. B. George (Ed.), *Nursing theories: The base for professional nursing practice* (4th ed., pp. 33–48). Norwalk, CT: Appleton & Lange.

Benner, P., & Wrubel, J. (1989). *The primacy of caring*. Menlo Park, CA: Addison-Wesley.

Boykin, A., & Schoenhofer, S. O. (2006). Anne Boykin and Savina O. Schoenhofer's nursing as caring theory. In M. E. Parker (Ed.), *Nursing theories and nursing practice* (2nd ed., pp. 334–348). Philadelphia, PA: F. A. Davis.

Bunkers, S. S. (2002). Nursing science as human science: The new world and human becoming. *Nursing Science Quarterly, 15*(1), 25–30.

Bunkers, S. S., Nelson, M. L., Leuning, C. J., Crane, J. K., & Josephson, D. K. (1999). The health action model: Academia's partnership with the community. In E. L. Cohen & V. DeBack (Eds.), *The outcomes mandate: Case management in health care today* (pp. 92–100). St. Louis, MO: Mosby.

Bunkers, S. S., & Putnam, V. (1995). A nursing theory based model of health ministry: Living Parse's theory of human becoming in the parish community. In *Ninth Annual Westberg Parish Nurse Symposium: Parish nursing: Ministering through the arts*. Northbrook, IL: International Parish Nursing Resource Center–Advocate Health Care.

Burns, N., & Grove, S. (2001). *The practice of nursing research: Conduct, critique, and utilization* (4th ed.). Philadelphia, PA: W. B. Saunders.

Butcher, H. K. (2006). Applications of Rogers' science of unitary human beings. In M. E. Parker (Ed.), *Nursing theories and nursing practice* (2nd ed., pp. 167–186). Philadelphia, PA: F. A. Davis.

Carter, L. C., Nelson, J. L., Sievers, B. A., Dukek, S. L., Pipe, T. B., & Holland, D. E. (2008). Exploring a culture of caring. *Nursing Administration Quarterly, 32*(1), 57–63.

Crews, J. (1972). Nurse-managed cardiac clinics. *Cardio-Vascular Nursing, 8*(4), 15–18.

Dayer-Berenson, L. (2011). *Cultural competencies for nurses: Impact on health and illness*. Sudbury, MA: Jones & Bartlett Learning.

Duffy, J. (1992). The impact of nurse caring on patient outcomes. In D. Gaut (Ed.), *The presence of caring in nursing* (pp. 113–136). New York, NY: National League for Nursing.

Duffy, J., & Hoskins, L. (2003). The Quality-Caring Model©: Blending dual paradigms. *Advances in Nursing Science, 26*(1), 77–88.

Dunphy, L. M. H. (2006). Florence Nightingale's legacy of caring and its applications. In M. E. Parker (Ed.), *Nursing theories and nursing practice* (2nd ed., pp. 39–57). Philadelphia, PA: F. A. Davis.

Engebretson, J. (1997). A multiparadigm approach to nursing. *Advances in Nursing Science, 20*(1), 21–23.

Falco, S. M. (1995). Faye Glenn Abdellah. In J. B. George (Ed.), *Nursing theories: The base for professional nursing practice* (4th ed., pp. 143–158). Norwalk, CT: Appleton & Lange.

Falco, S. M., & Lobo, M. L. (1995). Martha E. Rogers. In J. B. George (Ed.), *Nursing theories: The base for professional nursing practice* (4th ed., pp. 229–248). Norwalk, CT: Appleton & Lange.

Fawcett, J. (1997a). Conceptual models of nursing, nursing theories, and nursing practice: Focus on the future. In M. R. Alligood & A. Marriner-Tomey (Eds.), *Nursing theory: Utilization and application* (pp. 211–221). St. Louis, MO: Mosby.

Fawcett, J. (1997b). The structural hierarchy of nursing knowledge: Components and their definitions. In I. M. King & J. Fawcett (Eds.), *The language of nursing theory and metatheory* (pp. 11–17). Indianapolis, IN: Center Nursing Press.

Fawcett, J. (1999). The state of nursing science: Hallmarks of the 20th and 21st centuries. *Nursing Science Quarterly, 12*(4), 311–315.

Fawcett, J. (2000). *Analysis and evaluation of contemporary nursing knowledge: Nursing models and theories*. Philadelphia, PA: F. A. Davis.

Foster, P. C., & Bennett, A. M. (1995). Dorothea E. Orem. In J. B. George (Ed.), *Nursing theories: The base for professional nursing practice* (4th ed., pp. 99–123). Norwalk, CT: Appleton & Lange.

Furukawa, C. Y., & Howe, J. K. (1995). Virginia Henderson. In J. B. George (Ed.), *Nursing theories: The base for professional nursing practice* (4th ed., pp. 67–85). Norwalk, CT: Appleton & Lange.

Galbreath, J. G. (1995). Callista Roy. In J. B. George (Ed.), *Nursing theories: The base for professional nursing practice* (4th ed., pp. 251–279). Norwalk, CT: Appleton & Lange.

George, J. B. (Ed.) (1995). *Nursing theories: The base for professional nursing practice* (4th ed.). Norwalk, CT: Appleton & Lange.

Gesse, T., Dombro, M., Gordon, S. C., & Rittman, M. R. (2006). Wiedenbach, Henderson, and Orlando's theories and their applications. In M. E. Parker (Ed.), *Nursing theories and nursing practice* (2nd ed., pp. 70–78). Philadelphia, PA: F. A. Davis.

Gizar, J., Davidhizar, R., Purnell, L., Harden, J., Phillips, J., & Strickland, O. (2007). American Academy of Nursing Expert Panel Report: Developing cultural competency to eliminate health disparities in ethnic minorities and other vulnerable populations. *Journal of Transcultural Nursing, 18*(2), 95–102.

Hamric, A. B., & Reigle, J. (2005). Ethical decision making. In A. B. Hamric, J. A. Spross, & C. M. Hanson (Eds.), *Advanced practice nursing: An integrative approach* (3rd ed.). Philadelphia, PA: W. B. Saunders.

Holaday, B. (2006). Dorothy Johnson's behavioral system model and its applications. In M. E. Parker (Ed.), *Nursing theories and nursing practice* (2nd ed., pp. 79–93). Philadelphia, PA: F. A. Davis.

Isenberg, M. A. (2006). Applications of Dorothea Orem's self-care deficit nursing theory. In M. E. Parker (Ed.), *Nursing theories and nursing practice* (2nd ed., pp. 149–159). Philadelphia, PA: F. A. Davis.

Issel, L., & Kahn, D. (1998). The economic value of caring. *Health Care Management Review, 23*(4), 43–53.

Johnson, D. E. (1961). The significance of nursing care. *American Journal of Nursing, 61*(11), 63–66.

Kenney, J. W. (2006). Theory-based advanced nursing practice. In W. K. Cody (Ed.), *Philosophical and theoretical perspectives for advanced nursing practice* (pp. 295–310). Sudbury, MA: Jones and Bartlett.

Kim, H. S. (1997). Terminology in structuring and developing nursing knowledge. In I. M. King & J. Fawcett (Eds.), *The language of nursing theory and metatheory* (pp. 27–36). Indianapolis, IN: Center Nursing Press.

King, I. M. (1971). *Toward a theory for nursing: General concepts of human behavior.* Hoboken, NJ: Wiley.

King, I. M. (1990). *A theory for nursing: Systems, concepts, process.* Albany, NY: Delmar.

King, I. M. (2006). Imogene M. King's theory of goal attainment. In M. E. Parker (Ed.), *Nursing theories and nursing practice* (2nd ed., pp. 235–243). Philadelphia, PA: F. A. Davis.

Kleiman, S. (2006). Josephine Paterson and Loretta Zderad's humanistic nursing theory and its applications. In M. E. Parker (Ed.), *Nursing theories and nursing practice* (2nd ed., pp. 125–137). Philadelphia, PA: F. A. Davis.

Leininger, M. M. (2006). Madeleine M. Leininger's theory of culture care diversity and universality. In M. E. Parker (Ed.), *Nursing theories and nursing practice* (2nd ed., pp. 309–333). Philadelphia, PA: F. A. Davis.

Liners Kersbergen Brett, A. (1992). *Caring attributes the nurse administrator needs to receive in order to facilitate a caring environment.* Unpublished manuscript, University of Wisconsin Oshkosh.

Lobo, M. L. (1995). Florence Nightingale. In J. B. George (Ed.), *Nursing theories: The base for professional nursing practice* (4th ed., pp. 33–48). Norwalk, CT: Appleton & Lange.

Malinski, V. M. (2006). Martha E. Rogers' science of unitary human beings. In M. E. Parker (Ed.), *Nursing theories and nursing practice* (2nd ed., pp. 160–166). Philadelphia, PA: F. A. Davis.

McEwen, M., & Wills, E. M. (2006). *Theoretical basis for nursing* (2nd ed.). Philadelphia, PA: Lippincott Williams & Wilkins.

Meleis, A. I. (1992). Directions for nursing theory development in the 21st century. *Nursing Science Quarterly, 5*(3), 112–117.

Meleis, A. I. (1997). *Theoretical nursing: Development and progress* (3rd ed.). Philadelphia, PA: Lippincott.

Mitchell, G. J. (1999). Evidence-based practice: Critique and alternative view. *Nursing Science Quarterly, 12*(1), 30–35.

Mitchell, G. J., Schmidt Bunkers, S., & Bournes, D. (2006). Applications of Parse's human becoming school of thought. In M. E. Parker (Ed.), *Nursing theories and nursing practice* (2nd ed., pp. 194–216). Philadelphia, PA: F. A. Davis.

Monti, E. J., & Tingen, M. S. (1999). Multiple paradigms of nursing science. *Annals of Nursing Science, 21*(4), 64–80.

Nyberg, J. J. (1998). *A caring approach in nursing administration.* Boulder, CO: University Press of Colorado.

Orem, D. E. (2006). Dorothea E. Orem's self-care deficit nursing theory. In M. E. Parker (Ed.), *Nursing theories and nursing practice* (2nd ed., pp. 141–149). Philadelphia, PA: F. A. Davis.

Parker, M. E. (2006). Introduction to nursing theory. In M. E. Parker (Ed.), *Nursing theories and nursing practice* (2nd ed., pp. 3–13). Philadelphia, PA: F. A. Davis.

Parse, R. R. (1997). The language of nursing knowledge: Saying what we mean. In I. M. King & J. Fawcett (Eds.), *The language of nursing theory and metatheory* (pp. 73–77). Indianapolis, IN: Center Nursing Press.

Parse, R. R. (1999). The discipline and the profession. *Nursing Science Quarterly, 12*(4), 275–276.

Parse, R. R. (2006). Rosemarie Rizzo Parse's human becoming school of thought. In M. E. Parker (Ed.), *Nursing theories and nursing practice* (2nd ed., pp. 187–194). Philadelphia, PA: F. A. Davis.

Paterson, J. G., & Zderad, L. T. (1976). *Humanistic nursing.* New York, NY: Wiley.

Peden, A. R. (2006). Hildegard E. Peplau's process of practice-based theory development and its applications. In M. E. Parker (Ed.), *Nursing theories and nursing practice* (2nd ed., pp. 58–69). Philadelphia, PA: F. A. Davis.

Pharris, M. D. (2006). Margaret A. Newman's theory of health as expanding consciousness and its applications. In M. E. Parker (Ed.), *Nursing theories and nursing practice* (2nd ed., pp. 217–234). Philadelphia, PA: F. A. Davis.

Phillips, J. R. (1996). What constitutes nursing science? *Nursing Science Quarterly, 9*(2), 48–49.

Praeger, S. G. (1995). Josephine E. Paterson and Loretta T. Zderad. In J. B. George (Ed.), *Nursing theories: The base for professional nursing practice* (4th ed., pp. 301–315). Norwalk, CT: Appleton & Lange.

Ray, M. A. (1984). The development of a classification system of institutional caring. In M. Leininger (Ed.), *Care: The essence of nursing and health* (pp. 95–112). Thorofare, NJ: Slack.

Ray, M. A. (1989). The theory of bureaucratic caring for nursing practice in the organizational culture. *Nursing Administration Quarterly, 13*(2), 31–42.

Reed, P. (1997). Nursing: The ontology of the discipline. *Nursing Science Quarterly, 10*(2), 76–79.

Risjord, M. (2010). *Nursing knowledge: Science, practice and philosophy.* Chichester, England: Wiley-Blackwell.

Rogers, M. E. (1970). *The theoretical basis of nursing.* Philadelphia, PA: F. A. Davis.

Rogers, M. E. (1994). The science of unitary human beings. *Nursing Science Quarterly, 7*(1), 33–35.

Rolfe, G. (1993). Closing the theory practice gap: A model of nursing praxis. *Journal of Clinical Nursing, 2,* 173–177.

Roy, C., & Andrews, H. A. (1991). *The Roy adaptation model: The definitive statement.* Norwalk, CT: Appleton & Lange.

Roy, C., & Zhan, L. (2006). Sister Callista Roy's adaptation model and its applications. In M. E. Parker (Ed.), *Nursing theories and nursing practice* (2nd ed., pp. 268–280). Philadelphia, PA: F. A. Davis.

Schaefer, K. M. (2006). Myra Levin's conservation model and its applications. In M. E. Parker (Ed.), *Nursing theories and nursing practice* (2nd ed., pp. 94–112). Philadelphia, PA: F. A. Davis.

Schumacher, K. L., & Gortner, S. R. (1992). (Mis)conceptions and reconceptions about traditional science. *Annals of Nursing Science, 14*(4), 1–11.

Senge, P. M. (1994). *The fifth discipline: The art and practice of the learning organization.* New York, NY: Doubleday Business.

Sieloff, C. L., Frey, M., & Killeen, M. (2006). Application of King's theory of goal attainment. In M. E. Parker (Ed.), *Nursing theories and nursing practice* (2nd ed., pp. 244–267). Philadelphia, PA: F. A. Davis.

Silva, M. C. (1999). The state of nursing science: Reconceptualizing for the 21st century. *Nursing Science Quarterly, 12*(3), 221–226.

Sitzman, K., & Eichelberger, L. W. (2003). *Understanding the work of nurse theorists: A creative beginning.* Sudbury, MA: Jones and Bartlett.

Smith, M. C. (1994). Beyond the threshold: Nursing practice in the next millennium. *Nursing Science Quarterly, 7*(1), 6–7.

Stevenson, J. S., & Woods, N. F. (1986). Nursing science and contemporary science: Emerging paradigms. In G. E. Sorensen (Ed.), *Setting the agenda for the year 2000: Knowledge development in nursing* (pp. 6–20). Kansas City, MO: American Academy of Nursing.

Talento, B. (1995). Jean Watson. In J. B. George (Ed.), *Nursing theories: The base for professional nursing practice* (4th ed., pp. 317–333). Norwalk, CT: Appleton & Lange.

Touhy, T. A., & Birnbach, N. (2006). Lydia Hall: The care, core, and cure model and its applications. In M. E. Parker (Ed.), *Nursing theories and nursing practice* (2nd ed., pp. 113–124). Philadelphia, PA: F. A. Davis.

Watson, J. (1979). *Nursing: The philosophy and science of caring.* Boston, MA: Little, Brown.

Watson, J. (2006). Jean Watson's theory of human caring. In M. E. Parker (Ed.), *Nursing theories and nursing practice* (2nd ed., pp. 295–302). Philadelphia, PA: F. A. Davis.

Wheatley, M. J. (2006). *Leadership and the new science: Discovering order in a chaotic world* (3rd ed.). San Francisco, CA: Berrett-Koehler.

Chapter 2

Systems Thinking, Healthcare Organizations, Global Health, and the Advanced Practice Nurse Leader

Sandra Wiggins Petersen

> *The true professional is a person whose action points beyond his or herself to that underlying reality, that hidden wholeness, on which we all can rely.*
>
> —Parker Palmer

Introduction

Health care's tenuous outlook, both within the United States and globally, necessitates the rapid evolution of advanced practice nursing to a station of independent practice, autonomy, flexibility, and leadership. As the "powers that be" struggle to make sense of fragmented systems, a dwindling budget, significant global health issues, and an ever-expanding deficit, coupled with a clamoring for increased access to care for all, the Institute of Medicine (IOM), The Joint Commission, the Robert Wood Johnson Foundation (RWJF), the United Nations (UN), and other national and international authorities, along with the American Association of Colleges of Nursing (AACN) and the National Organization of Nurse Practitioner Faculties (NONPF), have called for a reconceptualizing of health professions education and development to meet the needs of the healthcare delivery system while maintaining quality, safety, and ethical practice. Meanwhile, nursing has been catapulted into the limelight as a solution to the burgeoning masses who are now accessing insurance benefits.

Transforming the healthcare system in the United States to meet the demand for safe, quality, and affordable care has necessitated a fundamental shift in thinking regarding the roles of many healthcare professionals, including advanced practice nurses. The 2010 Affordable Care Act represented the broadest healthcare overhaul since the 1965 creation of the Medicare and Medicaid programs, but the current healthcare workforce remains woefully unprepared to meet the need. Nurses, heretofore unable to fully participate in the resulting evolution of the U.S. healthcare system because of a variety of historical, cultural, regulatory, and policy barriers that limited nurses' ability to contribute to broad, meaningful change, are now being called on to lead the charge in primary care as well as wellness and prevention efforts.

Dubbed "Obamacare" by many, the Affordable Care Act has given tens of millions of previously uninsured Americans access to care. These individuals are now looking for primary care providers, and estimates reflect a shortage of providers ranging from a low figure of 52,000 to as many as 90,000 by 2025 and will worsen because of the aging population. It is no exaggeration to say that the success of the healthcare law, and indeed the U.S. healthcare system, rests on providers choosing to do something that is not always in their economic self-interest, given that reimbursements in primary care are low when compared with those of specialty care venues. Acceptance of advanced practice nurses as a viable solution to the primary care crisis has been slow in coming; even with these staggering figures, some state medical boards and medical advocacy groups have remained oppositional (Iglehart, 2013).

Causing even more alarm, the dearth of a systems approach to global health care became acutely evident with the recent Ebola crisis, with its rapid, unchecked spread to adjoining countries and other countries around the globe in which the United States has a large stake. The message by senior UN officials briefing an informal meeting of the General Assembly at UN headquarters on the public health crisis emanating from the Ebola virus outbreak was threefold: the need for resources for immediate response to the disease that has affected some 23,000 people, with 9,300 deaths; the need to begin planning for revival and recovery; and the need to implement systems to limit spread to other countries. Dr. David Nabarro, the Secretary-General's Special Envoy to the United Nations, noted in January 2015 that having strong surveillance capabilities on the ground to identify people with Ebola, confirming diagnosis, quickly arranging effective treatment, identifying people the patient was in contact with, and keeping those people under review for 21 days "is a really difficult task"—especially given that all these steps must be coordinated through 63 different government structures in an area the size of France (UN News Centre, 2015).

Despite the increased prominence and funding of global health initiatives by the United States and other countries, efforts toward expansion of contiguous health services across the globe have fallen short of the policy dictates in the United States and United Nations Millennium Development Goals (United Nations, 2015). Advanced practice nurses, as change agents, are needed to define the view of global health as a compilation of complex adaptive systems with path dependence, feedback loops, scale-free networks, emergent behaviors, and phase transitions and to uncover relevant lessons for the design and implementation of health policy and programs and strategies. The implications of the application of systems thinking include more attention to local context, incentives, and institutions; anticipating certain types of unintended consequences that can undermine efforts; and developing and implementing programs that engage key players through transparent use of data for ongoing problem solving and adaptation.

In 2008, the RWJF and the IOM launched a two-year initiative to address the need to assess and transform the nursing profession. Through the RWJF initiative, the IOM appointed the Committee on the Future of Nursing, with the purpose of producing a report that would make recommendations for an action-oriented blueprint for the future of nursing. Through its deliberations, the committee developed four key messages:

- Nurses should practice to the full extent of their education and training.
- Nurses should achieve higher levels of education and training through an improved education system that promotes seamless academic progression.
- Nurses should be full partners with physicians and other healthcare professionals in redesigning health care in the United States.
- Effective workforce planning and policy making require better data collection and an improved information infrastructure.

As part of its 2010 report, *The Future of Nursing: Leading Change, Advancing Health* (IOM, 2010), and its 2013 report, *The Future of Nursing:*

A Look Back at the Landmark IOM Report (IOM, 2013), the committee considered the obstacles that all nurses encounter as they take on new roles in the transformation of health care in the United States. Although nurses face challenges at all levels, the committee took particular note of the legal barriers in many states that prohibit advanced practice registered nurses (APRNs) from practicing to their full education and training. The committee determined that such constraints must be lifted for nurses to assume the responsibilities they can and should have during this time of great need. Advanced practice nursing, now with the support of many state legislators, state boards of nursing, and the federal government, coupled with additional funding for advanced practice education, is answering this call by preparing transformational leaders to shape evolving practice and the future of health care (IOM, 2010, 2013).

AACN lends credence to this evolution in the second essential of the doctor of nursing practice (DNP), which accompanied the call for moving the level of preparation necessary for advanced nursing practice roles from the master's degree to the doctorate level by 2015:

> *DNP graduates must understand principles of practice management, including conceptual and practical strategies for balancing productivity with quality of care. They must be able to assess the impact of practice policies and procedures on meeting the health needs of the patient populations with whom they practice. DNP graduates must be proficient in quality improvement strategies and in creating and sustaining changes at the organizational and policy levels. Improvements in practice are neither sustainable nor measurable without corresponding changes in organizational arrangements, organizational and professional culture, and the financial structures to support practice. DNP graduates have the ability to evaluate the cost effectiveness of care and use principles of economics and finance to redesign effective and realistic care delivery strategies. In addition, DNP graduates have the ability to organize care to address emerging practice problems and the ethical dilemmas that emerge as new diagnostic and therapeutic technologies evolve. (AACN, 2006)*

In 2011, NONPF showcased a description of core competencies; an emphasis on population focus was added in 2014, consistent with the IOM report for advanced practice nurses, inclusive of DNPs:

> *Nurse Practitioner graduates have knowledge, skills, and abilities that are essential to independent clinical practice. The NP Core Competencies*

are acquired through mentored patient care experiences with emphasis on **independent** *and* **interprofessional** *practice; analytic skills for evaluating and providing* **evidence-based, patient centered care** *across settings; and advanced knowledge of the health care delivery system. Doctorally-prepared NPs apply knowledge of scientific foundations in practice for quality care. They are able to apply skills in technology and* **information literacy,** *and engage in practice inquiry to improve health outcomes, policy, and healthcare delivery. Areas of increased knowledge, skills, and expertise include advanced communication skills, collaboration, complex decision making, leadership, and the business of health care. (NONPF, 2011, 2014)*

The advanced practice nurse must be able to discern issues quickly and effectively and contribute to strategic energy and system redesign. This phenomenon was perhaps best described by Senge (1990) in *The Fifth Discipline,* when he conveyed the development of the *mental model* as "turning the mirror inward; learning to unearth our internal pictures of the world, to bring them to the surface and hold them rigorously to scrutiny" (p. 9). "Learningful" conversations result in intense scrutiny that balances inquiry and advocacy and allows leaders to expose their own thinking effectively and make that thinking open to the influence of others. In 2003, and again in its 2010 *Future of Nursing* report, the IOM emphasized the necessity of such an approach in declaring the following competencies as foundational: patient-centered care, teamwork and collaboration, evidence-based practice, and quality improvement strategies.

In her treatise *Holistic Nursing: A Handbook for Practice,* Dossey (2008) reiterated a still-relevant plea:

> *Our time demands a new paradigm and a new language where we take the best of what we know in the science and art of nursing that includes holistic and human caring theories and modalities. With an integral approach and worldview we are in a better position to share with others the depth of nurses' knowledge, expertise, and critical-thinking capacities and skills for assisting others in creating health and healing. Only an attention to the heart of nursing, for "sacred" and "heart" reflect a common meaning, can we generate the vision, courage, and hope required to unite nurses and nursing in healing. This assists us as we engage in healthcare reform to address the challenges in these troubled times—local to global. This is not a matter of philosophy, but of survival. (p. 34)*

Systems Thinking: Dealing with Complexity and Chaos

The AACN essentials statement (2006) further noted,

> *Advanced nursing practice includes an organizational and systems leadership component that emphasizes practice, ongoing improvement of health outcomes, and ensuring patient safety. In each case, nurses should be prepared with sophisticated expertise in assessing organizations, identifying systems' issues, and facilitating organization-wide changes in practice delivery. In addition, advanced nursing practice requires political skills, systems thinking, and the business and financial acumen needed for the analysis of practice quality and costs.*

In his 2002 book *The Ingenuity Gap: Can We Solve the Problems of the Future?* Homer-Dixon presented evidence that the demand for ingenuity arising from the ever-increasing complexity of our world is far outstripping our capacity to supply it. Although in the past we have been able to find solutions—and, in Homer-Dixon's words, "throw huge amounts of energy at our problems" (p. 187)—to keep our ever-expanding complex systems glued together, in the future we will almost certainly find it necessary to accept some large breakdowns in human and natural systems and to develop radical new ways of running things. Homer-Dixon added, "There are a couple of areas where I sometimes despair about our capacity to deal with what lies ahead. One is our cognitive characteristics and the other is the self-reinforcing nature of our economic system" (p. 2). When Homer-Dixon referred to "cognitive characteristics," he underscored that societies adapt easily to small-scale, incremental change. It is this slow evolution that makes it possible for humanity to face each day and not feel as though our foundations have been shaken; it is part of self-preservation. And yet, Homer-Dixon said, this human capacity is "a real handicap when it comes to dealing with 'slow-creep' problems. We just don't see the change, and the thing about slow-creep problems is they may be slow-creep for a while, but then all of a sudden there's a non-linear shift and we find ourselves in a crisis" (p. 4).

The transformation of U.S. health care was not a "slow-creep" change. The nonlinear shift from a volume-based system to a value-based system has rocked the healthcare system and left legislators and providers frantically strategizing as to how to meet the needs of patients with newly acquired access to care. The goal of improving efficiency, access, and outcomes while reducing costs demands the realignment of stakeholder incentives and the development of a new payment structure that rewards those collective goals for all concerned. How well Homer-Dixon describes our current crisis in health care and the need for advanced practice nurses to be well versed in systems thinking and steeped in competency with regard to essential core skills!

Vision and Perspective: Keys to the Future of Advanced Practice

The evolution of the DNP advanced practice role as that of strategic systems thinker and visionary for health care lies largely within the profession's commitment to lifelong learning and the realization that people and organizations do not exist as islands unto themselves, but rather as part of a larger network, web, or matrix of systems that all function more or less independently, yet *inter*dependently. Burns's transformational theory (1978) described this matrix as a melding of social and spiritual values. He recognized it as a motivational lever that gives people an uplifting sense of being connected to a higher purpose, thus playing to the need for a sense of meaning and identity. Ultimately, one must realize the necessity of developing a dedication to disrupting the system as we know it, while at the same time retaining flexibility, balance, and a sense of social intelligence and responsibility.

Broadly, as we examine the healthcare landscape over the past two decades, common themes emerge. In general, the concern about dwindling access to health care—often linked to cost—that commanded much of the literature around the turn of the century has most recently been eclipsed by a general sense of alarm (perhaps panic) about the rising cost of health care and the inadequacy of globe-spanning systems to address burgeoning health concerns. These observations may have been influenced by rising health insurance rates, by the increasing healthcare needs of baby boomers reaching retirement, and by the release of a series of long-range healthcare cost projections. At one extreme are those who hotly contend that Americans have the "best healthcare system in the world," pointing to the freely available medical technology and state-of-the-art facilities that have become symbolic of the system. At the other extreme, however, are those who strongly criticize the American system as being fragmented and inefficient, pointing to the fact that America spends more on health care than any other country in the world, yet our nation still suffers from rampant lack of insurance, inconsistency in quality, and excessive administrative waste (Casoy, 2008).

In light of the new and growing evidence about the U.S. health disadvantage, the National Institutes of Health asked the National Research Council (NRC) and the IOM to convene a panel of experts to study the issue. The Panel on Understanding Cross-National Health Differences Among High-Income Countries, convened in 2013, examined whether the U.S. health disadvantage exists across the life span, considered potential explanations, and assessed the larger implications of the findings.

U.S. Health in International Perspectives

The United States is among the wealthiest nations in the world, but it is far from the healthiest according to the Panel on Understanding Cross-National Health Differences Among High-Income Countries (Woolf & Aron, 2013). Although life expectancy and survival rates in the United States have improved dramatically over the past century, Americans live shorter lives and experience more injuries and illnesses than people in other high-income countries. The U.S. health disadvantage cannot be attributed solely to the adverse health status of racial or ethnic minorities or poor people: even highly advantaged Americans are in worse health than their counterparts in other, "peer" countries.

In 2005, the Employee Benefits Research Institute (EBRI) first reported that the erosion of employer-based coverage was offset by increased enrollment in Medicaid, which was initially designed to provide a safety net for the lowest income Americans (EBRI, 2012). However, as the *Washington Post* noted in late 2008, Medicaid had become the subject of relentless funding cuts by budget-strapped states and congressional representatives who were ideologically opposed to welfare programs. As the program continued to be slashed, it was increasingly evident that Medicaid or other state-funded programs would be unable to offset the losses in employer-based insurance, resulting in more and more uninsured individuals. Thus, the insecurity of health care rose to an all-time high as thousands of people lost their health insurance as a result of a sagging job market. Health care, as a result, has become increasingly elusive, even for affluent Americans. Because any employee is just one pink slip away from becoming uninsured, it is clear that some solution in health care is not just important to achieve, but imperative.

In early 2014, the EBRI reported that more than 20%, or 1 in 5 Americans 50 or older, reported saving on health costs by switching to cheaper generic drugs, getting free samples, and stopping pills or reducing dosages, and nearly as many skip or postpone doctor appointments for the same reason. Many also questioned their providers regarding the costs of procedures before agreeing to have them performed, especially those with high-deductible insurance policies. In fact, the data suggest that spending by those near or in retirement has declined to match income, even when it may mean giving up critical care.

Specifically, the 2014 analysis found that more than 1 in 5 (21.5%) households reported making some changes in their prescription drugs to save money, and nearly as many (19.4%) said that they have either skipped or postponed doctor appointments to do so. The report found that these reductions were spread almost equally among households, whether they reported increasing or decreasing their annual spending. Even for those who reported that their spending was unchanged, 16.5% reported making prescription drug changes, while 11.7% reported skipping or postponing doctor visits to save money.

The study also found that about 1 in 10 of those in excellent health reported skipping or postponing doctor appointments to save money, while more than three times as many (36.5%) of those in poor health reported doing so. Similarly, nearly 1 in 3 (29.9%) of those in poor health reported making prescription drug changes to save money, which is nearly twice the number of those in excellent health.

Even with the recent unrest and disconcerting statistics, it is tempting to believe that the current design of the healthcare system is beyond repair. Yet, a look back reveals the countless metamorphoses of an externally different yet eternally fundamentally flawed entity. Thus, transformational DNPs can drive the avoidance of this abysmal cycle through full dissection and understanding of the underlying structure and root cause(s) of the dysfunction. Will value-based care and increased access create appropriate solutions? Is it acceptable to deny people health care based on their ability to pay? Is health care a basic need that should be provided to every American as a matter of course? Or does the solution lie somewhere between the two extremes? Regardless of the answer, we must ensure that the DNP is well armed to overcome the remarkably complex inertia of the American healthcare system and spearhead the effort to create a society in which health care is, at a minimum, cost effective, of reasonable quality, and readily accessible.

The Advanced Practice Path to Healthcare Solutions

Many of the healthcare problems that plague us today are complex, involving multiple factors that are at least partly the result of past actions taken to alleviate problems. Traditional approaches often attack single factors or problems with little regard for the impact on the whole.

Dealing with such problems is notoriously difficult, and the results of conventional solutions are frequently poor enough to create great discouragement about the prospects of ever effectively addressing them. One of the key benefits of the application of systems thinking to such massive, complex concerns is the ability to deal effectively with a variety of problems from a holistic viewpoint. The systems approach helps us raise our thinking to the level at which we create the results we want as individuals and organizations, even in those difficult situations marked by complexity, great numbers of interactions, and the absence or ineffectiveness of immediately apparent solutions (Bass, 1990).

In his book *The Fifth Discipline*, Senge (1990) described the process of systems thinking as "seeing the world anew." He noted, "There is something in all of us that loves to put together a puzzle, that loves to see the image of the whole emerge. The beauty of a person, or a flower, or a poem lies in seeing all of it. It is interesting that the words 'whole' and 'health' come from the same root as the Old English hal, as in 'hale and hearty.' So, it should come as no surprise that the unhealthiness of our world today is in direct proportion to our inability to see it as a whole" (pp. 42–43).

In considering the fragmented state of national health care, the astute DNP can readily see that systems thinking can likely be employed as the much-needed framework for seeing the diversity (and fragmentation) as a "whole." A systems approach provides the framework for seeing interrelationships and patterns of change rather than individual issues. The approach uses a focused sensitivity to the interconnectedness that gives social systems of extreme complexity their unique character.

Systems Thinking and Advanced Practice

Systems thinking has its roots in the field of system dynamics, honed most successfully in 1958 by Massachusetts Institute of Technology professor Jay Forrester, who acknowledged the need for a better way of testing new ideas in complex engineering problems and, additionally, realized its value in addressing issues within social systems, such as the provision of health care. Systems thinking allows people to gain an explicit understanding of social systems and improve them in the same way that people can use engineering principles to make explicit and improve their understanding of mechanical systems. Complexity can easily undermine responsibility and creativity and result in feelings of helplessness and hopelessness. To combat this, systems thinking across organizations offers a discipline for understanding the unique structures that undergird complex systems and, through that understanding, a way to effect change that is significant and enduring.

Schyve (2000) noted that systems thinking has already become ubiquitous in health care, largely due to continuous quality improvement initiatives in patient safety. Even 10 years ago, the idea of "looking at the whole" (the process) with regard to medical errors rather than at the individual might not have been acceptable. The advent of "blameless" cultures within this context provides a much less threatening venue than the former reliance on accusations of error. It is this systems thinking that has enabled many in health care to traverse beyond the old (and extremely ineffective) "name, blame, and shame" approach to patient safety and toward a more effective focus on human factors engineering and the systems within which doctors, nurses, pharmacists, and other healthcare professionals function. If systems thinking can be successfully applied to this one critical aspect of patient safety, could not the transformational advanced practice nurse leader consider an application of this strategy to the whole?

Adopting a Systems Perspective

Transformational leadership in advanced practice roles involves a willingness to take reasonable risks based on empirical data, a commitment to action, reflection of core values, and a drive for excellence at all levels. As leaders seek to hone their skills in their enthusiasm for creating the future, systems thinking must be an integral part of problem solving. Bass (1990) noted that more charismatic transformational leaders may achieve this alignment with systems thinking through evoking strong emotions that result in the identification of followers with the leader, perhaps through stirring appeals. Others may achieve the same result through quieter methods such as coaching and mentoring.

Nevertheless, the approach to any complex situation must begin with the deep insight that the problems and the hopes for improvement are inextricably tied to how the problem solvers think. Learning about a problem of great complexity requires a conceptual framework of "structural" or systems thinking to facilitate the ability to discover the underlying structural causes of poor performance (Wheatley, 2002). Lynham and Chermack (2006), in their theory of responsible leadership for performance (RLP), suggested a general, integrative theoretical framework of leadership that addresses the nature and challenges of leadership and is both responsible and focused on performance. Two core premises govern the framework. The first is that leadership is itself a system consisting of purposeful, integrated inputs, processes, outputs, feedback, and boundaries. The second is that leadership takes place within a performance system—that is, a system of joint, coordinated, and purposeful action. Leadership can therefore be conceived of as a system of interacting inputs, processes, outputs, and feedback that derives meaning, direction, and purpose from the larger performance system and environment within which it occurs. From this perspective, leadership is defined as a focused system of interacting inputs, process, outputs, and feedback wherein individuals or groups influence or act on behalf of specific individuals or groups of individuals to achieve shared goals and commonly desired performance outcomes within a specific performance system and environment.

As leaders come to understand the structures within systems that cause patterns of behaviors or patterns within relationships that result in problems (inputs), they see more clearly how to effect change and adopt mechanisms that will work successfully on a larger scale (outputs). Ouchi's (1981) "Theory Z" (sometimes called participative theory or "Japanese management") also speaks of an organizational performance-driven culture that mirrors the Japanese culture, in which workers are participative and capable of performing many and varied tasks. Theory Z emphasizes such things as broadening of skills, generalization versus specialization, and the need for continuous training of workers to address this need for redesign. Redesigning the way one addresses decisions or behaviors (throughputs) through careful analysis of as many problem patterns as possible on a small scale inherently leads to redesign of the larger system structure; only then can consumers of the system provide feedback to validate the effectiveness of the changes.

The Essence of Problem Solving

Senge (1990) noted that there are multiple levels of explanation in any complex situation. These include reactive, responsive, and generative explanations. As leaders begin to look for patterns within relationships, it is critical that these investigations remain focused on structure and patterns rather than on specific events.

Event explanations "lay blame" or result in a *reactive* stance to problems. To further explore this concept, let's take the example of the patient who has a fall. A reactive stance might be to immediately restrain the patient in response to that event. We assume in this instance that because the patient could move and has fallen, we must keep him from moving in the future. As one can quickly see, the reactive stance leaves no room for discussions about why the fall occurred or what could be done to improve the patient's fall risk, if one even exists. There are no discussions regarding quality of life for the patient, and certainly there are no explorations of root cause or how falls might affect other patients. This type of explanation is tied to a single event and is the most likely type to reinforce the flaws within a reactive system, maintaining the status quo. Little room is left for problem solving or quality improvement.

Approaching this same scenario from a *responsive* stance, we might look at patterns of behavior and ask whether the patient had incurred falls in the past. If he had multiple falls, at what times did the falls occur? We might also look at fall risk and prevention for this patient and ultimately for other patients within the system, tracking and trending in response. The responsive approach focuses on explaining patterns of behavior and envisioning long-term results and trends that can benefit the larger system. The responsive approach allows for quality improvement in response to data gathered through tracking and trending within a system, thus breaking the hold of reactivity and the "short-term fix."

Generative explanation, the most powerful of the three, focuses on finding the root cause(s) of patterns of behavior. In the case of the falling patient, for example, we might look at the types of situations in which the falls occur. We could ask, "Under what circumstances did the falls occur?" We could consider falls occurring during transfers; perhaps staff are not using appropriate transfer techniques or appropriate equipment. Perhaps there are critical steps missing from transfer procedures that result in the failure of the process. It is at this level of explanation that patterns of behavior can be changed—not just reacted to or responded to, but actually *changed*.

Ultimately, the systems perspective tells advanced practice leaders that we must look beyond individual mistakes, karma, or unrelenting bad luck to understand important issues. We must also look beyond personalities, politics, and events to observe and explain the structures that result in individual actions and use this knowledge to discern processes whereby certain types of events become more likely. Senge (1990) quoted Donella Meadows, who said, "A truly profound and different insight is the way you begin to see that the system causes its own behavior" (p. 68).

Systems Thinking, Advanced Practice, and the Learning Organization

"Experience is the best teacher" is a phrase that has been a mantra within the healthcare environment for many years. "See one, do one, teach one" has long been a part of nursing and medical education. We learn through taking an action and observing the consequences of that action; then we adjust and take a new and different action. Thus, learning is woven throughout the fabric of life and indeed throughout complex healthcare organizations—at least the ones that are successful. Lack of learning within an organization often results in its demise or in very poor performance.

In a large, complex organization, however, the primary consequences of our actions may well be in the distant future or in a distant but interrelated part of a larger system in which we operate. For this reason, we are often puzzled by the underlying causes of current problems within our organizations. We are unable to look at underlying structures or patterns of behavior that may have resulted in less than stellar outcomes. Instead, we are very likely to fixate on events and on "working harder" to try to resolve or troubleshoot current issues.

Early in 1992, Jeanie Duck of the Boston Consulting Group wrote about the "reductionist" approach to managing an organization and ferreting out issues. The reductionist management model has long been popular in the United States as a means of explaining and quickly addressing issues. Duck noted that the premise of reductionism is that to understand something, you reduce it to its simplest components and analyze the components in great detail. At the outset, the reductionist approach makes complex tasks (or problems) more manageable. However, the disadvantage to this approach is that the organization is no longer able to see the consequences of actions or decisions, and the connection to the larger system is lost. Learning organizations must successfully abandon reductionism. Once that occurs, leaders and employees within the organization can continually expand their capacity to create results. New and expansive patterns of thinking that foster interconnectedness within the organization are encouraged.

As the role of nursing leadership continues to expand, the advanced practice leader will no doubt be called on to foster the development of learning organizations and to function as a change agent to facilitate organizational functioning within larger complex systems. Adopting a sustained culture of learning enables an organization to maintain a competitive advantage in times of change and to inspire its workforce to achieve greater results and improved quality. Furthermore, organizations can draw on a learning culture to encourage innovation or manage change.

David Garvin, of Harvard Business School and QualityGurus.com fame, defined a learning organization as "skilled at creating, acquiring, and transferring knowledge, and at modifying its behavior to reflect new knowledge and insights" (Garvin, Edmondson, & Gino, 2008). This is best accomplished by first assessing the organization's culture, leadership, and tolerance for change. The organization must be open to developing a conceptual framework for systems thinking and a shared vision to make patterns clearer and effectively initiate change (Gill, 2015).

Advanced practice leaders have the responsibility for instilling the ideas of personal mastery in all employees as a basis for shared vision and connection throughout the organization. As a basis for change, personal mastery (Senge, 1990) is the discipline of continually clarifying and deepening one's personal vision, of focusing one's energies, of developing patience, and of seeing reality objectively and letting go of mental models (ingrained ideas) from the past. An organization's commitment to and capacity for learning can be no greater than those of its employees. The roots of this idea are detailed in both Eastern and Western spiritual traditions, as well as in some secular traditions. More and more healthcare organizations are tapping into this idea; healthcare entities around the country are now developing leadership residencies aimed at personal leadership growth as a valuable resource within the organization. The learning organization grows and changes as its people learn and develop personal mastery. Thus, becoming a learning organization can be viewed as a continual process involving employees at all levels.

As an organization focuses on personal mastery for employees, it progresses to team learning and a free flow of information and ideas that eventually, if carefully guided, leads to a shared vision for the organization and, ultimately, a more effective organization. James P. Lewis (2001) noted the impact of team learning and the shared vision in his book *Project Planning, Scheduling, and Control*. He cited the example of a non-learning organization that decided to implement an electronic charting system based on executive input only. Final decisions were based on the huge financial outlay already made, choice of product, and scope of implementation. Contract negotiations were completed at a high level without the involvement of clinicians. Not involving those on the front line (clinicians) in the early stages cost the organization financially and functionally when the unwieldy system caused patient care to be more difficult than it was before the implementation.

Senge (1990) noted, "To practice a discipline is to be a lifelong learner. You 'never arrive'; you spend your life mastering disciplines. You can never say, 'We are a learning organization,' any more than you can say, 'I am an enlightened person.' The more you learn, the more acutely aware you become of your ignorance" (p. 43). A learning organization is one that constantly provides its employees timely access to relevant, practical information that inspires innovation. It involves creating a culture in which learning is embedded and in which it is communicated to and understood by all that there are many places to seek information. As Margaret Wheatley (1992) expounded, "Innovation is fostered by information gathered from new connections; from insights gained by journeys into other disciplines or places; from active, collegial networks and fluid, open boundaries. Innovation arises from ongoing circles of exchange, where information is not just accumulated or stored, but created. Knowledge is generated anew from connections that weren't there before" (p. 113).

The Downside to Systems Thinking

Systems thinking has a proven track record as a means of addressing problems within complex systems and has been successfully applied in healthcare venues. However, the principles of systems thinking are not typically conveyed in basic healthcare education. Although the DNP competencies clearly proclaim these principles as essential, nurses at the undergraduate level are generally educated in the personal mastery of knowledge, skills, and abilities to provide assistance to sick, often frail and vulnerable, individuals or populations. The individual ethical creed to "do no harm" pertains primarily to the nurse as an individual assisting individuals, not to systems and processes.

Given this perspective, a systems thinking approach to healthcare reform presents challenges for the advanced practice leader. The general understanding is that a system is perfectly designed to produce what it produces; or, conversely, whatever we get from a system is what the system is designed to produce, regardless of whether the design of the system was planned or unplanned and whether the results were intended or unintended. Different individuals within the same structure tend to produce similar results. Therefore, when performance is poor or expectations are unmet, it is relatively easy to find someone or something to blame. The paradigm shift of interrelationships and interrelatedness reinforces the fact that systems may cause their own crises. Such crises are not the fault of individuals, nor the result of external factors, but inherent within the system or processes that fall short.

According to Lynham and Chermack (2006), systems are composed of many related components: people, equipment, processes, and data. Each component directly or indirectly has the potential to affect not only the function of the system but also the functions of other components within the system. Traditional nursing leaders tend to consider structure as an external constraint based on the performance of individual components; however, in human systems, it is the basic *interrelationships* among components, not structural constraint, that control behaviors. As a result, the purpose of a system then becomes to maximize the output of the system, not the output of each of its components. The silos of leadership that exist throughout health care generally focus only on their own decisions and may ignore how their decisions affect others, creating instability within the system as a result. Senge (1990) illustrated this concept in the example of the engineer who noted that one could build a car from the then "best" engine, drive train, suspension, and tires, but it would be unlikely to run. Every system, including those in health care, must *optimize*—rather than *maximize*—the performance of each of its components to bolster the system's production.

As noted in the IOM competencies, the production (output) of a healthcare system has multiple dimensions. The dimensions of safety, effectiveness, patient centeredness, timeliness, efficiency, and equity are often used to describe the output of the system (IOM, 2003). It is uncommon for the system to *maximize* the level of each of the multiple dimensions of its output; rather, the system must *optimize* the level of each dimension. This optimization, however, is a value judgment by those who design and manage the system and, to some degree, those who use the output of the system. These stakeholders in the healthcare system do not always agree on the relative priorities for the dimensions of the system's output, thus presenting a problem but also an opportunity for compromise that must be recognized by the astute leader.

Multifaceted, multilayered healthcare systems are all at significant risk of producing unintended consequences. Even apparently "inconsequential" changes in healthcare systems at any level will almost always produce unintended consequences. It is predictable that unintended consequences will likely emerge, but what those consequences will be, and whether they will be beneficial or destructive, is often unpredictable. At worst, well-intentioned changes could result in unintended harm. Margaret Wheatley (1992) espoused an interesting perspective on unintended consequences, seeing them as unintended opportunities to find new ways of looking at things and to redesign poor processes. In her book *Turning to One Another: Simple Conversations to Restore Hope to the Future*, written in 2002, Wheatley noted that failures within organizations are the signal that more connections need to be made within the organization; she contended that the solution lies within untapped conversations and undiscovered connections.

A Challenge to Advanced Practice Leaders: Operationalizing Systems Thinking

The evolution of the advanced practice leader is the by-product of concerted efforts to align personal behavior with values and to learn how to listen and to appreciate others' talents, abilities, and insights. Without this diligent effort dedicated to the development of the capacity to lead, a lack of personal charisma, personal mastery, information sharing, and mental mastery would render us ineffective in the pursuit of the shared vision and the transformational leadership so vital to the survival of health care in the future (Ouchi, 1981).

Once personal mastery is achieved, however, one must transcend the traditional activity of management as most of us know it and focus on wielding power within a system. This endeavor not only encompasses the balancing of structures within an organization or system but also is the embodiment of shared vision and empowerment, inducing people and resources to migrate from the current state to the desired state while seeking their own personal mastery (Senge, 2006). Although this sounds very noble, the reality is that as the current state approaches the desired state, promotion of the activity and motivation typically decline; this goes on until someone takes notice and raises the red flag of organizational panic and urges reactive decision making (which rarely produces good results). Therefore, the task of the leader becomes sustaining the effort long enough to close the gap between what *was* and the present while avoiding panic, reactivity, and, ultimately, disaster.

The Learning Organization and the Inquiring Mind: Sustaining the Effort

In *The Fifth Discipline*, Peter Senge (1990) described five basic disciplines that support shared vision and empowerment, placing systems thinking in the primary position. He called it "the fifth discipline" because it is the conceptual cornerstone that underlies all the other learning disciplines. As he noted, all are concerned with a shift of mind from seeing parts to seeing wholes, from seeing people as helpless reactors to seeing them as active participants in shaping their reality, from reacting to the present to creating the future.

When it comes to operationalizing and applying systems thinking concepts within the learning organization or across many organizations, Charles West Churchman (1913–2004), a pragmatic philosopher with a deep concern for the welfare of humanity, laid the groundwork for the most practical approach to creatively shaping the future. In the 1950s, he worked with Russell L. Ackoff and E. Leonard Arnoff to develop and describe the philosophical and methodological aspects of operations research, designed as an interdisciplinary approach to "real-world problem solving" (Ulrich, 1988/2009, 2012).

Early in 1971, Churchman adapted the design of what he called "inquiring systems"—systems capable of facilitating learning and organizational change. The purpose of these inquiring systems is to create knowledge, thereby "creating the capability of choosing the right means for one's desired ends" (Churchman, 1971, p. 200). Churchman's model for the design of inquiring systems provides the basis for sustaining evolving organizations. Churchman's theoretical work was driven by his unrelenting interest in determining whether it is "possible to secure improvement in the human condition by means of the human intellect" (Ulrich, 1988/2009). One of his significant contributions to the development of systems theory was his recognition that "problem solving often appears to produce improvement, but the so-called 'solution' often makes matters worse in the larger system" (Churchman, 1982, p. 19n). He argued that "simple, direct, head-on attempts to 'solve' system problems don't work and, indeed, often turn out to be downright dangerous" (Churchman, 1979, p. 4). No problem exists in isolation; rather, problems are inextricably linked to each other and to the environment, thus requiring an approach to the whole.

Underlying Concepts of Churchman's Systems Model

Churchman's inquiry systems model is centered on the *client* as the "complex of persons whose interests ought to be served" (Churchman, 1971, p. 48). Clients can be described by their value structure. Each client has a set of possible futures (i.e., goals or objectives) and a preference for one future over others. Clients have trade-off principles that reveal how much of one objective they would relinquish in order to achieve or increase another objective, establishing a means of "balancing" a given system.

Within Churchman's model, the *environment* is limitless. It consists of all things outside the system that may, in some direct, indirect, or even barely comprehensible way, affect—or be affected by—what happens within the system. Also within the model, a *decision maker* controls system resources. He or she "*co-produces* the future along with the environment, which he [or she] does not control" (Churchman, 1971, p. 47). The decision maker's preferred future may not be identical to that of other stakeholders (clients), and his or her trade-off principle may not be the same.

The system *planner* is the person who should at all times strive toward improvement of the human condition. Churchman (1971, 1979) envisioned a planner who seeks to identify the client's underlying principles and trade-off principles, to create measures of performance based on those principles, and to trace out all potential consequences of any given action. The planner's intentions are presumed to be "always good with respect to the client" (Churchman, 1971, p. 47), and the planner assumes the role of trying to ensure that the decision makers' value structure also supports that of the client. The *measure of performance* is, in simple form, the degree of attainment of a stated goal, purpose, or objective, sometimes measured by the probability or amount of attainment and sometimes by evaluating benefits and costs (Churchman, 1979).

Agents and factors both within and outside the system may be said to *co-produce* the measures of performance. By their influence, co-producers may either assist to actualize or prevent the achievement of the client's objectives. Following the work of Edgar A. Singer, Churchman stated that "something is a producer of an event if at least one description of the event would be different were the producer not there" (1979, p. 87). Churchman went on to note that "in the case of organizational decision making, the co-producers are many but often operate in subtle and non-formalized manners." Indeed, "part of an organization's 'unconscious' is the existence of co-producers who block the implementation of 'good' ideas, but are never mentioned" (p. 87).

The aforementioned roles belie Churchman's dedication to creating learning systems within organizations. Foremost in these systems is the recognition that decision makers must be as open-minded and creative as possible so that their problem identifications and proposed solutions reflect not merely the concerns of interest to the decision makers but also the implications of the problem and its solutions for the whole system—indeed, for the environment itself (Ulrich, 1988/2009; 2012).

To create a learning system, leaders, acting as planners, must move away from focusing on the obvious (e.g., data, hard facts). For planners who focus on the obvious—*goal planners*—"reality stops at the boundaries of the problem" (Churchman, 1979, p. 108). In contrast, *objective planners* attempt to reframe the obvious within the context of a larger problem. For the objective planner, "reality stops at the boundaries set by feasibility and to some extent by responsibility" (p. 106). Although this larger perspective moves the system in the direction of learning, Churchman pondered another level: *ideal planning*. Whereas goals are deemed short term and objectives long term, ideals are considered to stretch indefinitely into the future and to approach the essential question of how to improve the human condition. The ideal planner moves past the feasible and the realistic and attempts to define purposes that could hold if these restraints were removed. In the ideal system, planners and decision makers work not with the obvious and the tangible but with limitless imagination (Churchman, 1979; Ulrich, 2012).

Because the bounds of creativity can never fully be known, Churchman's model (1979) for inquiring systems is one constructed not of answers but of many questions. Inquiry—and its corollary, decision making—is conducted in a learning system through a process of unfolding questions. As each new aspect of the environment is considered, more layers of influence (co-production) or impact are discovered and must be addressed in turn. Churchman laid out a dialectical framework within which the questions are posed, stakeholders' interests are considered, the environment is limitless, and the ethics are those of the whole system. The inquiry model begins with the questions in **Table 2-1** and can be readily applied in problem solving (Churchman, 1971, pp. 79–80).

Table 2-1 Churchman's Problem-Solving Model

The Client

What is his or her purpose(s)?

What should be his or her purpose(s)?

How is the variety of his or her purposes unified under a measure of performance?

How should the variety of his or her purposes be unified under a measure of performance?

The Decision Maker

What is the decision maker able to use as resources?

What should the decision maker be able to use as resources?

What can the decision maker not control, which nonetheless matters—the environment?

What should the decision maker not control, which nonetheless matters—the environment?

The Planner

How is the planner able to implement his or her plans?

How should the planner be able to implement his or her plans?

[Ideally] What is the guarantor that his or her planning will succeed, that is, will secure improvement in the human condition?

[Ideally] What should be the guarantor that his or her planning will succeed, that is, will secure improvement in the human condition?

Reproduced from Churchman, C. W. (1979). *The design of inquiring systems* (pp. 79–80). New York, NY: Basic Books.

Within any human service organization dedicated to benevolent purposes, the DNP leader can readily see how Churchman's model could be used to provide organizational assessment and a blueprint for a holistic systems approach to problem solving. The complexities of healthcare issues lend themselves to the use of Churchman's design of inquiring systems and provide the transformational leader with a solid, methodical approach that promotes engagement by all parts of the organization.

If we consider the example of an organization that provides primary family care, the construction of a simple spreadsheet could readily identify key stakeholders whose purposes and counterpurposes the organization must consider in addressing problems. The spreadsheet might list each stakeholder as a *client* with particular needs and objectives—purposes—relating to optimal health care. For example, geriatric clients served by the practice might be identified as having several purposes, including a desire for fulfilling quality of life, for the attention of a cost-effective skilled medical provider, and for the cost-effective provision of medication. In Churchman's model, client purposes are both those things that the client desires (e.g., fulfilling quality of life) and those things that the client *should* have (e.g., safe, cost-effective care and medications).

Continuing with the example, a stakeholder may be represented by more than one client category. Young adult clients of the primary care practice, for example, may have purposes both as "parents" concerned about their children's health and as "patrons" who may themselves access the healthcare system. In addition, every stakeholder has the potential to act as a *co-producer* of the solution to the problem posed. He or she may do so by assisting the decision maker or by placing obstacles in the decision maker's path. It is important to note that the decision makers are also clients, in that they too have purposes to be served.

Maximizing the Efforts of Inquiry

As one completes the inquiry just described, it becomes easier to observe patterns within the desires and needs of clients at all levels of the system. These patterns become the basis for understanding the overall system; leaders, as a result, can target innovation (change) efforts more effectively. This is where the approach of systems thinking is fundamentally different from that of traditional methods of analysis. Instead of isolating smaller parts of a system (e.g., individual clients), systems thinking looks at the whole, considering larger numbers (patterns) of interactions to gain understanding.

If we continue our consideration of the primary care clinic described earlier, we might, for instance, through traditional analysis, make a change in practice that would benefit one group of clients but work to the detriment of another. Let's say that we decide to see all pediatric sick cases in the morning to accommodate working mothers and move geriatric chronic cases to the afternoon. We find, however, in examining feedback from the geriatric clients, that they are only able to get public transportation to appointments in the morning, with the latest senior bus picking up at 11:30 a.m. If the senior clients catch the earlier buses to make an afternoon appointment, they have a long wait time *and* are exposed to the sick children. Over time, if we continued with this plan (without the feedback), we would see that the benefits of this innovation would quickly begin to evaporate, and our organization and patients would suffer.

Avoiding this global failure is a key advantage of systems thinking. By closely examining all the interactions created by a decision, potential backfires within the system can be detected and, it is hoped, avoided (see **Figure 2-1**). In the example case, a compromise of selected days for

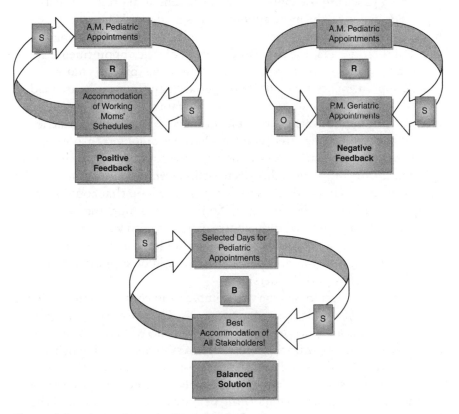

Figure 2-1 Advanced Practice Nurse Leader

pediatric morning appointments might achieve a balance of the needs of all patients accessing the system. Examination of feedback leads to innovation that is a better fit for the big picture and to results that create substantial, lasting benefits.

The arrows in a causal loop diagram are usually labeled with an "S" or an "O." "S" means that when the first variable changes, the second one changes in the same direction (for example, as you schedule more pediatric appointments in the mornings, the number of mothers who desire to make these appointments goes up too). "O" means that the first variable causes a change in the opposite direction in the second variable (for example, the more pediatric appointments scheduled in the morning, the fewer geriatric appointments occur in the afternoon because of exposure to sick children and long wait times for transportation).

In causal diagrams, the arrows join to form loops, with each loop labeled with an "R" or a "B." "R" means reinforcing and refers to causal relationships within the loop that create exponential growth or collapse. For instance, the more appointments made in the morning, the happier working mothers become; because the mothers are happier, they tell their friends, and more and more pediatric appointments are made, and so on, in an upward spiral. By the same token, as more pediatric appointments are made, fewer geriatric appointments are made overall. Pediatric patients are taking up the morning slots, so there are few morning appointments available for older patients. The geriatric patients do not like the afternoon slots because of long transportation wait times and exposure to sick children. This could cause a downward spiral in the business and a dire decrease in revenue for the practice. The "B" means balancing and refers to factors in the loop that could keep things in equilibrium. For example, if only selected mornings—one or two per week—are reserved for pediatric patients with working mothers, geriatric patients can continue to be accommodated at times they prefer. The result is a sustainable process that would be supported by both groups of patients (stakeholders).

Causal loop diagrams can be very complex and contain many different "R" and "B" loops, all connected with arrows. The use of these diagrams can offer leaders and their teams valuable perspectives on what is happening within an organization. This type of systems thinking helps avoid reactive decisions and explores the possibilities of negative outcomes for the business before they happen. For example, by understanding the relationship between morning pediatric appointments and the exposure of frail elderly clients to long wait times, a poor business decision can be avoided.

Summary: The DNP Systems Thinker

Advanced practice leadership must acknowledge the healthcare system as an open system, affected by and, to some degree, dependent on larger systems of which it is a part. We have learned the value of studying and changing the microsystems of health care—the people, equipment, and data at the level of direct patient care. But these microsystems are subsystems within macrosystems such as hospitals, nursing homes, and clinics. These macrosystems, in turn, are part of the megasystem of American health care, which itself is a component of the even larger economic, political, and social metasystems of society as a whole and, ultimately, a part of global systems.

Employing a systems approach to seeking solutions in health care will ultimately alter the role of the various disciplines within health care. This reconsideration of roles will become the purview of advanced practice leaders at all levels. These advanced systems thinkers will ultimately lead the way as we seek to begin the inquiries expressed by the following questions: What are the human vulnerabilities with respect to our capacity to keep up with new knowledge, to remember, or to analyze large amounts of data? How might the principles of distributed cognition (interaction and feedback) and information-sharing technology protect us from these vulnerabilities? How might system redesign as a result of a shared vision protect us from making fatal design errors? What are the human vulnerabilities with respect to our thinking, emotions, and actions?

The challenges ahead require that the advanced practice leader be well prepared in the application of systems thinking to the healthcare environment. Through careful analysis of the structure of both microsystems and macrosystems, how their performance is best measured, and how they interrelate, one can make a determination of their vulnerabilities and strengths within the context of a structural explanation. Detection of behavioral patterns in underlying structure may assist in optimizing system components to maximize results of the system. Systems thinking may further provide the tools for identifying and monitoring for unintended consequences and illuminate the possible interventions to prevent harm from such consequences.

References

American Association of Colleges of Nursing. (2006). *The essentials of doctoral education for advanced nursing practice.* Retrieved from http://www.aacn.nche.edu/publications/position/DNPEssentials.pdf

Bass, B. (1990). *Bass and Stogdill's handbook of leadership: Theory, research, and managerial applications* (3rd ed.). New York, NY: Free Press.

Burns, J. M. (1978). *Leadership*. New York, NY: Harper & Row.

Casoy, F. (2008, December 26). The case for universal healthcare. Written statement for the American Medical Student Association. *The Washington Post.*

Churchman, C. W. (1971). *The design of inquiring systems: Basic concepts of systems and organization*. New York, NY: Basic Books.

Churchman, C. W. (1979). *The systems approach and its enemies*. New York, NY: Basic Books.

Churchman, C. W. (1982). *Thought and wisdom*. Seaside, CA: Intersystems Publications.

Dossey, B. M. (2008). Integral and holistic nursing: Local to global. In B. M. Dossey & L. Keegan (Eds.), *Holistic nursing: A handbook for practice* (5th ed., pp. 17–41). Sudbury, MA: Jones and Bartlett.

Duck, J. (1992). *The seduction of reductionist thinking*. Boston, MA: Boston Consulting Group.

Employee Benefits Research Institute. (2005). Uninsured unchanged in 2004, but employment-based health coverage declined. *EBRI Notes, 25*(5). Retrieved from http://www.ebri.org

Employee Benefits Research Institute. (2012). 1 in 5 older Americans cutting back on health care to save money. *EBRI Notes, 33*(1). Retrieved from http://www.ebri.org

Employee Benefits Research Institute. (2014). How does household expenditure change for older Americans? *EBRI Notes, 35*(9). Retrieved from http://www.ebri.org

Forrester, J. (1958). Industrial dynamics: A major breakthrough for decision makers. *Harvard Business Review, 36*(4), 37–66.

Garvin, D., Edmondson, A., & Gino, F. (2008). Is yours a learning organization? *Harvard Business Review, 86*(3), 109–116.

Gill, S. (2015). Learning culture: A workplace environment for success, parts 1 & 2. *The Business Thinker.* Retrieved from http://businessthinker.com/?s=Learning+Organization

Homer-Dixon, T. (2002). *The ingenuity gap: Can we solve the problems of the future?* New York, NY: Vintage Books.

Iglehart, J. (2013). Expanding the role of advanced nurse practitioners—Risks and rewards. *New England Journal of Medicine, 368*, 1935–1941.

Institute of Medicine. (2003). *Health professions education: A bridge to quality.* Washington, DC: National Academies Press.

Institute of Medicine. (2010). *The future of nursing: Leading change, advancing health.* Retrieved from http://www.iom.edu/Reports/2010/The-Future-of-Nursing-Leading-Change-Advancing-Health.aspx

Institute of Medicine. (2013). *The future of nursing: A look back at the landmark IOM report.* Retrieved from http://www.iom.edu/Global/Perspectives/2013/The-Future-of-Nursing.aspx

Lewis, J. (2001). *Project planning, scheduling, and control: A hands-on guide to bringing projects in on time and on budget.* New York, NY: McGraw-Hill.

Lynham, S. A., & Chermack, T. J. (2006). Responsible leadership for performance: A theoretical model and hypotheses. *Journal of Leadership and Organizational Studies, 12*(4), 73–88.

National Organization of Nurse Practitioner Faculties. (2011). *Nurse practitioner core competencies.* Retrieved from http://www.nonpf.com/displaycommon. cfm?an=1&subarticlenbr=14

National Organization of Nurse Practitioner Faculties. (2014). *Nurse practitioner core competencies content.* Retrieved from http://c.ymcdn.com/sites/ nonpf.site-ym.com/resource/resmgr/Competencies/NPCoreCompsContent FinalNov20.pdf

Ouchi, W. (1981). *Theory Z: How American business can meet the Japanese challenge.* Reading, MA: Addison-Wesley.

Schyve, P. M. (2000, September). *Testimony of Paul M. Schyve, Panel 5: State coalitions and public policy advocates.* Written statement. National Summit on Medical Errors and Patient Safety Research. Retrieved from http://www.quic .gov/summit/wschyve.htm

Senge, P. (1990, 2006). *The fifth discipline: The art and practice of the learning organization.* New York, NY: Doubleday.

Ulrich, W. (2009, March 26). *An appreciation of C. West Churchman* (Rev. ed.). Retrieved from http://www.wulrich.com/cwc_appreciation.html (Original work published 1988 as C. West Churchman—75 years. *Systems Practice, 1*(4), 341–350).

Ulrich, W. (2012). CST two ways: A concise account of critical systems thinking. *Ulrich's Bimonthly (Formerly "Picture of the Month").* Retrieved from http:// wulrich.com/downloads/bimonthly_november2012.pdf

United Nations. (2015). *The Millenium Development Goals Report.* Retrieved from http://www.un.org/millenniumgoals/2015_MDG_Report/pdf/MDG%20 2015%20rev%20(July%201).pdf

UN News Centre. (2015, February 18). *Ebola: UN envoy likens final phase of response to "looking for needles in haystacks."* Retrieved from http://www.un.org/apps/ news/story.asp?NewsID=50118&Kw1=ebola&Kw2=&Kw3=#.VRB2L50o7IU

Wheatley, M. (1992). *Leadership and the new science: Discovering order in a chaotic world.* San Francisco, CA: Berrett-Koehler.

Wheatley, M. (2002). *Turning to one another: Simple conversations to restore hope to the future.* San Francisco, CA: Berrett-Koehler.

Woolf, S., & Aron, L. (2013). The US health disadvantage relative to other high-income countries: Findings from a National Research Council/Institute of Medicine report. *Journal of the American Medical Association, 309*(8), 771–772.

Chapter 3

Clinical Scholarship and Evidence-Based Practice

Catherine Tymkow

> *True scholarship consists in knowing not what things exist, but what they mean; it is not memory but judgment.*
>
> —James Russell Lowell

Any discussion of scholarship and evidence-based practice (EBP) and the doctor of nursing practice (DNP) role must first begin with some essential questions. These include questions as basic as the following: What is scholarship? Are EBP and clinical scholarship the same thing? How does clinical scholarship differ from the traditional definition of scholarship? Why do we need nursing scholars in practice settings? What is the role of the DNP in clinical scholarship? What are the knowledge resources, tools, and methods necessary to implement and support clinical scholarship and EBP?

These questions are important ones to consider as healthcare organizations and schools of nursing redefine and expand nurses' roles. If nursing is to maintain a full partnership with medicine in the delivery of health care, the education of nurse leaders and nurses in advanced practice roles must be at a comparable level with other doctorally prepared healthcare practitioners such as MDs, PharmDs, and PsyDs. The merging of nursing leadership skills, evidence-based decision making, and expert clinical care will ensure that nursing has a strong and credible presence in an ever-changing and complex healthcare system. In a presentation by former president Faye Raines to the American Association of Colleges of Nursing (AACN), the leader noted that "the DNP degree more accurately reflects current clinical competencies and includes preparation for the changing healthcare system" (Raines, 2010, p. 5).

The DNP degree is a terminal practice degree and is now considered by many healthcare organizations as the preferred degree for nursing leaders involved in the delivery and organization of clinical care and healthcare systems. The result has been a proliferation of DNP programs throughout the United States. Since the first edition of this book, the number of DNP programs and DNP graduates has increased exponentially. In a recent survey, the AACN reported that there are now 269 DNP programs in 48 states, with 59 more in the planning stages. Between 2012 and 2013, enrollment in DNP programs was 4,688 students, and there were 2,443 graduates during those same years. Currently, 18,000 students are enrolled in DNP programs nationwide—an increase of 26.2%, as noted in the fall 2014 survey of nursing programs (AACN, 2015). The DNP's academic preparation—with a strong curricular base in advanced practice principles, experiential learning, intra- and interprofessional collaboration, and application of the best clinical research evidence—can best fulfill nursing's goals for leadership in practice and clinical education. In addition, clinical scholarship, including critical inquiry, analysis, synthesis, creativity, and translational research, must be a distinguishing feature of the DNP's role and expertise.

The purpose of this chapter is to define and explore the meaning of clinical scholarship; to distinguish EBP from other forms of scholarly activity; to describe the unique role of the DNP in scholarship; and to provide an overview of the language, methodological tools, strategies, and thought processes that are necessary to ensure that nursing's scholarship is useful, significant, and of the highest quality. Entire books are dedicated to research processes, methodologies, and EBP. This is not the intent of this chapter; rather, it is to explore concepts, provide resources, and whet the reader's appetite for more in-depth information on the topic.

What Is Clinical Scholarship?

In Sigma Theta Tau International's (1999) *Clinical Scholarship Resource Paper*, Melanie Dreher, chair of the task force, wrote that "clinical scholarship is about inquiry and implies a willingness to scrutinize our practice" (Dreher, 1999, p. 26). In addition, "clinical scholarship is not clinical proficiency . . . unless we are questioning the reason for its use in the first place . . . ; and neither is it clinical research, although it is informed by and inspires research" (p. 26). Finally, she noted that "clinical scholarship is an intellectual process. . . . It includes challenging traditional nursing interventions, testing our ideas, predicting outcomes, and explaining both patterns and exceptions. In addition to observation, analysis, and synthesis, clinical scholarship includes [translation], application and dissemination, all of which result in a new understanding of nursing phenomena and the development of new knowledge" (p. 26).

The AACN's Position Statement on *Defining Scholarship for the Discipline of Nursing* (1999) defined scholarship as "those activities that systematically advance the teaching, research, and practice of nursing through rigorous inquiry that: 1) is significant to the profession, 2) is creative, 3) can be documented, 4) can be replicated or elaborated, and 5) can be peer-reviewed through various methods" (p. 1). According to the National Organization of Nurse Practitioner Faculties (NONPF), scholarly projects can be varied but should meet the needs of a group, community, or population versus an individual. Examples include, but are not limited to, translating research in practice, quality improvement, implementing and evaluating EBP guidelines, and collaborating on legislative change using evidence (NONPF, 2007).

These definitions and examples are congruent with the evolving definition of scholarship in academia since Boyer's (1990, 1997) groundbreaking work, *Scholarship Reconsidered: Priorities of the Professoriate*. Ernest L. Boyer was an American educator, chancellor, and president of the Carnegie Foundation for the Advancement of Teaching (Carnegie Foundation for the Advancement of Teaching, 1996). Since the publication of *Scholarship Reconsidered* (1990), a new and expanded role for scholarship has emerged in academia that makes the previously mentioned definitions of scholarship more compatible with the goals and processes of practice disciplines. The traditional definition of scholarship in academia did not account for the nuances and rigors of clinical practice knowledge and its application for problem solving and interactive, human engagement (AACN, 2006). Boyer's model (1990, 1997), however, is well suited to scholarship in nursing practice. In Boyer's view, scholarship is not linear; rather, there is a constant, reciprocal, iterative relationship between each of its four aspects. It embraces the concepts of discovery (building new knowledge through research and careful inquiry to refine existing knowledge), integration (interpreting knowledge through dissemination in various forms), application (using knowledge for problem solving, service, and growth), and teaching (developing and testing instructional materials to advance learning, including the formation and sustaining of an engaging environment for learning between teacher and student) (Boyer, 1990, 1997; Stull & Lanz, 2005).

The AACN's *The Essentials of Doctoral Education for Advanced Nursing Practice* (2006) embodies much of Boyer's criteria in the specification of the eight core essentials and specialty-focused competencies as the basic underpinnings to be integrated into the DNP curriculum (AACN, 2006).

Essential 3 of the core elements is "clinical scholarship and analytic methods for evidence-based practice" (AACN, 2006). In this document, the authors stated that "scholarship and research are the hallmarks of doctoral education" (p. 11), and, further, that "research doctorates are designed to prepare graduates with the research skills necessary to discover new knowledge in the discipline. However, DNPs engaged in advanced nursing practice provide leadership for EBP. This requires competence in knowledge development activities such as the translation of research in practice, the evaluation of practice, activities aimed at improving the reliability of health care practice and outcomes, and participation in collaborative research" (DePalma & McGuire, as cited in AACN, 2006, p. 11). Therefore, DNP programs focus on the translation of new science, its application, and its evaluation. In addition, DNP graduates generate evidence to guide practice.

As DNP programs have proliferated, the curriculum has evolved to include more focus on research translation and EBP. An Internet review of the curricula from several national DNP programs indicates that most curricula include courses that provide graduates with the skills needed to participate in whatever level of research is appropriate to their setting and scholarship goals. Such courses include, for example, theory or scientific foundations for knowledge development, research and/or applied methods, statistics, and translating evidence into practice.

Evidence-Based Practice and Clinical Scholarship: Are They the Same?

Scholarship is an evolutionary process that raises the level of the profession through participation in the generation of new knowledge and through scientific and social exchange. "The difference between evidence based nursing practice and scholarship or applied nursing research is that evidence based practice is practice driven" (French, 1999, p. 77). Whereas scholarship was often viewed by many practicing professionals as an add-on, optional activity, EBP has become a necessity in our current information-based, technological age. Computers have given everyone access to both good and bad information. The defining feature of EBP is the linking of current research findings with patients' conditions, values, and circumstances. In addition, it involves "the conscientious, explicit, and judicious use of current best evidence for making decisions about the care of individuals" (Sackett, Richardson, Rosenberg, & Haynes, 1997, p. 2). Nursing's unique addition to this process must offer a more holistic approach that adds artful practice and ethical standards to the empirics of evidence (Fawcett, Watson, Neuman, Hinton Walker, & Fitzpatrick, 2001).

The work of clinical scholars has increased during the past two decades. A review of published nursing articles from 1986 to 2015 in the Cumulative Index to Nursing and Allied Health Literature (CINAHL) database resulted in 153 published articles with clinical scholarship as the focus. When "evidence-based practice" was added to the search terms, an additional 20 articles were found. When "evidence-based practice" alone was used as the search term, the search returned 10,774 articles that were nursing focused.

Holleman, Eliens, van Vliet, and van Acterburg (2006) extensively reviewed six databases, including CINAHL, PubMed, Scirus, Invert, Google, and the Cochrane databases, focusing on the years between 1993 and 2004. In their meta-analysis of the literature on promotion of EBP and professional nursing associations, the authors found 179 articles that addressed EBP activities. Of the 179 articles, 47 dealt with EBP as structural measures (policy, role, quality indicators), 103 as competence- and attitude oriented (journals, conferences, workshops, research committees, etc.), and only 29 as behavior oriented (care models, guidelines).

Since the prior versions of this chapter, there has been progress in closing the gap between nursing science discovery and application or implementation in practice. Broome, Riner, and Allam (2013) specifically noted the increase of clinical investigations and practice/provider-based studies published by DNP-prepared authors from the years 2005–2012. A total of 300 articles in 59 journals were found. Of the 300 articles found, 175 met the study criteria. However, the authors recommended "greater integration of translational science models into DNP curricula to achieve the goal of publishing scholarly products that use evidence to improve practice or patient outcomes" (p. 429).

The principles of EBP were an outgrowth of the work of Dr. Archie Cochrane, a British epidemiologist who criticized the medical profession for not using evidence from randomized clinical trials as a basis for clinical care. He believed that the evidence from these trials should be systematically reviewed and constantly updated to afford patients the best quality care (Cochrane Collaboration, 2004). EBP includes an emphasis on the efficacy of treatments or interventions based on the results of experimental comparison between untreated control groups, treatments, or both. The core principles include: (1) formulating the clinical question; (2) identifying the most relevant articles, research, and other best evidence; (3) critically evaluating the evidence; (4) integrating and applying the evidence; and (5) reevaluating the application of evidence and making necessary changes. **Table 3-1** presents the hierarchy of evidence for practice.

Table 3-1 Hierarchy for Evaluating Evidence for Practice	
Level 1 (strongest)	Systematic reviews/meta-analysis of all randomized controlled trials (RCTs); clinical practice guidelines based on RCT data
Level 2	Evidence from one or more RCTs
Level 3	Evidence from a controlled trial; no randomization
Level 4	Case control or cohort studies
Level 5	Systematic reviews of descriptive/qualitative studies
Level 6	Single descriptive or qualitative study
Level 7 (weakest)	Opinions of authorities/experts

Note: All levels assume a well-designed study.

This article was published in *The practice of nursing research: Appraisal, synthesis, and generation of evidence*, 7th ed., Grove, S.K., Burns, N. & Gray, J.R., p. 30, Copyright Elsevier 2013.

The definition of "evidence-based practice" has been adapted to include provisions for the provider's experience and the patient's values. It is through the incorporation of intuition, observation, theory, research, intelligent analysis, and judgment based on the data that nurses provide care that is truly individualized, reflective, and evidence based. With an increased knowledge of the theory and the tools necessary to critique and translate research into practice, the DNP is in a prime position to affect the delivery of care and to aggregate and translate evidence that can be disseminated to improve overall care and outcomes in myriad clinical areas. The translation and dissemination of clinical knowledge constitute the core of clinical scholarship.

What Is the Role of the Doctor of Nursing Practice in Clinical Scholarship?

In advanced practice, scholarship should be integrated with practice as a purposeful, systematic, and conscious endeavor. The emphasis is on inquiry, outcomes, and evidence to support practice (Sigma Theta Tau International Clinical Scholarship Task Force, 1999). Because of their education, advanced practice nurses (APNs), particularly DNPs, are expected to have mastery of essential information so that the teaching of staff, patients, and communities becomes a key function of the role. The dynamic nature of health care requires that DNPs be up to date on new information and that they be able to discern nuances in research findings so as to translate those findings in understandable ways that improve care and practice. This requires constant critique, integration, and synthesis of new information from various sources into formats that can be disseminated to patients, colleagues, and others.

What distinguishes the role of the DNP from that of other advanced practice degree holders? The answer is not a simple one; the difference is, in fact, a combination of knowledge, expert skill, and the integration of *best* research to advance the practice and the profession. This skill comes from additional formal education, experience, and the translation, application, and evaluation of research in practice. Although most practicing nurses are exposed to "research" and "evidence" in practice, the DNP must not only embrace the process but also implement the findings in ways that ultimately change or improve practice and outcomes. Scholarship is the dissemination of those findings in publications, presentations, and Internet offerings that can be used by others. As envisioned in *The Essentials of Doctoral Education for Advanced Nursing Practice* (AACN, 2006), the DNP program prepares graduates to:

1. Use analytical methods to critically appraise existing literature and other evidence relevant to practice.
2. Design and implement processes to evaluate outcomes of practice, practice patterns, and systems of care within a practice setting, healthcare organization, or community against national benchmarks to determine variances in practice outcomes and population trends.
3. Design, direct, and evaluate quality improvement methodologies to promote safe, timely, effective, efficient, equitable, and patient-centered care.
4. Apply relevant findings to develop practice guidelines and improve practice and the practice environment.
5. Use information technology and research methods appropriately to:
   - Collect appropriate and accurate data to generate evidence for nursing practice.
   - Inform and guide the design of databases that generate meaningful evidence for nursing practice.
   - Analyze data from clinical practice.
   - Design evidence-based interventions.
   - Predict and analyze outcomes.
   - Examine patterns of behavior and outcomes.
   - Identify gaps in evidence for practice.
6. Function as a practice specialist/consultant in collaborative, knowledge-generating research.
7. Disseminate findings from evidence-based practice to improve healthcare outcomes. (p. 12)

These objectives encompass the essential skills, tools, and methods necessary to implement and support clinical scholarship and EBP. They can be distilled into six categories: (1) translating research in practice, (2) quality improvement and patient-centered care, (3) evaluation of practice, (4) research methods and technology, (5) participation in collaborative research, and (6) disseminating findings from EBP. Each of these areas is discussed in the following sections.

Translating Research in Practice

The use of evidence to support clinical practice is not a new phenomenon. Medical professionals have relied on data from science, empirical observation, case reviews, and other means for centuries (Monico, Moore, & Calise, 2005). However, as electronic access to sources of data has increased, the amount of evidence now available as a basis for clinical practice has become overwhelming. In addition, the use of translational science has increased and includes a number of processes, including knowledge translation, quality improvement, adoption of innovation, implementation science (applied research) for quality, and safety improvement (May, 2013; Newhouse, Bobay, Dykes, Stevens, & Titler, 2013).

The key to making best practice decisions is using the best quality evidence—evidence that is scientifically based and that has been replicated with success in repeated research and application. Unfortunately, although knowledge and availability of EBP have increased in the last decade, EBP remains underutilized as a tool to improve patient outcomes (Newhouse et al., 2013). Implementation science provides the tools—methods, interventions, and variables—that facilitate decision-making toward practice change (May, 2013; Newhouse et al., 2013).

Stevens (2011) specified three primary knowledge sources for EBP: valid research evidence, clinical expertise, and patient choice. Currently, evidence generated from large-scale randomized controlled trials is considered the gold standard for application in interventions (Fawcett & Garrity, 2009). Depending on the clinical situation and the patient's personal preference, other sources of evidence may be appropriate. These sources may include meta-analyses of all relevant randomized controlled trials; EBP guidelines from systematic reviews of randomized controlled trials, case control, or cohort studies; expert opinion; and nursing theory (Fawcett & Garrity, 2009; O'Mathuna, Fineout-Overholt, DiCenso, & Johnston, 2011).

To understand research evidence that may be used in practice, the following sections on qualitative and quantitative research offer a brief description of the processes and questions to be considered in the evaluation of such research. Exhaustive coverage of every research method is beyond the scope of this chapter. However, the definitions, discussion, and examples are meant to illustrate how different types of research might be applied or used in practice and how their rigor and adequacy as evidence for practice should be evaluated.

Understanding, Distinguishing, and Evaluating Types of Research Evidence

Qualitative Research Evidence

Qualitative research is based on four levels of understanding:

1. What is the nature of reality? (Ontology)
2. What constitutes knowledge? (Epistemology)
3. How can we understand reality? (Methodology)
4. How can we collect the evidence? (Methods)

(Porter, 1996, as cited in Maggs-Rapport, 2001)

Types of Qualitative Research Studies Qualitative research is important in that it allows the nurse to consider the context of a situation while connecting with patients and noting individual differences. In addition, it permits nursing's unique perspective to be valued and considered critically when making clinical decisions. In her discussion of qualitative research and evidence-based nursing (EBN), Zuzelo (2007) proposed that "nursing needs to ensure that qualitative research is as much a part of the considered evidence as quantitative evidence is" (p. 484).

There are several kinds of qualitative research studies, including critical social theory, ethnographic studies, grounded theory research, historical research, phenomenological studies, and philosophical inquiry. Each of these methods is discussed briefly to provide an overview of the scope and potential uses of qualitative evidence and to provide a basis for evaluating the use of qualitative studies as a basis for changes in practice.

Critical Social Theory *Critical social theory* uses multiple research methods as a basis for promoting change in areas where power imbalances exist (N. Burns & Grove, 2009). According to Horkheimer (1895–1973), Marcuse (1898–1979), Adorno (1903–1969), and Habermas (1929–), critical social theory is based on the belief that individuals should seek freedom from domination (Maggs-Rapport, 2001). Habermas in particular believed that people must understand the nature of "constraining circumstances" before they can be liberated from them (Maggs-Rapport, 2001). Another critical social theorist, Giddens (as cited in Maggs-Rapport, 2001), believed that we can understand why people act in certain ways only if we can appreciate the meanings of their actions.

The DNP might use data from critical social theory to identify meaning or patterns of concern where certain societal cultural norms exist in the form of barriers that affect particularly vulnerable populations such as the elderly, the incarcerated, abused women, and the chronically ill. Analysis would necessarily include an examination of the underlying conditions, a critique of the social phenomena, and the discovery and revelation of the social and political injustices embedded in the experience of the population in question that could lead toward removal of barriers (Maggs-Rapport, 2001).

Ethnographic Research *Ethnographic research* is used to describe the nature or characteristics of a culture to gain insight into the lifeways or behaviors of a group. Distinguishing features are immerged in the participant's way of life (Polit & Hungler, 1997), and the information gathered speaks for itself rather than being interpreted or explored for additional meanings (Maggs-Rapport, 2001). Field notes based on researcher observations over time describe daily interactions with subjects.

In one ethnographic study, Kovarsky (2008) compared clients' and families' personal experiences of outcomes and interventions with written professional discourse, technical reports, and other conceptualizations of evidence in practice. Of note was "the dismissal of subjective, phenomenally oriented information that functioned to marginalize and silence voices . . . of clients when constituting proof of effectiveness" (Kovarsky, 2008, p. 47). Further, "the current version of EBP needs to be reformulated to include subjective voices from the life-worlds of clients as a form of evidence" (p. 47). As one example of an ethnographic approach, Kovarsky proposed the personal experience narrative as a measure of qualitative outcomes and intervention analysis (p. 48). Citing a study by Simmons-Mackie and Damico (2001), Kovarsky described an ethnographic interview with a patient experiencing poststroke aphasia. When asked to comment on life before her stroke, K. [the patient] said,

> *"Before teacher . . . now I don't know . . . .what." and "uh . . . uh . . . -always, always . . . uh . . . busy, busy, busy, . . . teachin . . . teachin . . . always, I love it. . . . it's me . . . But now . . . here (points to mouth) talk, not uh . . . teaching." When asked about a typical day, she shrugged and said "nothing . . . here (points to television)" and later added "eat . . . and (points to newspaper) and shows (points to television)." (Simmons-Mackie & Damico, 2001, as cited in Kovarsky, 2008, p. 51)*

These statements illustrate an altered level of life activity that cannot be appreciated in objective technical descriptions of outcomes of disease processes and their sequelae.

The ethnographic narrative is a method of subjective evidence gathering that can enhance the specificity and richness of other research methodologies, including evidence gained from logical positivist approaches such as randomized controlled trials. In particular, DNPs in public health or community health could use this method in conjunction with other, more traditional forms of evidence to gain a better real-world understanding of the populations they serve.

Grounded Theory Research *Grounded theory research* is focused on the influence of interactional processes (identification, description, and explanation) between individuals, families, or groups within a social context (Strauss & Corbin, 1994). It is an observational method used to study problems in social settings that are "grounded" in the data obtained from those observations (Glaser & Strauss, 1967; Grove, Burns, & Gray, 2013). Grounded theory is an applicable framework for study of myriad contexts, situations, and settings because it bridges the gap between empirical observation and the generation of theory by providing a structured method of sampling procedures and coding observations for explaining social phenomena or generating new theory (Annells, 1996; Barnes, 1996; Glaser & Strauss, 1967; Hammersley, 1989).

For example, a study of the implementation of EBN in Iran (Adib-Hajbaghery, 2007) sought to distinguish factors influencing the implementation of EBP in Eastern countries (versus Western countries), particularly Iran. A brief description of this study using the grounded theory approach is presented here. Data collection consisted of purposive sampling of 21 nurses (nine staff and six head nurses in differing clinical settings) with experience in nursing greater than 5 years. An interview questionnaire consisted of open-ended questions, such as "What is the basis of care you give your patients?" (p. 568), "In your opinion, what is the basis of evidence based nursing?" (p. 568), and "Can you describe some instances in which you used scientific evidence in nursing?" (p. 568). "Issues were clarified and interviews were audiotaped, transcribed verbatim and analyzed consecutively" (Adib-Hajbaghery, 2007, p. 568). A total of 36 hours of observations and interviews were carried out concurrently and involved observations of those interviewed and others working on the units.

According to the procedure identified by Strauss and Corbin (1998), each interview was analyzed before the subsequent interview took place, and the results were coded in three ways: open coding (breaking down, examining, comparing, conceptualizing, and categorizing), axial coding (putting data back together in new ways by linking codes to contexts, consequences, and patterns of interactions), and selective coding (identifying core categories and systematically relating and validating relationships) (Adib-Hajbaghery, 2007). To confirm the credibility of the data, participants were given a full transcript of their responses and a list of codes and themes to determine whether the codes and themes matched their responses.

To establish validity, two peer researchers also checked codes and themes using the same procedure as the researcher. The results were that two main categories emerged from the research: (1) the meaning of EBN; and (2) factors in implementation of EBN, including the themes of possessing professional knowledge and experience, having opportunity and time, becoming accustomed, self-confidence, the process of nursing education, and the work environment and its expectations (Adib-Hajbaghery, 2007).

The process and results of grounded theory research and analysis provide rich data for application in practice when paired with evidence from other sources. This is especially true when there is little clinical trial evidence to support the affective dimension of care or practice.

Historical Research *Historical research* is a description or analysis of events that have shaped a discipline. Although historical research may not be used directly in practice, it provides the foundation for examination of the discipline and for providing future directions (Fitzpatrick & Munhall, 2001; Grove et al., 2013). Often history is handed down in written documents. The Library of Congress's (n.d.) American Memory Collection has original writings, newspaper clippings, photos, and other documents that provide a realistic account of the influence and actions of famous women in history, including nursing leaders. Pictures and other documents showcase the original work of early nurse leaders such as Lavinia Dock (1858–1956), Margaret Sanger (1879–1966), Clara Barton (1821–1912), and Mary Breckinridge (1881–1965), which provides a basis for advanced nursing practice and can be used by DNPs in education to provide a historical perspective for practice.

Another source of historical research is oral history. Using both written documents and oral history, Libster and McNeil (2009) traced the history and meaning of a religious tradition of care of the sick and poor by the Sisters of Charity. Wall, Edwards, and Porter (2007) used oral history and a method of textual analysis to determine how retired nurses made sense of their educational experiences. Decker and Iphofen (2005) described a method of oral history research to discover knowledge about, and change within, a profession, particularly as it relates to EBP. Tropello (2000) used oral history technique in her dissertation, "Origins of the Nurse Practitioner Movement: An Oral History." The purpose was to gain a better understanding of current advanced nursing practice roles through an exploration of the original movement. Eight participants in the original movement were the primary sources, and the information obtained and transcribed from taped interviews was enhanced by supportive papers, correspondence, and other documents, including secondary sources. One conclusion of the study was that the politics of the 1960s, which emphasized greater freedoms for women and a focus on social programs, helped alleviate healthcare manpower shortages (Tropello, 2000). This movement has paved the way for additional professionalization in nursing, including the evolution of the DNP curriculum. Started as a research project, it became part of the core curriculum under the continuing education division of the School of Nursing at the University of Colorado. The program used a nursing–physician team approach to aid families with limited access to primary providers (Tropello, 2000).

For DNPs to prescribe their future, they must have a clear understanding of and appreciation for their history so that they can build on and shape EBP in ways that preserve the essence of nursing. The National League for Nursing and Sigma Theta Tau International have excellent historical resources. Several of the audiotapes, videotapes, and other historical resources produced by these and other nurse theorists whose original work and theory development continue to provide frameworks for advancing nursing practice were referenced by Allen (1996) in a special report, "Celebrating Nursing History: What to Keep."

Phenomenological Research   The aim of a *phenomenological (hermeneutic) study* is to understand a phenomenon through the recognition of the meaning of an experience or occurrence. Phenomenology focuses on discerning the real truth of a phenomenon rather than arguing a point or developing abstract theory (Hallett, 1995). Researchers explore an experience as it is lived by the participants in the study. The phenomenon of interest may include any number of experiences, such as death, divorce, pain, or cancer. The researcher collects data and interprets the experiences as they are lived (Grove et al., 2013). One example of a phenomenological study by Marineau (2005) involved perceptions of telehealth support by an APN for patients discharged from the hospital with acute infections.

Empirical data were insufficient in patients who had previously been enrolled in a quantitative pilot study of telehealth. Therefore, eidetic phenomenology, which compares variations in imagination after an event to capture patients' lived experiences after discharge, was used. Theme categories were: initial response, engaging in care, and experiencing the downside. Of the 10 participants in the trial, only one had a negative experience. The study was seen as useful in adding to the understanding of the transitional process of care (Marineau, 2005).

In another phenomenological approach, Maggs-Rapport (2001) used van Manen's (1990) social scientific approach to look at women's immediate response to the phenomenon of egg sharing (donation of one woman's eggs to another woman) after consultation with a clinician, and their lived experiences of egg sharing in return for free fertility treatment. The in-depth open-ended interviews of this technique established a conversational relationship about the meaning of the experience and produced a narrative that "enriches the understanding of the phenomena" (Maggs-Rapport, 2001, p. 374). Before each description can be transformed into phenomenological language, meaning units must be made of each description (Giorgi, 2000). However, only a small number of descriptions are necessary for the nature of the phenomenon to become apparent (Giorgi, 2000; van Manen, 1990).

Phenomenological techniques with a strong nursing orientation include those of Crotty (1996) and Munhall (1994, 2007). Other studies that utilized the phenomenological approach in advanced practice include those about the analysis of patient experiences of low back pain (Volker & Limerick, 2007); advanced nursing practice in rural areas (Conger & Plager, 2008); the meaning of U.S. childbirth for Mexican immigrant women (Imberg, 2008); the lived experience of the APN's transition to nurse educator (Bailey, 2012); how family practice physicians, nurse practitioners (NPs), and physicians assistants (PAs) incorporate spiritual care into practice (Tanyi, McKenzie, & Chapek, 2009); the leadership and management role of the DNP in the care of older persons in the United States (Stoekel, 2010); sociophenomenology and conversation analysis, and interpreting video lifeworld healthcare interactions (Bickerton, Procter, Johnson, & Medina, 2011); and hospital nurses' lived experience of power (Fackler, Chambers, & Bourbonniere, 2015). Phenomenological studies contribute to the evidence base by enhancing our understanding of the true meaning of patients' experiences and the broader dimensions of a problem, thus aiding in a more holistic perspective in practice.

Philosophical Inquiry *Philosophical inquiry* is used to explore the nature of knowledge, values, meaning, and ethical factors related to a question of interest. Although philosophical inquiry is related to theory, it is not the same as theory, which is more specific and concrete (Pesut & Johnson, 2007). Citing Edwards (2001), Pesut and Johnson (2007) described three "strands" that compose philosophical inquiry: (1) philosophical presupposition, which involves identifying and analyzing presuppositions in nursing (an example might be a concept analysis of nursing practice or advanced practice); (2) philosophical problems, such as what constitutes knowing in a particular situation, or ethical analyses, such as the ethics of caring in situations in which nurses' and patients' values conflict; and (3) scholarship, in which nurse theorists' works are examined from a philosophical perspective. In this case, as noted by N. Burns and Grove (2009), the researcher would "conduct an extensive search of the literature, examine conceptual meaning, pose questions and propose answers including the implications for those answers" (p. 26).

In a practical application of philosophical inquiry, Dorn (2004) described a model, caring-healing inquiry for holistic nursing practice, to guide nursing research and quality improvement in a tertiary hospital. The model, which integrated the values of the hospital, provided the basis for nurses (mostly APNs) to describe their contributions to care through research and practice improvement in a partnership between a hospital and university nursing program. Facilitated by a nurse-researcher faculty member, the group served as an advisory group for program planning, development and clinical innovation.

In a more recent example, Alimohammadi, Taleghani, Mohammadi, and Akbarian (2014) used philosophic inquiry to explore the meaning of "human being" in the eastern Islamic tradition. Included were implications for practice and patient care. Knowledge about the process of philosophical inquiry and a focus on value analysis, as demonstrated in these examples, provides DNPs with a basis for facilitating ethical decision making in practice.

Evaluating Qualitative Research Evidence What are the evaluative questions? Regardless of the type of research design, the general criteria for evaluation of qualitative studies are as follows:

1. *Question, purpose, and context:* Is the research question clear, the primary purpose and the focus of the study stated, and the context described?
2. *Design:* Was the design appropriate; were the units of analysis and sampling strategy described, and the sampling criteria clear?

3. *Data collection:* What types of data were collected? Were data collection processes systematic and adequately described? How were logistical issues addressed?
4. *Data analysis:* Was data analysis systematic and rigorous? What controls were in place? What analytical approach or approaches were used? How were validity and confidence in the findings established?
5. *Results:* Were results surprising, interesting, or suspect? Were conclusions supported by data and explanation (theory)? Were the authors' positions clearly stated?
6. *Ethical issues:* How were ethical issues and confidentiality addressed?
7. *Implications:* What is the worth/relevance to knowledge and practice?

(Gifford, Davies, Edwards, Griffin, & Lybanon, 2007; Patton, 1990; Russell & Gregory, 2003)

Qualitative research questions and methods provide an avenue for truly knowing patients and practicing both the "art" and "science" of nursing. These are the hallmarks of nursing that nurses at every level must retain and that DNPs must foster as role models to ensure that "best practice" does not exclude the best of nursing's perspective.

Quantitative Research Evidence

Steps in the Quantitative Research Process Two important aspects of any quantitative research project are that the project builds on prior results or evidence and provides a basis for future research and discovery (Grove et al., 2013). **Figure 3-1** shows the steps in the quantitative research process.

The *research problem* is often derived because there is a gap in knowledge that needs to be addressed or described. Research problems or questions often arise from direct observations made in practice. The *purpose* of the study is to address the problem. To better understand the problem, an extensive *literature review* must be done in order to develop an understanding of the nature and scope of the problem and to determine what research has already been done. A framework, map, or theoretical base made up of concepts is developed to provide structure and help the researcher make sense of the findings. The *research objectives, questions,* or *hypotheses* set the study limits in terms of who will be studied, what question(s) will be addressed, and what relationships among variables exist.

The remaining steps are to define the variables in conceptual terms (theoretical meaning) and operational terms (how the variables will be measured or manipulated); explain assumptions (those things we take for granted to be true, whether proved or not); and then select the research design, including the population to be included, the methods

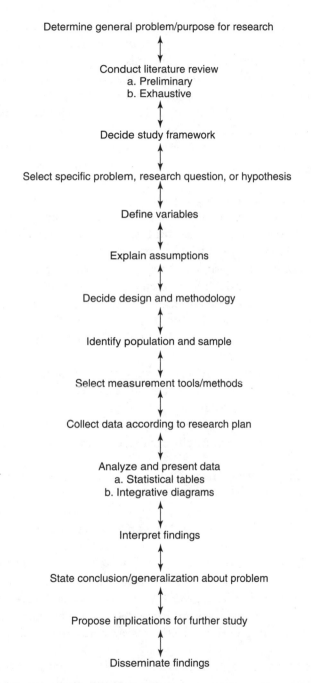

Figure 3-1 The Quantitative Research Process
Modified from Grove, S.K., Burns, N., & Gray, J.R. (2013). *The practice of nursing research: Appraisal, synthesis, and generation of evidence* (7th ed., p. 39). St. Louis, MO: Elsevier Saunders.

of measurement, the plan for data collection, and data analysis. Implementing the plan follows, including piloting the study, collecting and analyzing the data, and evaluating and interpreting the research findings, including identifying study limitations (any issue within the study that serves to limit its generalizability beyond the population or sample studied) and applicability for practice. The final step is to communicate the research findings. A brief description of the research process steps and methodological considerations follows. The reader is directed to a research book for a complete description of each of the steps in this process.

Categories and Selection of a Design Quantitative research may be categorized as experimental, quasi-experimental, or nonexperimental (descriptive or correlational). Quantitative research may be either basic research (as in laboratory studies) or applied (as in clinical research). In an experimental or quasi-experimental study, the researcher actively manipulates the independent variable (treatment or intervention) to see the effect on the dependent variable. In an experimental study, the variables and the setting are highly controlled. In a nonexperimental design, the researcher may simply want to describe or explain a phenomenon or predict a relationship (Grove et al., 2013).

Quantitative designs may also be retrospective (the proposed cause and effect have already occurred), prospective (the cause, but not the effect, has occurred), cross-sectional (examines groups in various stages of development), or longitudinal (the same subjects are studied over a period of time). None of the categories are mutually exclusive (Schmidt & Brown, 2015).

Population and Sample The *population* is everyone or everything that meets the criteria for inclusion. The criteria for inclusion may be narrow or broad depending on the size and scope of the study and the specific research question to be addressed. The *sample* is a subset of the population and the process for how the subset will be selected. This may be random (all have a better than zero chance of selection), nonrandom (convenience), cross-sectional (groups studied over time), or stratified (divided to ensure representation from groups when some variables are known). Often the population and the sample are determined by the method and how accessible the population is to the researcher (Grove et al., 2013).

Measurement Instruments Measurement instruments are tools used by the researcher to answer the operational questions posed in research studies. These tools may be questionnaires, tests, indicators of health status, and a variety of other measurement techniques.

Data Collection and Analysis Plan Most data collected in quantitative research studies are coded numerically so they can be systematically analyzed and interpreted through the use of statistics. A plan for data collection and analysis is an important part of the research process and is crucial to meaningful interpretation of results.

Pilot Study A pilot study, a smaller version of a proposed study, is an important part of the research implementation plan. It allows the researcher to refine methodology, instruments, and data collection procedures before the full study is launched (Grove et al., 2013). This cursory overview of the research process provides the basis for evaluating evidence from research. The following sections describe considerations for evaluating research evidence for use in practice.

Interpreting and Evaluating Quantitative Evidence Interpretation involves "1) examining the results from data analysis, 2) exploring the significance of findings, 3) identifying study limitations, 4) forming conclusions, 5) generalizing the findings, 6) considering the implications for nursing, and 7) suggesting further studies" (Grove et al., 2013, p. 48). Once the researcher has synthesized, interpreted, and evaluated the quantitative evidence, implications for further study, practice, or both should be discussed.

When a quantitative study is appraised for use in practice, three questions are generally considered: Is the study valid? Is the study reliable? Is the study applicable in the identified case?

Is the Study Valid? Specifically, were the methods used scientifically sound? Are the independent (manipulated variable) and dependent variables (observed result) clearly identified? Is the study free from bias or confounding variables?

Bias is a standard point of view or personal prejudice, especially when there is a tendency "to affect unduly or unfairly, or to impose a steady negative potential upon" [a result or process] (Bias, 2003, p. 135). It is an influence or action that distorts or "slant[s findings] away from the true or expected" (Grove et al., 2013, p. 197). In research, bias (sometimes called systematic variation) may occur when participants' characteristics specifically differ from those of the population (Grove et al., 2013). This is always possible because volunteers are used for samples. It is less likely to occur, however, if the sampling strategy is well planned and followed and there is random assignment to groups. Bias may also occur if the instruments or measurement tools are faulty or if the data or statistics are inaccurate.

Selection Bias When a researcher decides to prospectively compare two types of strategies for educating nursing students, such as online instruction and traditional classroom instruction, *selection bias* may occur if the students are allowed to select which group they enter. Students who select online teaching may be very different from those who choose the traditional classroom experience. Random assignment to the groups minimizes the risk of selection bias.

Gender Bias Another form of bias is *gender bias*. Gender bias occurs in research when one gender is used more than the other to study research interventions, thus impacting generalizability of results. In nursing, gender bias is prevalent, with most studies "over-sampling" women (Polit & Beck, 2008). In an update of their 2005–2006 study, the authors sampled 300 studies over the 2010–2011 period in four research journals. One third of studies and 74% of all participants were female. Less bias was seen in studies authored by males (Polit & Beck, 2013, pp. 78–79). Timmerman (1999) outlined a procedure for ensuring that research decisions avoid gender bias. The procedure includes critically analyzing the literature, testing gender-specific differences, and identifying researchers' personal biases. The following example of binge-eating behaviors between men and women illustrates the point. Timmerman (1999), citing Hawkins and Clement (1984) and Spitzer et al. (1992), stated, "We know that men tend to binge less frequently, consume less during binges and are less distressed by their binge eating behavior than women" (p. 642). And, "In this case, the literature provides justification for either separately studying binge eating behavior in men and women, or, if the sample has both men and women, analyzing the data separately for men and women" (Timmerman, 1999, p. 642). **Table 3-2** lists some gender-based studies. Additional gender-based studies can be found online through the Office on Women's Health of the U.S. Department of Health and Human Services.

Confounding Variables *Confounding* occurs when a third variable, either known or unknown, produces the relationship with the outcome instead of the research intervention itself. Or, stated differently, confounding may occur when comparing two groups that may be different in additional ways from the treatment being studied (Leedy & Ormrod, 2010). Randomizing participants to either the intervention or study group helps to eliminate the possibility of confusion because there is an equal chance that extraneous variables will appear equally in both groups, thus minimizing the confounding effect.

Table 3-2 Gender-Based Studies	
Celik, Lagro-Janssen, Widdershoven, & Abma (2011)	Bringing gender sensitivity into healthcare practice: A systematic review
Diaz-Granados et al. (2011)	Monitoring gender equality in health using gender-sensitive indicators: A cross-national study
Dunlop & Beauchamp (2011)	Engendering choice: Preferences for exercising in gender-segregated and gender-integrated groups and consideration of overweight status
Gelb, Pederson, & Greaves (2011)	How have health promotion frameworks considered gender?
Griffieon & Halsey (2014)	Gender differences in immediate hypersensitivity reactions to vaccines: A review of the literature
Lauffenburger, Robinson, Oramasionwu, & Fang (2014)	Racial/ethnic and gender gaps in the use of and adherence to evidence-based preventive therapies among elderly Medicare Part D beneficiaries after acute myocardial infarction
Mark et al. (2014)	The impact of sex and gender on adaptation in space
Merryfeather & Bruce (2014)	The invisibility of gender diversity: Understanding transgender and transsexuality in nursing literature
Oliver, Martin, Richardson, Kim, & Pisu (2013)	Gender differences in colon cancer treatment
Yuh-Min, Yueh-Ping, & Min-Ling (2015)	Gender differences in the predictors of physical activity among assisted living residents
Zeeman, Aranda, & Grant (2014)	Queer challenges to evidence-based practice

One type of confounder is the effect of *history*. The history effect occurs when an event outside the researcher's control occurs at the same time as, or during, the period of the intervention. For example, in a study of patients with hypertension, a researcher may be interested in the impact of a low-salt diet on hypertension levels. The plan is to take a baseline blood pressure and then start patients on the low-salt diet. However, if, during the study period, some of these same patients also began a rigorous exercise routine and others did not, a confounding effect would be present. In this case, the intervening exercise program would make it difficult to attribute the outcome solely to the effect of the intervention. Adding a control group whose members adhered to a low-salt diet and

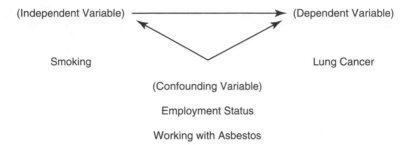

Figure 3-2 Interrelationships Among Smoking, Working in an Asbestos Coal Mine, and Risk for Lung Cancer in a Cohort/Case Control Study
Used with permission of IDRC Canada, www.idrc.ca

exercise routine or using statistical tests to control for this confounding variable would minimize the threat to validity in this study.

In another example of confounding, a researcher was interested in comparing lung cancer and smoking incidence in various regions of the country. In this study, a particular region was seen to have a significantly higher rate of lung cancer death among smokers (15 times higher) than other regions of the country. The confounding factor was that these smokers had also worked in asbestos coal mines for many years. When the researchers controlled for the variable of working with asbestos by removing the confounder, the rate of cancer due to smoking was nearly the same as that in other regions of the country. **Figure 3-2** shows the relationship among the independent variable (smoking) and confounding variable (working in an asbestos coal mine) in relationship to the dependent variable (lung cancer) (International Development Research Center, 2009).

Is the Study Reliable? The *reliability* of a study is based on questions such as the following: Does the instrument or test measure what it is supposed to measure? Does it do this consistently? Do the items on the instrument consistently measure the same characteristic? How much consistency is there between raters? (Fain, 2009; Grove et al., 2013). Reliability is measured through the use of a reliability coefficient (r) and ranges from 00.0 (lowest) to 1.00 (highest). Therefore, the closer a reliability score is to 1.00, the higher the reliability. In most cases, a coefficient of 0.80 or higher is considered acceptable if the instrument has already been tested and has been used frequently. If an instrument is new, a reliability coefficient of 0.70 may be acceptable depending on the purpose of the study (Griffin-Sobel, 2003). Reliability also focuses on stability (test–retest reliability—whether an instrument yields the same results for the same two people on two different occasions), homogeneity (internal consistency—the extent to which all the items within a single instrument yield similar results), and equivalence (interrater reliability—the extent to which two or more individuals evaluating the same product or performance give identical judgments) (Fain, 2009; Leedy & Ormrod, 2010).

A simple example of reliability is seen in the selection of timing devices used in sports events. Timing devices must work consistently every time so that competitors are ensured an equal chance of winning. An example of interrater reliability is that of a classroom situation in which two evaluators are trained to use the same tool with a Likert scale to measure student performance on oral presentations.

Are the Results of the Study Applicable in the Identified Case? Once the science of a study has been appraised and the reliability of results assessed, the next important questions are: Do the results apply to the case of interest? Are the populations in the study and in the proposed population for application similar? If the populations studied are not similar, the significance of results in the study has little value for real-life implementation in a given clinical situation.

Is the effect size sufficient so that application of the study intervention will make a significant difference? The *effect size* is calculated by determining the mean difference between two groups (intervention and control) and dividing by the standard deviation. It is not the same as the statistical significance, but rather is the size of the difference between two groups. The effect size is often used in meta-analysis for combining and comparing estimates from different studies to determine the effectiveness of an intervention. "An effect size is exactly equivalent to the Z-score of a normal standard deviation. For example an effect size of 0.8 means that the score of the average person in the experimental group is 0.8 standard deviations above the average person in the control group, and hence exceeds the scores of 79% of the control group" (Coe, 2002, p. 2). Thus,

$$\text{Effect size} = \frac{\text{Mean of experimental group} - \text{Mean of control group}}{\text{Standard deviation}}$$

Generally, in evaluating any quantitative study, additional questions include the following: Why was the study done? How was the sample size decided? How were the data analyzed? Were there any surprises or unexpected events that occurred during the study? How do the results of this study compare with others? (Melnyk & Fineout-Overholt, 2015).

The standard of care for practice is increasingly based on scientific evidence. Finding the most current research based on well-conducted clinical trials is an important first step. But how do we evaluate that evidence in practice? Several statistical measures help in the evaluation of study results. **Table 3-3** briefly describes some commonly used statistical tests. An excellent guide to biostatistics is also available from *MedPage Today* online (Israni, 2007).

What happens if the evidence conflicts with patients' values and preferences? What if our own experience conflicts with the evidence? The key is that the evidence must be relevant to the problem and tested through

Table 3-3 Clinical Statistical Measures

Clinical Statistic	Description
Odds ratio (OR)	The odds of risk for a person in the experimental group having an adverse outcome compared with a person in the control group. An odds ratio of 1 means the event is equally likely in both groups. An odds ratio greater than 1 means the event is more likely in the intervention group than the control group. An odds ratio less than 1 means the event is less likely in the intervention group than the control group. Used most in case control and retrospective studies.
Relative risk ratio (RR)	The risk of an outcome in the intervention/treatment group (Y) compared with the control group (X). RR = Y/X. A relative risk of 1 means there is no difference between the two groups. A relative risk of less than 1 means a smaller potential for the effect to occur in the intervention group than in the control group. Used most in randomized controlled trials and cohort studies.
Relative risk reduction (RRR)	The percentage of reduction in the treatment group (Y) compared with the control group (X). RRR = 1 − Y/X? 100%.
Absolute risk reduction (ARR)	The difference in risk between the control group (X) and the intervention group (Y). ARR = X − Y.
Number needed to treat (NNT)	The number of patients that must be treated over a given period of time to prevent one adverse outcome. NNT = 1/(X − Y).

Modified from Long, C. O. (2015). Weighing in on the evidence. In N. A. Schmidt & J. M. Brown (Eds.), *Evidence-based practice for nurses* (p. 427). Burlington, MA: Jones & Bartlett Learning.

application. In addition, some scholars (Fawcett et al., 2001; Kitson, Harvey, & McCormack, 1998; Rycroft-Malone et al., 2004) insisted that evidence as defined by medicine is too narrowly focused and does not recognize the complexities of nursing practice. Others recommended that the definition include the influence of context in the application of evidence (Scott-Findley & Pollack, 2004). This would include findings from qualitative research.

Regardless of the definition, however, once evidence is implemented, the results must be evaluated. Did the evidence support better decision making? Was the patient's care improved? In what ways were care or outcomes improved? If they were not improved, why not? (Melnyk & Fineout-Overholt, 2011).

Determining and Implementing the Best Evidence for Practice

A distinguishing feature of EBN is that nurses treat and work *with* patients rather than "work on them" (McSherry, 2002). In addition, nursing's approach is more holistic, so that "effectiveness of treatment" is but one indicator; cost-effectiveness and patient acceptability also matter (McSherry, 2002). According to the Agency for Healthcare Research and Quality (AHRQ, 2002), three benchmark domains must be considered when evaluating evidence: quality, quantity, and consistency. *Quality* refers to the absence of biases due to errors in selection, measurement, and confounding biases (internal validity). *Quantity* refers to the number of relevant, related studies; total sample size across studies; size of the treatment effect; and relative risk or odds ratio strength (causality). *Consistency* refers to the similarity of findings across multiple studies regardless of differences in study design. These considerations make it essential that all types of evidence be considered when delivering individual care and implementing systems of care. Based on these domains of evidence, a critical appraisal of types of studies can be facilitated and evaluated to determine the best approach for practice (Melnyk & Fineout-Overholt, 2011).

Quality Improvement and Patient-Centered Care

In patient care, a process that facilitates continuous improvement is central to an environment that produces changes in practice, is patient centered and focused on care, and is both evidence based and of high quality. The process must be based on a commitment by all those involved to change practice, and this commitment must be made in advance so that the research findings are applied early on in the process (French, 1999). As changes are made, they must be continuously evaluated for their impact on care and care systems. The EBP process is consistent with total quality improvement, and often the same resources can be used for both processes.

The steps in the quality management, monitoring, and evaluation processes are based on the work of William Edwards Deming, an American author, professor, statistician, and consultant best known for his work in improving manufacturing production efficiency during World War II. Deming believed that quality is based on continuous improvement of processes and that when work is focused on quality, costs decrease over time (Deming, 1986).

As an APN, the DNP must be constantly attuned to and knowledgeable about changes in practice to ensure that current best practice is maintained. Considering the context of empirical evidence and patients' preferences and using processes and frameworks that aid translation evaluation help to ensure quality.

Conceptual Frameworks for Evidence and Practice Change

Two conceptual frameworks that help in the promotion and translation of evidence into practice are the PARIHS (promoting action on research implementation in health services) model (Rycroft-Malone et al., 2002) and the AGREE (appraisal of guidelines for research and evaluation) model (AGREE Collaboration, 2001). The PARIHS model, which is based on the work of Kitson et al. (1998, 2008), suggests that the integration of evidence is based on three factors: the nature of the evidence, the context of the desired change, and the mechanism of facilitating change. This evidence, and its translation for practice, includes practice guidelines and other forms of evidence specific to patient outcomes. The use of randomized controlled trials was central to implementation of this model. The model was revised by Rycroft-Malone et al. (2002) to include research information, clinical experience, and patient choice. In the new conceptualization, which involves continuous improvement of patient care, evidence based on one's "professional craft" or experience was part of the evidence contribution (Rycroft-Malone et al., 2004, p. 83).

Further work by Doran and Sidani (2007) identified gaps in the PARIHS model that led to an intervention framework that specifically addressed indicators for evaluating nursing services, systems, performance measures, and feedback to design and evaluate practice change. The intervention framework incorporates the work of Batalden and Stoltz (1993) and Batalden, Nelson, and Roberts (1994), which identified four categories of information in making care improvements. This information included "clinical (e.g. signs and symptoms), functional (e.g. activities of daily living), satisfaction (e.g. perceived benefit of care) and cost (i.e. both direct and indirect cost to the health care system and the patient)" (Doran & Sidani, 2007, p. 5). **Figure 3-3** depicts Doran and Sidani's (2007) outcomes-focused knowledge translation intervention framework.

The purpose of the AGREE instrument, as defined by the collaborators, "is to provide a framework for assessing the quality of clinical practice guidelines" (AGREE Collaboration, 2001, p. 2). As further described, quality means that potential biases are addressed and that the recommendations are valid and feasible for practice. In addition, as described in AGREE, "this process involves taking into account the benefits, harms, and costs of the recommendations, as well as the

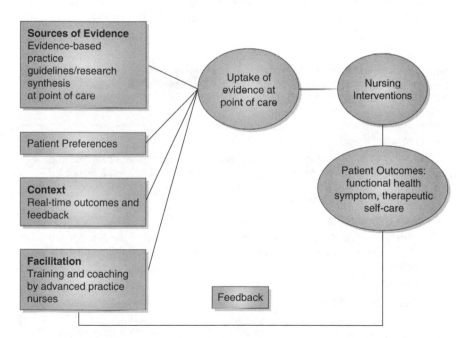

Figure 3-3 Outcomes-Focused Knowledge Translation Intervention Framework
Doran, D. M., & Sidani, S. (2007). Outcomes-focused knowledge translation: A framework for knowledge translation and patient outcome improvement. *Worldviews on Evidence-Based Nursing,* 4(1), 3–13.

practical issues attached to them. Therefore, the assessment includes the judgments about the methods used for developing the guidelines, the content of the final recommendations, and the factors linked to their uptake" (AGREE Collaboration, 2001, p. 2). The AGREE instrument consists of 23 items organized in six domains: scope and purpose (items 1–3), stakeholder involvement (items 4–7), rigor of development (items 8–14), clarity of presentation (items 15–17), applicability (items 18–21), and editorial independence (items 22–23). The complete instrument and user guide are available for download from the Internet.

The nursing faculty at one family NP program, the Lienhard School of Nursing at Pace University, used the AGREE instrument to teach family NP students how to critically appraise clinical practice guidelines (Singleton & Levin, 2008). In this program, students practice critiquing single studies, systematic reviews, and clinical practice guidelines. **Tables 3-4 and 3-5** present an exemplar of a learning activity using the AGREE instrument.

In another application of the AGREE instrument, Zadvinskis and Grudell (2010) used the guideline to appraise the National Kidney Foundation Kidney Disease Outcomes Quality Initiative Clinical Practice

---

Table 3-4 Learning Activity for the Critical Appraisal of Clinical Practice Guidelines

Steps

1. Preparatory reading:

   Slutsky, J. (2005). Using evidence-based practice guidelines: Tools for improving practice. In B. M. Melnyk & E. Fineout-Overholt (Eds.), *Evidence-based practice in nursing and healthcare: A guide to best practice* (pp. 221–227). Philadelphia, PA: Lippincott Williams & Wilkins.

2. Focus for assignment:

   Academy of Breastfeeding Medicine (2004). *Breastfeeding the near term infant (35–37 weeks gestation)*. New Rochelle, NY: Academy of Breastfeeding Medicine.

3. Work in teams.

4. Obtain the guideline.

5. Use the AGREE instrument to critically appraise the guideline.

6. Report back.

Reprinted with permission from SLACK Incorporated: Singleton, J., & Levin, R. (2008). Strategies for learning evidence-based practice: Critically appraising clinical practice guidelines. *Journal of Nursing Education, 47*(8), 380–383.

Table 3-5 Sample Domain and Items from the AGREE Instrument for Critical Appraisal of Clinical Practice Guidelines, with Rating Scale

Scope and Purpose

The overall objective(s) of the guideline is (are) specifically described.

The clinical question(s) covered by the guideline is (are) specifically described.

The patients to whom the guideline(s) is (are) meant to apply are specifically described.

Rating Scale

Strongly agree 4 3 2 1 Strongly disagree

Reprinted with permission from SLACK Incorporated: Singleton, J., & Levin, R. (2008). Strategies for learning evidence-based practice: Critically appraising clinical practice guidelines. *Journal of Nursing Education, 47*(8), 380–383.

Guideline for Chronic Kidney Disease. **Table 3-6** shows the scoring tool and mean guideline scores across the AGREE appraisal domains for the National Kidney Foundation outcomes.

The Johns Hopkins Nursing Evidence-based Practice Model (JH-NEBP), another evidence-based model, was developed as a collaborative effort between Johns Hopkins Hospital and the Johns Hopkins School of Nursing (Johns Hopkins Center for Health Services and Outcomes Research, 2012). The model is explained in six sections. Section I introduces the concept, the evolution of EBP, and the role of critical thinking in EBP. Section II describes the components of the model, which uses the PET process—practice question, evidence, and translation. Section III further explores the PET process in developing EBP projects. Section IV describes the environment necessary for the success of EBP. Section V provides examples of EBP projects. Section VI contains tools used for EBP at Johns Hopkins. A table of contents and sample, including levels of evidence from the model and guidelines, can be downloaded from the Nursing Knowledge International website. In addition, two evidence appraisal tools, JHNEBP research and nonresearch evidence appraisal tools are downloadable through the American Nurses Association website (ANA, 2015). The JHNEBP model and guidelines have "leveled objectives" for nursing students at the baccalaureate, graduate, and doctoral levels. At the doctoral level, the focus is on reviewing, rating, synthesizing, evaluating, and translating evidence at an advanced level (Newhouse, Dearholt, Poe, Pugh, & White, 2008). An example of one evidence-based project, developed by the Neuroscience Nursing Practice Committee, is a question related to the correct procedure for establishing nasogastric

Table 3-6 Mean Guideline Scores Across Domains of the Appraisal of Guidelines, Research and Evaluation in Europe (AGREE) Instrument for National Kidney Foundation Kidney Disease Outcomes of Quality Initiative (NKF KDOQI) Clinical Practice Guidelines for Chronic Kidney Disease

AGREE Domains	Scores
Domain 1—scope and purpose	
1. The overall objective(s) of the guideline is (are) specifically described.	4.0
2. The clinical question(s) covered by the guideline is (are) specifically described.	3.9
3. The patients to whom the guideline is meant to apply are specifically described.	4.0
Standardized domain 1 score (scale, 0–100)	98.0
Domain 2—stakeholder Involvement	
4. The guideline development group includes individuals from all relevant professional groups.	3.7
5. The patients' views and preferences have been sought.	1.0
6. The target users of the guideline are clearly defined.	3.9
7. The guideline has been piloted among target users.	1.7
Standardized domain 2 score (scale, 0–100)	52.4
Domain 3—rigor of development	
8. Systematic methods were used to search for evidence.	3.9
9. The criteria for selecting the evidence are clearly described.	4.0
10. The methods used for formulating the recommendations are clearly described.	3.9
11. The health benefits, adverse effects, and risks have been considered in formulating the recommendations.	3.9
12. There is an explicit link between the recommendations and the supporting evidence.	3.7
13. The guideline has been externally reviewed by experts prior to its publication.	3.9
14. A procedure for updating the guideline is provided.	1.4
Standardized domain 3 score (scale, 0–100)	87.0
Domain 4—clarity and presentation	
15. The recommendations are specific and unambiguous.	3.9
16. The different options for management of the condition are clearly presented.	3.9
17. Key recommendations are easily identifiable.	3.7
18. The guideline is supported with tools for application.	3.1
Standardized domain 4 score (scale, 0–100)	88.1

AGREE Domains	Scores
Domain 5—applicability	
19. The potential organizational barriers in applying the recommendations have been discussed.	1.3
20. The potential cost implications of applying the recommendations have been considered.	2.6
21. The guideline presents key review criteria for monitoring and/or audit purposes.	3.6
Standardized domain 5 score (scale, 0–100)	49.2
Domain 6—editorial independence	
22. The guideline is editorially independent from the funding body.	1.7
23. Conflicts of interest of guideline development members have been recorded.	3.6
Standardized domain 6 score (scale, 0–100)	54.8

Each item is rated on a 4-point scale ranging from 4 (strongly agree) to 1 (strongly disagree), with 2 mid points: 3 (agree) and 2 (disagree). The scale measures the extent to which a criterion (item) has been fulfilled.

Zadvinskis, I. M., & Grudell, B. A. (2010). Clinical practice guideline appraisal using the AGREE instrument: Renal Screening. *Clinical Nurse Specialist, 24*(4), 209–214. © Wolters Kluwer Health/Lippincott Williams & Wilkins.

tube placement in adult patients. Using the PICO (patient, intervention, comparison, and outcomes) format and levels of evidence, the existing protocol that required insufflations of air was discontinued. A table of the process and levels of evidence is shown in the Johns Hopkins model instructor's guide (Dearholt & Dang, 2012), available on the Internet.

Designing and Implementing Processes to Evaluate Outcomes of Practice and Systems of Care

As nursing moves practice decisions from those based on tradition to those based on empirical evidence, the APN, particularly the DNP, is in the best position to effect and assess change within the clinical setting. Why? EBP and quality management are both practice-driven processes (French, 1999). Each is informed by experience and outcomes that can be directly seen and measured. In most cases, the observations that arise during daily practice provide the basis for questions, which can be empirically tested and their results implemented and evaluated. The findings of previous research studies can be replicated in a variety of settings with resources that are already in place.

The curriculum of DNP programs includes specialty-focused competencies delineated by specialty nursing organizations, and the core essentials include courses and application experiences in research methods and statistical analysis (AACN, 2006). This education, coupled with advanced clinical knowledge, provides the DNP with the requisites necessary to design and collaborate in studies that can make a practical difference in the delivery of clinical care (French, 1999; Reavy & Tavernier, 2008). Listed in **Table 3-7** are some recent examples of clinical studies concerning advanced practice nursing interventions and outcomes designed by DNPs.

The Essentials of Doctoral Education for Advanced Nursing Practice (AACN, 2006) states that "DNP graduates must understand principles of practice management, including conceptual and practice strategies for balancing productivity and quality care" (p. 4). In addition, "they must be able to assess the impact of clinical policies and procedures on meeting the health needs of the patient populations with whom they practice" (p. 4). In addition, "they must be proficient in quality improvement strategies and in creating and sustaining changes at the organizational and policy levels" (p. 4).

Quality Improvement Initiatives to Promote Safe, Timely, Effective, Efficient, Equitable, and Patient-Centered Care

The design of quality improvement initiatives must be empirically based and dependent on sources of knowledge that include research evidence; clinical experience; reasoning; authority; quality improvement data; and the patient's situation, values, and experience (Brown, 2005). These are the tools that can help the DNP decide whether the clinical guidelines and scientific evidence are consistent with the context, values, and desires of the patient (Glanville, Schirm, & Wineman, 2000).

For the past century, most outcome measurement has focused on the outcomes of medical care, particularly negative outcomes. However, during the past several years, there has been a greater focus on positive indicators of nursing care delivery (Melnyk & Fineout-Overholt, 2011). The development of nurse-sensitive patient outcomes (NSPOs) was an outgrowth of public demand for greater accountability by healthcare providers.

Some examples of nurse-sensitive indicators of quality include health-promoting behaviors (Mitchell, Ferketich, & Jennings, 1998), compliance/adherence (Ingersoll, McIntosh, & Williams, 2000), quality of life (Ingersoll et al., 2000), support systems available to assist with caregiver

Table 3-7 Selected DNP Scholarly Publications: Evidence-Based Research Interventions and Outcomes

Author/Year	Design, Sample, Setting	Framework/Intervention/Measures	Goal/Aim	Outcomes/Findings
Bundy, E. Y., & Murphy, L. S. (2014)	QI; retrospective audit; outpatient clinic; n = 42 medical records.	In-service based on literature review and retrospective chart audit for use of system-based asthma action plan (AAP).	Improve use and completion of AAP post-in-service.	Statistically significant proportional outcomes following in-service, use of AAP and procedure change.
Graling, P. R. (2011)	EBP; quality improvement; N = 283 surgical care providers = 287 at large university hospital.	Framework for Knowledge Transfer of Patient Safety (AHRQ); Universal Protocol (The Joint Commission, 2009) Attitude Questionnaire (SAQ); team education; implementation of safety checklist.	Enhance perioperative teamwork; decrease safety events; improve compliance with Universal Protocol (The Joint Commission, 2009).	Statistically significant differences were found in safety climate and working differences overall; safety events decreased by 50%; compliance with the safety checklist increased in 2010; resources have now been allocated for perioperative safety initiatives.
Hande, K. A. (2013)	EBP; QA; retrospective audit of 90 charts (30 randomly selected for each of 3 providers).	Total Quality Management (TQM/CQI); Plan, Do, Study, Act (PDSA); EBP measures modified colorectal prevention data collection form and TQE Benchmark.	Assess adherence to colorectal cancer prevention (CRC-P) benchmarking; improve CRC-P; close gaps in detection; report improvement.	Identified practice changes; analyzed root causes; actions for improvement. Redesign of CRC-P practices.

continues

Table 3-7 Selected DNP Scholarly Publications: Evidence-Based Research Interventions and Outcomes *(continued)*

Author/Year	Design, Sample, Setting	Framework/Intervention/Measures	Goal/Aim	Outcomes/Findings
Krebbeks, V. P., & Cunningham, V. M. (2013)	Development of a rural DNP-managed hepatitis C clinic; patients with positive HCV antibody or active HCV virus.	Effect and Process Theory (evaluation); DNP model for rural clinic; concepts and culture of rural nursing; DNP/hepatologist collaboration.	Quality; cost effective; culturally sensitive care.	Planned: QOL; treatment compliance; medication adherence; virus eradication.
Santucci, S. (2011)	EBP; community needs assessment and gap analysis; convenience sample of 50 adults; underserved southeastern U.S. community.	Health belief model with prevention constructs. Policy change in Community Rapid Testing Program to allow referral of HIV positive patients to hospital-based ID clinic for f/u and prevention; data on system change variables, e.g., tests/results, referrals, were entered weekly in database.	Close gap to secondary prevention service to decrease HIV morbidity, mortality, and transmission.	New system expedited care to marginalized groups; change decreased time to test results/referral for treatment from 6–8 weeks to 1–2 weeks.

burden (Craft-Rosenburg, Krajicek, & Shin, 2002), trust in care provider (Ingersoll et al., 2000), and length of stay (Hodge, Asch, Olson, Kravitz, & Sauve, 2002). **Table 3-8** presents additional examples of evidence-based outcome indicators.

The success of EBP depends on asking the right questions at the right time, critically analyzing results of other studies for fit in a given situation, observing for differences in responses, and evaluating outcomes. In this regard, quality improvement evaluation is important in advanced practice to ascertain the impact of interventions and their effect on cost-effective care. DNP and APN interventions are appropriately evaluated on the basis of physiological, psychosocial, functional, behavioral, and knowledge-focused effectiveness (Glanville et al., 2000). The evaluation process involves the selection of appropriate measurement instruments. Glanville et al. (2000) made the point that instruments that measure effectiveness in care processes are not the same as those that measure outcomes. For example, a tool that measures risk for patient infections is not the same tool as one that actually tracks infection rates in a group of postsurgical patients. Similarly, in process management, the focus is on which components produce or contribute to practice variations that may ultimately affect, but are not the same as, outcomes (Ingersoll, 2005).

Some basic provisions for an effective outcomes model are to keep the outcomes as short as possible; to use outcomes, not activities or processes;

Table 3-8 Selected Evidence-Based Outcome Indicators for Advanced Practice Nursing

Outcomes	Examples and Indicators
Patient satisfaction	Ambulatory care: Survey
Risk	Morbidity and mortality: Summary
	Patient falls: Reports
	Medication errors: Medication administration records (MARs); comprehensiveness of exams
Knowledge	Blood pressure medication: Blood pressure control
Condition-specific	Postoperative pain: Pain management scale
	Diabetes management: Blood glucose levels
Infection control	Surgical procedures: Hand washing; nosocomial infection rates
Compliance	Fluid restriction: Daily weights
	Prenatal and postpartum visits

and to use singular, not compound, outcomes (Duignan, 2006). Components of an effective outcomes management model include the following:

> 1) identification of the problem, 2) scanning the existing evidence and standards of care, 3) identification of benchmark targets, 4) determination and selection of outcomes measuring and monitoring tools, 5) development of specific guidelines to drive care delivery processes, 6) assessment of existing processes, 7) measurement and monitoring of processes and outcomes of care, 8) reporting findings to key stakeholders and decision makers, and 9) refining care delivery processes and data collection techniques based on findings. (Ingersoll, 2005, pp. 314–315)

A significant time commitment is required for designing systems for promoting safe, timely, patient-centered care. However, the benefits are efficiency and effectiveness. Since the Institute of Medicine (IOM) studies, patient safety has been a primary focus of quality improvement initiatives. Safety issues are of concern in every care setting—primary, secondary, and tertiary. A review of the literature from 2005 to 2015 in the CINAHL databases produced over 1,000 (CINAHL) nondissertation nursing studies that involved quality improvement projects with safety as a focus. Of these, 214 studies included the word "evidence" in the title, and 7 included "advanced practice nursing" in the title. Study topics included pharmacotherapy, environment, technology, acute care, pediatrics, critical care, intravenous infusions, long-term care and home health, rural health, diabetes, health education, chronic obstructive pulmonary disease, Alzheimer's, mental health treatment in children, head injury and neuroscience issues, electronic medical records, pregnancy, diabetes, and behavioral health. When search terms included "advanced nursing," a number of studies dealt with issues of timeliness (51 studies in CINAHL), effectiveness (427 studies in CINAHL), and equitable care (9 studies in CINAHL)—all of which are important dimensions of quality that need to be addressed, especially as they affect safety and quality outcomes. Patient-centered care was addressed in over 50,000 studies in the CINAHL database studies. However, few studies included "DNP" in the title of the article. Direct care providers, particularly DNPs, must take a lead role in continuing the effort to improve care delivery systems that benefit patients, families, and providers of care.

Using Practice Guidelines to Improve Practice and the Practice Environment

As Goolsby, Meyers, Johnson, Klardie, and McNaughton (2004) have noted, "clinical practice guidelines are protocol-driven, step-wise recommendations for diagnosing and treating specific conditions, or patient populations" (p. 178). Clinical decision making is grounded in the use of clinical research, expert opinion, and clinical practice guidelines. Further, clinical practice guidelines "minimize differences in practice patterns and the risk of misdiagnosis or treatment failures" (Goolsby, Meyers, et al., 2004, p. 178).

In one example, Cooke et al. (2004) described a program at one hospital that used a quality of life model and research department "linking agents" acting as in-service providers and unit consultants for EBP to encourage and link EBP, critical thinking, and practical application. Unfortunately, practice guidelines are not always used for a variety of reasons. Time, communication, involvement, resources, patient expectations, and perceived priority are all facilitators of or barriers to the implementation of EBP guidelines (Abrahamson, Fox, & Doebbeling, 2012; DiCenso, Cullum, & Ciliska, 1998; Gagan & Hewitt-Taylor, 2004; Graham, Graham, & Davies, 2013; Lopez-Bushnell, 2002; McCaughan, Thompson, Cullum, Sheldon, & Thompson, 2002; Rutledge & Bookbinder, 2002). Nevertheless, the use of practice guidelines and published articles on their use has increased substantially since the first edition of this chapter. For the 10-year period from 2004 to 2014, using the search terms "practice guidelines," "use," and "advanced practice," there were 48,072 articles in CINAHL—over 3 times the number in the prior 10 years.

Evaluation of Practice

He who every morning plans the transaction of the day and follows out that plan, carries a thread that will guide him through the maze of the most busy life. But where no plan is laid, where the disposal of time is surrendered merely to the chance of incidence, chaos will soon reign.

—Victor Hugo

Planning for evaluation is as important as the change itself and must be a systematic process. Evaluation is an ongoing process that must start early in a project and be continual. Evaluating practice and changes in practice is essential to the successful implementation of any quality improvement or EBP initiative. Classification schemes allow for an organized approach to evaluating outcomes. Outcomes may be classified according to population served (e.g., pediatric, adult, geriatric), time (long term, medium term, or short term), or type (care related, patient related, or performance related) (Rich, 2015).

Using Benchmarks to Evaluate Clinical Outcomes and Trends

One method of evaluating practice is to evaluate practice patterns against national benchmarks to determine variances in clinical outcomes and population trends. Benchmarking is the process of comparing performance with an external standard to motivate improvement (AHRQ, 2013). Organizations that regularly collect data on outcomes in health care are state boards of health and the Centers for Medicare and Medicaid Services (CMS). The Joint Commission and the Magnet Recognition Program (American Nurses Credentialing Center, 2005) also have performance measurement standards that are based on quality indicators. In addition to these organizations, many hospitals and healthcare facilities have memberships in organizations that benchmark indicators of quality in specialty services. Benchmarking is especially important since the passage of the Patient Protection and Affordable Care Act (2010). One interesting example was a study that compared NP and PA practices and productivity in outpatient oncology clinics at national comprehensive cancer network institutions. NPs were seen to be marginally more productive in seeing follow-up patients, whereas PAs conducted slightly more procedures. Both providers were seen as a useful addition to oncology practices in these centers (Hinkel et al., 2010).

Nursing services are an important aspect of outcome evaluation and reporting at any healthcare institution because nurses make up such a large part of the healthcare workforce. Effectiveness of nursing care is determined by nurse-sensitive indicators. Nursing administrators are responsible for maintaining evaluation systems and reporting nurse-sensitive outcomes. As leaders in clinical care and outcome evaluation, DNPs must be in the forefront of designing outcome evaluation plans for advanced practice.

DNPs in advanced practice roles are also included in medical outcome working groups within their scope of practice. The American Medical Association Physician Consortium for Performance Improvement (AMA-PCPI) has performance measures available for 31 topics or conditions (Gallagher, 2009). The general approach to measurement includes six steps: "1) identifying the opportunities for improvement, 2) involving representation from medical specialties and other care disciplines, 3) linking measures to an evidence base, 4) supporting clinical judgment and patient preferences, 5) testing measures, and 6) promoting a single

Table 3-9 Websites for Healthcare Outcome Information

Organization	Website
Academy Health	http://www.academyhealth.org
Agency for Healthcare Research and Quality	http://www.ahrq.gov
Centers for Medicare and Medicaid Services	http://www.cms.gov
Institute for Healthcare Improvement	http://www.ihi.org
International Society for Pharmaco-economics and Outcomes Research	http://www.ispor.org
Johns Hopkins Center for Health Services and Outcomes Research	http://www.jhsph.edu
The Joint Commission	http://www.jointcommission.org
National Cancer Institute	http://www.cancer.gov/
National Committee for Quality Assurance	http://www.ncqa.org
National Quality Forum	http://www.qualityforum.org/Home.aspx
University of Iowa College of Nursing	http://www.nursing.uiowa.edu/excellence/evidence-based-practice-guidelines
University of Arizona Health Outcomes and Pharmacoeconomics Research (HOPE)	www.pharmacy.arizona.edu

Modified from Rich, K. A. (2015). Evaluating outcomes of innovations. In N. A. Schmidt & J. M. Brown (Eds.), *Evidence-based practice for nurses* (p. 491). Burlington, MA: Jones & Bartlett Learning.

set of measures for widespread use and multiple purpose" (Gallagher, 2009, p. 185). **Table 3-9** contains a brief listing of websites for healthcare outcomes and data.

Database Design to Generate Meaningful Evidence for Nursing Practice

A systematic process for patient care and practice data is essential to guide practice. This requires the development of standardized databases to guide outcomes research for practice. Clinical databases from computerized medical records and disease registries are the result of documentation of care or research protocols. Outcome data are also available from birth logs, death records, discharge summaries, and clinical pathways.

Most important, the outcome must be measurable, and the data must relate to the care processes or interventions (Arthur, Marfell, & Ulrich, 2009).

Another useful resource for evidence-based outcomes is the National Guideline Clearinghouse (NGC), an initiative of the AHRQ, the American Medical Association (AMA), and America's Health Insurance Plans. Users can subscribe to the NGC weekly email update service. The site provides information about new and updated guidelines from the Centers for Disease Control and Prevention (CDC), the National Institute for Clinical Excellence, the Program for Evidence-Based Care, and others. Conference information is also available from the NGC, as well as nutrition, chemicals, and drug advisory information.

The Cochrane Collaboration Review is another source that provides reprints online of the newest intervention reviews. The *Review* lists authors and their affiliations; an abstract, including background, objectives, search strategies, selection criteria, data collection, and analysis; authors' conclusions; and a plain-language summary. The library contains sections for clinicians, researchers, patients, and policy makers. The Cochrane Library, a collection of medical and healthcare databases, is available online through Wiley InterScience. Podcasts are also available.

These and other evidence-based resources are effective tools to aid in the efficient delivery of evidence-based care. **Table 3-10** provides a brief description of other available databases. The use of these resources is valuable when combined with the best empirical knowledge and judgment. The true measure of their effectiveness is in the evaluation of the outcomes of management and care decisions, and delivery processes.

As nursing takes on larger, more autonomous roles in the delivery of health care through advanced practice, the need for accountability will continue to increase. DNPs, with their knowledge of clinical practice, research, and informatics, can best represent advanced practice nursing by participating in and guiding the development of databases that are relevant to the care that DNPs and APNs provide. Becoming involved in professional organizations that have quality initiatives is an excellent way for DNPs to become knowledgeable in research that contributes to quality care and the profession.

New since the last edition of this chapter is the Doctors of Nursing Practice, Inc., an organization whose purpose is to promote global networking, curricular and program enhancement, and research collaboration. The organization offers conferences, practice updates, and scholarship of particular interest to DNPs. In addition, the ANA and specialty organizations such as the Oncology Nursing Society, the

Table 3-10 Evidence Databases

Source	Content
American College of Physicians (ACP) Journal Club	Articles reporting original studies and systematic reviews.
ACP JournalWise	Personalized journal alerting service sends messages to a smartphone or email inbox according to subscriber interest and specialties.
AHRQ	Guidelines and technology assessments on selected topics from 12 evidence-based practice centers.
AHRQ (SHARE)	A five-step process for shared decision making that includes exploring and comparing the benefits, harms, and risks of each option through meaningful dialogue about what matters most to the patient.
AIDSLINE	Indexes the published literature on HIV and AIDS. The index includes journal articles; monographs; meeting abstracts; and papers, newsletters, and government reports (Fain, 2009).
Bandolier	Reviews literature; offers subjects by medical specialty.
CANCERLIT	Includes cancer literature from journal articles, government reports, technical reports, meeting abstracts and papers, and monographs.
CDC Sexually Transmitted Disease Treatment Guidelines	Includes Web-browsable sources with crosslinks.
Cochrane Database of Systematic Reviews	"Reviews individual clinical trials and summarizes systematic reviews from over 100 medical journals" (Fain, 2009, p. 277).
DynaMed	Point-of-care resource to support clinical decision making.
EPPI Centre	Evidence for Policy and Practice Information and Coordinating Centre, Institute of Education, University of London.
Essential Evidence Plus (formerly InfoPOEMs)	Includes reviews and commentary of recently published articles by the *Journal of Family Practice*.
Evidence-Based Practice at the University of Iowa	Includes an evidence-based practice toolkit, information about recent evidence-based practice projects, and an evidence-based practice model and resources.
HSTAT	Health Services Technology Assessment Text, full-text guidelines.
Johns Hopkins Evidence-Based Practice Center	Includes systematic reviews of evidence.

continues

Table 3-10 Evidence Databases *(continued)*	
Source	**Content**
MD Consult	Includes full-text access to journal articles, text-books, practice guidelines, patient education hand-outs, and drug awareness information. MD Consult is a good, quick source for background information on a topic.
MEDLINE	A compilation of information from Index Medicus, Index to Dental Literature, and the International Nursing Index. It includes published research in allied health, biological sciences, information sciences, physical sciences, and the humanities.
MedPage Today	Includes daily research updates, news by specialty, policy news, continuing medical education (CME), and surveys. Includes an excellent tool, MedPage Tools Guide to Biostatistics, that can be used as a reference guide when reading research articles.
Prescriber's Letter	Includes evidence-based information on new drug developments, with links to articles and continuing education offerings.
PubMed	Provides source for queries and evidence-based filters for MEDLINE.
School of Health and Related Research (ScHarr)	Comprehensive up-to-date evidence on the Web.
The Joanna Briggs Institute	International institute that provides resources for evidence-based practice for healthcare professionals in nursing, medicine, midwifery, and allied health.
The National Guideline Clearinghouse (NGC)	Provides nonintegrated evidence-based practice clinical guidelines and recommendations on selected topics from a number of organizations.

Modified from Fain, J. A. (2009). Understanding evidence-based practice. In *Reading, understanding and applying nursing research* (3rd ed., pp. 276–278). Philadelphia, PA: F. A. Davis. Used with permission.

National Quality Forum, the AHRQ, and the CMS provide avenues for collaboration and dissemination of information on quality and nurse-sensitive outcomes (Grove et al., 2013).

Information Technology, Databases, and Evidence for Practice

Digital technologies, including computers, handheld devices, and Internet software applications, have changed the face of clinical care, making them a necessary tool for research and EBP. They provide efficiency in the inputting of statistical data and the retrieval of the most current information on relevant clinical trial outcomes, supportive research, and accepted practice protocols. It is essential to pay attention to the kinds of data that are retrieved and how they are used to make clinical decisions and evaluate practice.

Collecting Appropriate and Accurate Data

Data and observations from practice can be augmented and strengthened through evidence from clinical trials. Several electronic databases provide access to clinical trial data and other peer-reviewed research and outcome data. However, clinical trial data and data from other aggregate sources do not always address the outcomes that can be uniquely attributed to APN/DNP practice. For APN/DNPs to assess and demonstrate their effectiveness, data are needed that reflect what they do. Although the primary goal of outcome data and analysis is to improve care, DNPs in direct practice may be asked to justify their roles in terms of factors such as cost, time, patient outcomes, and revenue generation, among other indicators (S. Burns, 2009).

Most institutions rely on aggregated data to determine nursing outcomes. Unfortunately, most aggregated data do not show the APN/DNP's specific contribution to the outcomes (S. Burns, 2009). For this reason, it is important that measures be selected that truly reflect the APN/DNP role. This means developing role-sensitive indicators and collecting data that are specific to those indicators in a systematic way. Indicators such as satisfaction with APN/DNP care related to a particular program or procedure that the APN/DNP initiates, controls, or coordinates are better than trying to extrapolate the APN/DNP's role in a multidisciplinary effort. Time savings or clinical outcomes related to a change in practice coordinated by the APN/DNP may also be role sensitive.

A well-designed assessment plan uses a model that considers organizational factors, employee behavior, patient characteristics, patient experience, and outcomes (Minnick & Roberts, 1991, Figure 4-1, as cited in Minnick, 2009). Instruments for measuring outcomes are also a necessary component in the assessment process. A systematic search of the databases mentioned in Table 3-10, such as AHRQ, PubMed, and CANCERLIT, may be helpful as a starting place for appropriate measurement tools.

Analyzing Data from Clinical Practice

Data from practice are rich and can be analyzed in a number of ways, depending on the nature of the research question. Computer-based statistical tools such as absolute risk (AR) and absolute risk reduction

(ARR) calculations, relative risk (RR) and relative risk reduction (RRR) calculations, number needed to treat (NNT), survival curves, hazard ratios, and sensitivity and specificity are helpful measures for assessing risk of disease in studies of different cohort groups and in aiding clinical decision making. In an excellent article in the *Journal of the American Academy of Nurse Practitioners*, Goolsby, Klardie, Johnson, McNaughton, and Meyers (2004) analyzed the implementation of clinical practice guidelines and their outcomes in a hypothetical patient situation. The analysis includes a review of commonly used statistical concepts, including some of those just mentioned, with examples of their application in interpreting and reporting research. O'Mathuna et al. (2011) also provided a detailed section on statistical measures and their meaning in a chapter entitled "Critically Appraising Quantitative Evidence for Clinical Decision-Making."

Designing Evidence-Based Interventions

Selecting and defining the problem is one of the most critical steps in the design of any evidence-based intervention. The problem statement provides the direction for the study design and is usually stated at the beginning. Essential to good design is adequate background information that includes a rationale for pursuing an intervention, evidence from research that has already been done on the topic, and the goals to be achieved (Fain, 2013). Depending on the problem to be addressed, evidence-based interventions may be generated from quantitative research, qualitative research, outcome studies, patient concerns and choices, or clinical judgment.

Models serve as good frameworks for design. Several models that were originally designed for research utilization were the historical precursors to EBP. Four well-known models for research utilization and EBP are: the Conduct and Utilization of Research in Nursing (CURN) model (Horsely, Crane, & Bingle, 1978), the Kitson model (Kitson et al., 1998), the Stetler/Marram model (Stetler, 1994; Stetler & Marram, 1976), and the Iowa Model of Research Utilization (Titler et al., 1994). As EBP has evolved, these models have been adapted, and other models have been developed. Some later models include the Advancing Research and Clinical Practice through Close Collaboration (ARCC) model (Melnyk & Fineout-Overholt, 2002), the Rosswurm and Larrabee model (1999), the Iowa Model of Evidence-Based Practice to Promote Quality Care (Titler, 2002), and the Johns Hopkins model (Newhouse et al., 2008). Each of these models has been successful in disseminating research or in facilitating change toward EBP. **Figure 3-4** shows a schematic of the Iowa model.

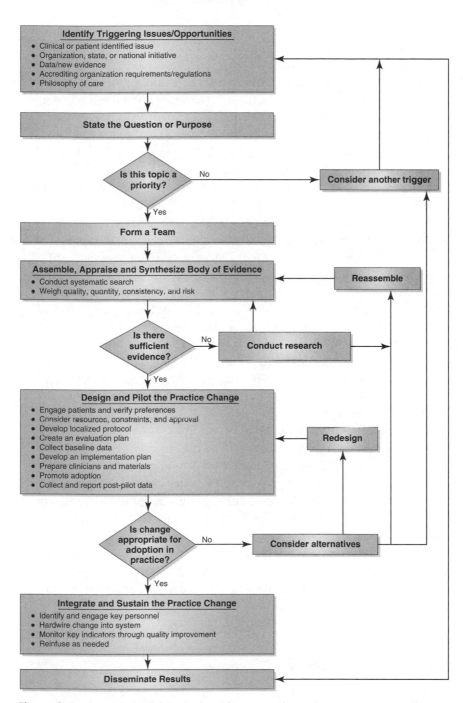

Figure 3-4 The Iowa Model Revised: Evidence-Based Practice to Promote Excellence in Health Care

Used/Reprinted with permission from the University of Iowa Hospitals and Clinics. Copyright 2015. For permission to use or reproduce the model, please contact the University of Iowa Hospitals and Clinics at (319)384–9098.

It is beyond the scope of this chapter to detail the specifics of each model. However, although there are nuances and structural differences, all the models support some form of practice change through the systematic review of research and other evidence, such as clinical practice guidelines, to create a culture of research conduct and research utilization. Certainly, the first step in the design of any practice intervention is to define the clinical practice questions. Once that is accomplished, critical questions include the following: What patients will be affected? What treatment or intervention or practice change is involved? What old practice would need to be discontinued? What outcomes are expected? (Collins et al., 2008).

The next step is to review the evidence, basing the analysis on the hierarchy of evidence (see Table 3-1) and a search of all relevant databases (e.g., Cochrane, CINAHL, NGC, PubMed). Once the evidence has been verified, assessing applicability to the population and environment is crucial. Questions to be considered may include the following: Will implementing this practice increase patient safety? Are there ethical or legal considerations? Will other departments or providers be affected? How will the change affect practitioner time? How will patients react to the change? The next step is to develop a plan for the change. Who are the key stakeholders? How will they be apprised and included? Who has final sign-off authority? Is a pilot study indicated before full-scale implementation? Finally, determine the methods of education and communication. How much time, money, and personnel resources will be needed?

When implementing the plan, the following questions should be considered: Who is responsible for coordinating the effort? What contingency plans are in place in the event that a change must be made? Who is managing issues that may arise? Will evaluation of implementation be ongoing? How will feedback be generated? Who will conduct the evaluation? What is the method of analysis? What are the measurement tools? How will results of the evaluation be presented? (Collins et al., 2008). Carey, Buchan, and Sanson-Fisher (2009) outlined some specific strategies to promote guideline implementation. **Table 3-11** summarizes their recommendations. Although the examples reference general practitioner (GP) practice, the strategies and constructs are applicable to DNP/APN practice.

Predicting and Analyzing Outcomes

Often in clinical practice, the occurrence of one event in time may be the basis for predicting a future event. In such instances, a predictive relationship is established. In this case, the practitioner or researcher is

Table 3-11 Strategies to Promote Guideline Implementation: Theoretical Constructs and Examples of Application

Strategy	Relevant Constructs	Key Illustrative Examples
		Phase 1
Concrete and specific recommendations	Knowledge, executability, decidability	Concrete and specific recommendations were more likely to be adopted by general practitioners (GPs) than vague, nonspecific recommendations. Observational study. (Grol et al., 1998)
Identify priorities	Goal setting, action planning	Of 228 primary care patients with cardiovascular disease risk factors who made an action plan to identify behavioral change goals, 53% also reported making behavioral change related to their action plan. Descriptive study. (Handley et al., 2006)
Set targets for implementation	Goal setting	
Present a rationale	Beliefs, attitudes, perceived relative advantage	Recommendations compatible with current values were more likely to be adopted by GPs than those perceived as controversial or incompatible with values. Observational study. (Grol et al., 1998)
Highlight clinical norms	Normative beliefs, attitudes, modeling/verbal persuasion	An intervention to improve myocardial infarction care that involved using local medical opinion leaders to influence peers through small-group discussions, informal consultation, and revisions of clinical protocols was compared with performance feedback alone. Hospitals in both groups improved from baseline to follow-up on indicators of quality; however, the improvement was greatest for those allocated to the peer intervention. Randomized controlled trial. (Soumerai et al., 1998)
Orient to the need of the end user	Complexity	Among the guideline characteristics most commonly endorsed to promote use by GPs was "clarity, simplicity and availability of a short format." Descriptive study of 391 GPs. (Watkins, Harvey, Langley, Gray, & Faulkner, 1999)
Skills training	Skills, knowledge, self-efficacy	Continuing medical education (CME) improves knowledge, skills, attitudes, and patient outcomes. CME that is interactive, uses multimedia, uses live media, and involves multiple exposures is more effective than other types. Systematic review. (Marinopoulos et al., 2007)

continues

Table 3-11 Strategies to Promote Guideline Implementation: Theoretical Constructs and Examples of Application *(continued)*

Strategy	Relevant Constructs	Key Illustrative Examples
		Phase 1
Social influences	Normative beliefs, attitudes, modeling, verbal persuasion	The use of local opinion leaders in hospital settings can be effective in promoting evidence-based practice. Systematic review of 12 studies (Doumitt, Gattelliari, Grimshaw, & O'Brien, 2007)
Environmental influences	Cues to action, environmental triggers	Guideline adherence improved due to the implementation of a computerized clinical decision aid that gave clinicians real-time recommendations for venous thromboembolism prophylaxis. Time series study (Durieux, Nizard, Ravaud, Mounier, & Lepage, 2000)
Patient-mediated	Knowledge, skills, and attitudes of patients	Patient request for a new drug and patient acceptability were cited as contributing to decisions to prescribe a new drug in approximately 20% of cases. Descriptive study (Prosser, Almond, & Walley, 2003)
Feedback	Positive/negative reinforcement; goal setting; skill development	Audit and feedback are effective strategies for improving care, particularly when baseline adherence to the recommended practice is low. Systematic review of 118 studies (Jamtvedt, Young, Kristofferson, O'Brien, & Oxman, 2006)
Incentives	Positive/negative reinforcement	Five of six studies examining physician-level incentives and seven of nine studies examining provider-group-level incentives demonstrated partial or positive effects on quality indicators. Systematic review (Peterson, Woodward, Urech, Daw, & Sookanan, 2006)
Pilot testing with iterative refinement of implementation strategies	Perceived advantages; beliefs; trialability	Breakthrough collaborative model intervention that involved a series of iterative plan-do-study-act cycles was found to be effective in improving care for chronic heart failure. Quasi-experimental, controlled study (Asch et al., 2005)

Carey, M., Buchan, H., & Sanson-Fisher, R. (2009). The cycle of change: Implementing the best-evidence clinical practice. *International Journal for Quality in Health Care, 21*(1), 37–43. Reproduced with permission.

looking for a correlation between the two events that may predict the outcome of a future intervention or occurrence that could be designed to affect or influence the independent variable. Although correlational prediction is not the same as cause and effect, it is stronger than a purely descriptive study (Melnyk & Cole, 2011). This type of study would be appropriate if, for example, the DNP was interested in how a person's initial attitude toward insulin affected compliance with the regimen 3, 6, or 12 months after the therapy began.

Correlation statistics would be used to measure the relationship between the two variables. The results of the correlation could later be used to design interventions, such as educational strategies or follow-up programs, that would help those with negative attitudes toward therapy learn, adapt, and achieve more positive outcomes. Correlational statistics are also used to measure the strength of relationship between two variables. A direct correlation is seen in correlation coefficients between the values of 0 (no correlation) and 1 (large positive correlation) and means that when there is a large change in the value of one predictor, there is a large change in the value of the other predictor; likewise, a small change in one predictor is accompanied by a small change in the other predictor. A relationship that has a correlation coefficient of 0.5 is stronger than 0, but less than 1.0. Conversely, in a negative correlation—between 0 (no correlation) and –1 (large negative correlation)—large changes in the value of one predictor would be accompanied by small changes in the other, or small changes in one would be accompanied by large changes in the other. Therefore, a negative correlation coefficient of –0.6 shows a stronger negative relationship between two variables than a coefficient of 0, but not as strong as a coefficient of –1.0 (Lanthier, 2002).

An example of this kind of analysis is shown in a correlation study on salary and income levels. **Table 3-12** shows salary levels and corresponding years of education. **Figure 3-5** shows an example of a correlation scatter plot, with years of education on the *y* axis and income on the *x* axis. Each point on the plot shows one person's answers to the questions regarding years of education and income. In a positive correlation such as this, the line is always in the upward direction. In another example, **Table 3-13** and **Figure 3-6** show a negative relationship between grade point average (GPA) and number of hours spent watching television. The scatter plot (Figure 3-6) shows the direction of the line when the correlation is negative. In these cases, the researcher is measuring conditions that already exist and looking for relationships—either positive or negative.

Participant	Income	Years of Education
#1	125,000	19
#2	100,000	20
#3	40,000	16
#4	35,000	16
#5	41,000	18
#6	29,000	12
#7	35,000	14
#8	24,000	12
#9	50,000	16
#10	60,000	17

Table 3-12 Salary and Years of Education

Lanthier, E. (2002). Correlation. www.nvcc.edu/home/elan thier/methods/correlation.htm. Copyright 2002 by Elizabeth Lanthier, PhD. Reproduced with permission.

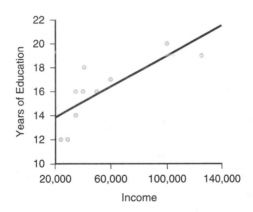

Figure 3-5 Regression Scatter Plot, Salary, and Education in Years
Lanthier, E. (2002). Correlation. www.nvcc.edu/home/elanthier/methods/correlation.htm.
Copyright 2002 by Elizabeth Lanthier, PhD. Reproduced with permission.

Examining Patterns of Behavior and Outcomes

Although much of the research and evidence for practice is focused on cause and effect, patterns of behavior, dispositions, and attitudes are also outcomes that require examination. Behavioral theories can be

Table 3-13 Grade Point Average and TV Use		
Participant	**GPA**	**TV Use (hrs/wk)**
#1	3.1	14
#2	2.4	10
#3	2.0	20
#4	3.8	7
#5	2.2	25
#6	3.4	9
#7	2.9	15
#8	3.2	13
#9	3.7	4
#10	3.5	21

Lanthier, E. (2002). *Correlation samples.* www.nvcc.edu/home/
elanthier/methods/correlation.htm. Copyright 2002 by Elizabeth
Lanthier, PhD. Reproduced with permission.

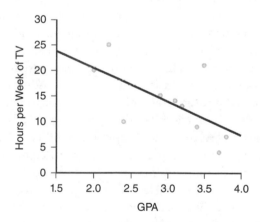

Figure 3-6 Regression Scatter Plot, Hours of Television Use, and Grade Point Average
Lanthier, E. (2002). *Correlation samples.* www.nvcc.edu/home/elanthier/methods/correlation.htm.
Copyright 2002 by Elizabeth Lanthier, PhD. Reproduced with permission.

classified as intrapersonal (individual), interpersonal (relational), and
community based. The stages of change model (Prochaska & DiClemente, 1986), the health belief model (Rosenstock, 1966), and the theory
of reasoned action (Fishbein & Ajzen, 1980) are useful in examining behaviors and their relationship to outcomes.

One way of examining data is through the use of aggregated data derived from large data sets. Organizations such as AHRQ, the CDC, the National Institute for Child Health and Development, and the National Institutes of Health (NIH) have large national data sets from various sources, such as quality of life surveys, hospital discharge data, and infection control data. The data sets can be accessed or purchased to allow researchers to develop clinical, behavioral, or interventional outcome questions that can be statistically analyzed. The advantage of this kind of analysis is that the data sets are large enough to provide an adequate sample and effect size from which to generalize intervention effects. AHRQ also maintains a database of comparative effectiveness reviews that synthesizes information from the most current studies on numerous diseases through the Evidence-Based Practice Centers (AHRQ, 2015b).

In addition to aggregated evidence, clinical trial data, and comparative effectiveness reviews, some innovative healthcare systems are bringing "'practice-based evidence' to the bedside or work setting in aggregate form so that providers have the most up-to-date information available on outcomes before evidence based interventions are begun" (Lambert & Burlingame, 2009, p. 1). As an example, this kind of decision support has been trialed in the Mental Health Services Centers for the state of Utah. The state partnered with an outcomes measurement vendor (OQ, LLC) to provide aggregated evidence from clinical trials and laboratory research that resulted in a 5-minute self-report outcome measurement for patients in any setting—outpatient, inpatient, or residential. Adult patients use a handheld personal digital assistant, computer kiosk, or paper survey to report information to clinicians based on the domains of symptomatic distress, interpersonal relations, and functional ability. Adolescents and parent/guardians provide information on age-normed questionnaires. The scoring is derived from empirically tested software that alerts the provider that a patient is at risk for a less than optimal outcome from treatment and gives the care provider options for consideration using a clinical decision support tree. According to the designers, the advantage of this kind of tracking is that the system provides immediate evidence-based support for direct patient care. Furthermore, it provides a method for storing data for future review, evaluation, and benchmarking (Lambert & Burlingame, 2009). Recent studies by researchers such as Bischoff and Hinjosa (2015) and Garrett and Klein (2008) have shown that use and expansion of this kind of system to document and support advanced clinical practice and scholarship in public health and other settings "support[s] the application of current standards, and knowledge for clinical decision making" (Stroud, Erkel, & Smith, 2005).

Identifying Gaps in Evidence for Practice

In a systematic analysis of reviews published by the Joanna Briggs Institute between 1998 and 2002, high-quality evidence to support nursing interventions was not evident (Averis & Pearson, 2003). Further, the report identified considerable gaps in the evidence base available for nurses in relation to 22 discrete areas of practice that were examined in the analysis. Since the impetus to improve patient safety generated by the IOM reports *To Err Is Human* (Kohn, Corrigan, & Donaldson, 2000), *Crossing the Quality Chasm* (IOM, 2001), and *Health Professions Education: A Bridge to Quality* (IOM, 2003), significant gains have been made in the availability of support for EBP through educational restructuring and systems support. A literature search of recent articles in CINAHL produced some 70 nursing articles identifying synthesis articles, systematic reviews, and meta-analyses of nursing interventions, including those based on randomized controlled trials. Of those found, 70% were written within the last 10 years. However, when meta-analysis and "advanced practice" or "DNP" nursing interventions were added to the search terms, only five additional articles were found in PubMed and CINAHL that were actually systematic reviews or meta-analyses. Of those, two dealt with interventions related to nursing education. Therefore, considerable gaps in the evidence for practice remain.

Research by nurses and family physicians suggests that a translational model to fill the gaps is necessary (Armson et al., 2007; Gumei, Tiedje, & Oweis, 2007). One such model, developed in Canada, uses a small, self-formed group-discussion format within local communities. The impetus for this model was the need to stay competent in view of the vast amount of medical information currently available. In these groups, a facilitator guides physicians' discussion using sample patient cases and prepared modules on selected clinical topics. The group discussions have been ongoing for 15 years and have attracted international interest (Armson et al., 2007; Kelly, Cunningham, McCalister, Cassidy, & MacVicar, 2007). Nurses engage in similar forums in hospital grand rounds within their professional specialty organizations and at regional and national conferences. However, collaborative engagement needs to be broader and more systematic. DNPs are in an excellent position to initiate this kind of practice-based dialogue in community-based practice settings.

The AMA, the AACN, the NONPF, and other professional nursing organizations in each specialty all have agendas for advancing research and evidence for practice in their respective areas. As examples, the American Academy of Nurse Practitioners, Nurse Practitioner Associates for Continuing Education, and the Practicing Clinicians Exchange provide excellent forums for translating current research into practice and for networking with peers about research and clinical outcome information.

The Joint Commission, the National Database of Nursing Quality Indicators, and individual hospital report cards may be used as sources of research or outcome analysis to identify gaps in care delivery or in patient or staff education in particular institutions or practice groups. Examples include adverse events, smoking cessation, rates of adherence to best practice, blood glucose control, patient satisfaction rates, time spent with patients, tests ordered, and number of consultations (care related); knowledge, functional status, and access to care (patient related); and collaboration, technical quality, exam comprehensiveness, and adherence to guidelines (performance related) (Kleinpell, 2009). Within these and other categories, the gaps may be identified through the development of a specific plan based on target areas of APN practice. Planning questions should include the following: What exactly can be measured? How can it be measured? What will be done with the information? When should it be done? (Kleinpell, 2007, 2013). **Figure 3-7** shows a sample timeline for outcome assessment.

As advanced practice nursing continues to evolve into the DNP role, it will be imperative that direct care providers, senior-level nurse executives, and doctorally prepared nurse educators take lead roles in quality improvement to positively affect patient safety (O'Grady, 2008). Identifying, testing, and disseminating information about nurse-sensitive quality indicators is essential to close the gap in quality care delivery.

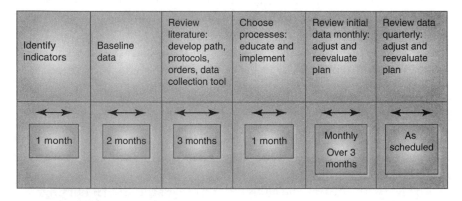

Figure 3-7 Timeline for Outcome Assessment for APN Practice

Modified from Kleinpell, R. M. (2007, May). APNs: Invisible champions. *Nursing Management*, 38(5), 18–22.

All APNs prepared at the clinical doctorate level must be involved in this effort.

Participation in Collaborative Research

It is a credit to the profession of nursing and its leaders that there are several EBP centers in the United States: the ANA National Center for Nursing Quality, Sigma Theta Tau International, the National Institute of Nursing Research at the NIH, and centers at many of the major university schools of nursing. However, as O'Grady (2008) noted, turf battles have limited collaboration. On the macro level, "APN organizations along with governmental and private research enterprise must come together to develop a research plan that identifies the most critical research questions" (O'Grady, 2008, p. 12). On the micro and macro levels, APNs individually and as a group must "demonstrate specific clinical performance and patient outcomes" (p. 12). This means "clearly distinguishing APNs in the context of interdisciplinary practice" (p. 12). Individual studies can demonstrate gaps in care in smaller samples, but the time has come for a more comprehensive and collaborative agenda for research that focuses on such issues as roles, function, outcomes, access improvements for vulnerable populations, interdisciplinary collaboration impacts, cost-effectiveness, safety, and other indicators. To discover gaps in care that are of concern to APNs/DNPs, nurses must have representatives from their ranks on research decision-making bodies. The AHRQ is positioned to take the lead in outcomes research, whereas the NIH focuses on biomedical aspects of disease management (O'Grady, 2008). To have their voices heard and their studies funded and disseminated, DNPs must use the power of their professional organizations and garner positions on national and international research collaboratives.

Participating in collaborative research is an excellent way for APNs to resolve clinical dilemmas and highlight their expertise through well-constructed questions that interest scientists and engage professional peers within and outside nursing. The dynamic nature of scientific evidence and the speed with which it is now possible to generate new knowledge through the use of technology demand that all care providers combine their expertise to interpret, plan, and evaluate the outcomes of interventions based on these new discoveries. Collaboration "implies collective action toward a common goal in a spirit of trust and harmony" (D'Amour, Ferrada-Videla, San Martin-Rodriguez, & Beaulieu, 2005, p. 116). Examples of interprofessional education programs to better integrate teaching, research, and professional activities among the healthcare and related disciplines are increasing. Some best practice models are those of the University of Washington School of Medicine (Seattle), Rosalind Franklin University of Medicine (North Chicago, Illinois), and the University of Florida (Gainesville) (Bridges, Davidson, Odegard, Maki, &Tomkowiak, 2011). The models incorporate didactic, community-based, and simulation experiences with interprofessional team-building and service learning in a variety of ways. Even within nursing, specialization demands collaboration between peers and patients to resolve complex clinical dilemmas if patients are to be treated holistically instead of as a collection of organ systems. In fact, as Nolan (2005) noted, patients must be included as "shapers of knowledge and action" (p. 503).

Nursing now has a body of knowledge, separate and unique from that of medicine, that provides the basis for unique contributions to science and to the care of individuals. At the same time, "nursing scholarship remains contextual and contingently situated" (Fairman, 2008, p. 10). Nurses have shown in practice that they are creative and capable of managing changing circumstances and dynamic cultural milieus, thus ensuring that APNs with both research and clinical skills are in a prime position to function as practice consultants in collaborative knowledge-generating research (AACN, 2006). This role is illustrated in the following example.

A DNP was a voluntary member of an advisory board of a suburban primary healthcare network that provided care to uninsured patients. The members of the board were very interested in ascertaining information about the effectiveness of the organization and its efforts to provide cost-effective, timely primary care. A question of particular interest was: Are emergency department visits decreased by offering this service? If they are, how much cost is actually saved? The DNP collaborated with the organization's administrator and developed an initial research question and a preliminary plan for presentation to a grant funding agency. The DNP researched the literature and took the preliminary plan to her institution's research group; with the help of a colleague from the college's health administration program, the DNP designed a study that was submitted to a grant funding agency specializing in grants to medical centers and community health agencies. The agency did not fund the grant that year. However, the following year, the original proposal was reframed as a cohort study, "Emergency Room Usage among Uninsured Patients with Access to a Primary Care Provider" (Tymkow, Shen, & MacMullen, 2006) and resubmitted as a subproject of a much larger NIH grant that was funded. A primary aim of the larger National Center on Minority Health and Health Disparities grant was to build capacity for research in healthcare disparities through mentoring by senior-level researchers (Samson, 2006). The DNP who was a mentee became the primary investigator and worked with two coinvestigators on this project.

In another example of collaborative research, Oman, Duran, and Fink (2008) described a collaborative EBP project to institute evidence-based policy and procedure development at the University of Colorado Hospital using the hospital's evidence-based multidisciplinary practice model. The model established the evidence base through valid and current research and through other forms of evidence or benchmark data, including cost-effectiveness analysis; pathophysiology; retrospective or concurrent chart review; quality improvement and risk data; international, national, and local standards; infection control data; patient preferences; and clinical expertise. The more sources that are added to the research core, the stronger the evidence. However, all sources are contributory to the evidence.

The Evidence-Based Practice Council used the levels of evidence of Stetler (1994) to guide the process of gathering evidence. As described by Oman et al. (2008), because there was nothing addressing policy and procedure in the literature, the members identified steps and created an algorithm to describe the process. Once developed, the algorithm was piloted on the units using six nurse champions, mentored by a researcher. The champions and researcher reviewed an orthostatic vital sign policy that was scheduled for update. After obtaining 12 research-based articles, eight clinical articles, one national guideline, and anecdotal recommendations, the group was divided into subgroups, and each person was assigned two reports to review using a standardized critique form. Each nurse was responsible for reading the articles, completing the critique form (with levels of evidence), and presenting the findings at a journal club. The policy being reviewed was checked for references and levels of evidence by the research scientist. A comparison of agreement between the policy author and reviewers was then determined, and the percentage of agreement between reviewer and author tabulated. Only clinically based policies were reviewed. This process is a good example of how collaboration between practice and education could be merged in any number of areas.

Whether collaboration involves clinical research or quality improvement, DNPs in clinical and leadership roles are key stakeholders in the process. As identified in the IOM report *Crossing the Quality Chasm* (IOM, 2001), communication and collaboration are requisites to the achievement of quality systems and patient outcomes. These skills are also a necessary part of a culture of collaboration that begins in educational programs and continues in the professional work setting. Collaborative efforts may include small unit-based or practice-based efforts or large system-wide initiatives. These efforts have been driven by consumer demand for excellence, accountability, and transparency in quality care, patient safety, and patient satisfaction (Freshman, Rubino, & Chassiakos, 2010). In any collaborative initiative, three levels of expertise are required: system leadership, including the authority to implement change; clinical technical expertise (guidance and know-how); and day-to-day leadership (details of the system) (Baker, Reising, Johnson, Stewart, & Baker, 1997, as cited in Freshman et al., 2010).

Disseminating Findings from Evidence-Based Practice

A primary reason for disseminating research is to use the findings to improve practice and health outcomes. Communicating the results of research and EBP trials is the culminating step of the research and research utilization processes. It is one of *the* most important steps in research and the application of research in practice because it is the communication of research findings that provides the basis for meaningful critique, development of new questions, and testing of research evidence in practice (Lyder & Fain, 2009).

The methods used to communicate evidence from practice trials are similar to those used for communicating research findings: journal publications, podium or poster presentations, Internet webinar sessions, media communications, journal clubs, and community presentations. However, the forums for dissemination may be broader because the audience of interest may be more diverse, including those with practice, research, and community development interests. In addition, the choice of method for communicating information depends on a number of important factors. For example, a journal publication may be personally advantageous to the author, but the time from submission to actual publication and dissemination may delay utilization of important evidence-based treatments in practice. Oral reports at national conferences may facilitate timelier dissemination. Webinars may be the fastest way to disseminate information but may not reach all the desired audiences. Journal clubs are useful forums for discussions of research findings in academic settings. Reports of community-based studies to advisory boards or media venues may also become the basis for further research and political support that help nonprofit and other community organizations. Nevertheless, because theory, research, and practice must be constantly intertwined, the circular and reciprocal relationship among these elements must be apparent regardless of where the research is presented (McEwen & Wills, 2014).

Preparing a Journal Publication

Preparing a journal article for publication is time consuming and at times tedious, but the rewards of feeling that you have made a contribution and seeing your work in print are worth the effort. Once the topic for an article has been established, the next step is selecting the journal. Peer-reviewed journals have the most rigorous review criteria. Therefore, publication in one of these journals is considered to be more credible. The actual content will be determined by the editorial guidelines of the journal, which may be found in the "Information for Authors" section of the journal. In most cases, the guidelines may also be obtained from the journal's website. Generally, the submission requirements cover technical details such as page length, margins, font style and size, reference format, use of graphics and figures, and method of submission. It is very important to follow the submission requirements because many journals will not review articles that are not submitted in the correct format.

Once submitted, articles in peer-reviewed journals are blind (anonymously) reviewed by several reviewers. It is not uncommon for the review process to last several weeks or months; articles may be rejected, accepted with revisions, or accepted. It is common to have articles returned for revision. The key to success is to be persistent, correct those things that can be corrected, give an explanation for those that cannot, and return the submission in the agreed-on time frame.

Preparing a Research Presentation

Regardless of where or how evidence is reported, the essential element is that it combines the knowledge and values of the study patients or population with practitioner expertise and the best in available and current research evidence. Reporting evidence also requires knowledge of the audience and their needs. Specifically, the presenter must ask: What is the specific content to be addressed? How will the audience use the information? What is the knowledge level of those who are to receive the information? What is the time allowed for the presentation? What audiovisual resources are available for the presentation? Once these questions

Table 3-14 Outline for Research Presentation
I. Introduction
II. Purpose of the study
III. Theoretical framework
IV. Hypothesis
V. Design
A. What kind of study
B. Intervention
C. Sample
1. Population
2. Inclusion/exclusion criteria
D. Instruments
VI. Analysis
A. Method
B. Types of statistical tests used
VII. Findings
VIII. Discussion
IX. Implications
A. Research
B. Clinical practice

have been answered, specific learning objectives should be developed in order to guide and organize the presentation.

An outline for presentation of research study findings is shown in **Table 3-14**. Important points of each aspect of the study can be displayed in a PowerPoint presentation to help keep the presentation within the designated time frame and allow the audience to stay focused on the important elements. Some useful websites for building PowerPoint presentations are listed in **Table 3-15**.

Preparing a Poster Presentation

Disseminating information from scholarship—original research, practice innovations, clinical projects—through poster presentations has become an accepted medium for the exchange of ideas in a more personal and less formal environment than the podium presentation.

Table 3-15 Resources and Websites for Developing Multimedia and PowerPoint Presentations

PosterPresentations.com (Scientific Template)	http://www.posterpresentations.com
Indiana University-Purdue University, Indianapolis, Center for Teaching and Learning	http://ctl.iupui.edu/Resources/ Documenting-Your-Teaching/ Resources-for-Poster-Presentations
Michigan State University, Office of Faculty and Organizational Development, Poster Presentations	http://fod.msu.edu/oir/ poster-presentations
University of Texas Health Science Center, Learn about poster presentations	http://library.uthscsa.edu/2011/12/ poster-presentations/
University of North Carolina, Academic Poster Presentations	http://gradschool.unc.edu/academics/ resources/postertips.html

It is both efficient and effective. Presenters and participants have the freedom to engage in a dialogue that allows for education, clarification, and networking. Posters also allow for the formatting of data in creative ways. As Berg (2005) noted, "imagery can be substituted for words and this is a powerful way to convey information" (p. 245). Like any presentation, posters require preparation. The following steps are essential.

Plan Ahead

A good poster presentation takes considerable time. The planning stage is a most important step. In this stage, considerable thought should be given to the message you are trying to convey. What is the purpose? The format for a research presentation will be different from that of a practice innovation. Is the conference only for nurses, only for APNs, or for a multidisciplinary audience? How much background information or detail do you need to include? Is the audience generally familiar with the topic? If they are, do not include familiar details, but if they are not, do not make the information so specific that those who are not familiar with the topic will be put off. Avoid using abbreviations that only a select audience will understand.

These and other considerations specific to the venue should be addressed during the planning stage (Berg, 2005; Hardicre, Devitt, & Coad, 2007).

Decide on Layout and Format

A good poster presentation is focused on a single message, uses graphics to tell the story, and is orderly with an obvious sequence (Hess, Tosney, & Liegel, 2013). Most people read top to bottom, left to right. This is the usual sequence for poster layout. Generally, the layout for a research poster presentation is as follows: title, abstract, introduction, methods, results, discussion, and acknowledgments. If the presentation is a practice innovation, the layout will be different. The innovation is usually in the center, with explanatory text at the periphery or below the diagram or explanation of the protocol or change (Hardicre et al., 2007). References are also included, as in the research poster. The poster should be easy to read from a distance of 4 to 6 feet (Halligan, 2005; Hess et al., 2013). Section heads should be at least 40 pt and supporting text 32 pt (Halligan, 2005, p. 49). Titles should be short, with letters 2 to 3 inches high (Berg, 2005).

Determine the Content

If the purpose of the poster is to display a research project, it will not be the same as one designed to describe a clinical innovation. The content of the research poster should follow the format established by the conference guidelines. If the study is funded by an outside or government agency, some grant-funded studies require specific wording of the acknowledgment; this should be determined during the poster planning. If an abstract is required, it should include the main purpose of the study, be clearly worded, and be succinct. A key component is to keep it simple because posters "show," they do not "tell" (Miracle, 2008).

Clinical project content will vary according to the specific topic and scope. The title for either a research study or clinical innovation should be creative, but, most important, it should accurately reflect the content of the project. The title banner should also include authors and affiliations in order of authorship and/or contribution to the effort. In many instances, the organization's logo will be included as well (Hardicre et al., 2007).

Prepare a Brief Presentation

"The poster is a story board of information" (Jackson & Sheldon, 1998, as cited in Hardicre et al., 2007, p. 398). However, it also gives the presenters an opportunity to present themselves. As with any kind of communication, you want to convey confidence and knowledge. Preparing a short presentation script or handouts for participants allows you to organize your thoughts and prepare for possible questions. The handouts are always welcomed by participants, who are inundated with information during a conference. Be sure to include your name and contact number or attach a business card so that participants may contact you with questions. This is a very effective networking tool (Miracle, 2008).

Media Communications

Communicating with large audiences is often facilitated through professional media communications. This kind of communication is essential when there is a major event or change, such as a policy to be initiated. It is usually best to engage the resources of a professional organization to make the preliminary contact and to aid in constructing the message.

Journal Club Presentations

Another way to facilitate the communication of evidence-based research is through journal club presentations. Journal clubs are not new, especially in academic and many professional settings. However, using them to facilitate EBP is a more recent development, especially as a forum for clinical guideline development (Kirchoff & Beck, 1995, as cited in McQueen, Miller, Nivison, & Husband, 2006). In a small survey study of the use of journal clubs to determine changes in practice, McQueen et al. (2006) found that journal clubs were effective in "1) focusing staff on clinical evidence in discussions, 2) increasing confidence as they became more aware of evidence, and 3) bridging the evidence-practice gap" (p. 315).

Additionally, with the aid of the Internet, evidence-based articles or studies can be posted in advance and facilitated online, thus increasing the possibility of wider participation. In one pilot study of this format, nurses in New Zealand branded the journal club's website and the articles for discussion. An article is posted for one month and removed on the Friday before the following month's posting (Trim, 2008). **Table 3-16** presents an outline of a journal club.

Whether live or Internet based, journal clubs provide a mechanism for promoting professional debate, increasing confidence, and, most important, improving practice and quality care (Sheratt, 2005, as cited in McQueen et al., 2006). With their educational background and advanced skills, DNPs are in an excellent position to implement this kind of strategy in a collaborative, interdisciplinary format.

Table 3-16 Online Journal Club

Outline of the Journal Club

1. A specific clinical question is chosen.

2. All evidence-based literature related to the question is derived from online databases.

3. A reference list of all literature for review is generated.

4. High-level-evidence, randomized controlled trials, and systematic reviews are critiqued and given more weight than quasi-experimental case studies and opinions.

5. Participants critically appraise the relevant literature before attending the journal club.

6. Journal club discussions center on the critical appraisal of evidence found for clinical interventions.

7. Implications for practice and further research are discussed, with key findings recorded in minutes.

8. A resource folder that includes a reference list of resource critiques, guidelines for practice, treatment resources, standardized assessments, disease management strategies, and gaps in evidence is created.

9. A system for ongoing evaluation of outcomes and changes in practice is developed and communicated.

Modified from McQueen, J., Miller, C., Nivison, C., & Husband, V. (2006). An investigation into the use of a journal club for evidence-based practice. *International Journal of Therapy and Rehabilitation, 13*(7), 313. Modified with permission.

Summary

Scholarship and EBP are not the same, but each has elements that support the other. Scholarship involves research and application, as does EBP. Whereas scholarship may be a joint or singular effort, EBP requires teamwork and collaboration. The outcome of scholarship is a scholarly product, a new way of thinking, or a change in awareness about a subject or phenomenon—an end in itself. EBP is based on the scholarship of research and evidence gathering and synthesis. It is a means for improving care for patients or effecting a change in a system that results in better care for patients, providers, and communities. It is a transformation of knowledge to new levels of understanding and integration. Changing to a model of EBP does not just happen; it requires the integration of a number of skills, such as the use of good research and the synthesis of best information and other "evidences," including patient choice and professional expertise. Dissemination of information gleaned from synthesis and translation in practice is essential for successful change. Using the knowledge of research methods to discover and interpret the best evidence for practice gives the DNP the tools to transform care.

References

Abrahamson, K. A., Fox, R. L., & Doebbeling, B. N. (2012). Facilitators and barriers to clinical practice guideline use among nurses. *American Journal of Nursing, 112*(7), 26–36.

Adib-Hajbaghery, M. (2007). Factors facilitating and inhibiting evidence-based practice in Iran. *Journal of Advanced Nursing, 58*(6), 566–575.

Agency for Healthcare Research and Quality. (2002). *Systems to rate the strength of scientific evidence: Summary* (Technical Report No. 47). Retrieved from http://www.ahrq.gov

Agency for Healthcare Research and Quality. (2013). *Module 7. Measuring and benchmarking clinical performance.* Retrieved from http://www.ahrq.gov/professionals/prevention-chronic-care/improve/system/pfhandbook/mod7.html

Agency for Healthcare Research and Quality. (2015b). *The SHARE approach.* http://www.ahrq.gov/professionals/education/curriculum-tools/shareddecisionmaking/

AGREE Collaboration. (2001). *AGREE instrument.* Retrieved from http://www.agreetrust.org/?o=1085

Alimohammadi, N., Taleghani, F., Mohammadi, E., & Akbarian, R. (2014). The nursing metaparadigm concept of human being in Islamic thought. *Nursing Inquiry, 21*(2), 121–129. Advance online publication. Retrieved from http://www.ncbi.nlm.nih.gov/pubmed/23786534

Allen, M. (1996). *Celebrating nursing history: What to keep.* Retrieved from http://nahrs.mlanet.org/home/resources

American Association of Colleges of Nursing. (1999). *Defining scholarship for the discipline of nursing.* Retrieved from http://www.aacn.nche.edu/Publications/positions/scholar.htm

American Association of Colleges of Nursing. (2006). *The essentials of doctoral education for advanced nursing practice.* Retrieved from http://www.aacn.nche.edu/DNP/pdf/Essentials.pdf

American Association of Colleges of Nursing. (2015). *New AACN data confirm enrollment surge in schools of nursing.* Retrieved from http://www.aacn.nche.edu/news/articles/2015/enrollment

American Nurses Association. (2015). John Hopkins Nursing evidence-based practice. *Nursing World.* Retrieved from http://www.nursingworld.org/Research-toolkit/Johns-Hopkins-Nursing-Evidence-Based-Practice

American Nurses Credentialing Center. (2005). *Magnet Recognition Program overview.* Retrieved from http://www.medscape.com/partners/ancc/public/ancc

Annells, M. (1996). Grounded theory method: Philosophical perspectives, paradigms of inquiry, and postmodernism. *Qualitative Health Research, 6*(3), 379–393.

Armson, H., Kinzie, S., Hawes, D., Roder, S., Wakefield, J., & Elmslie, T. (2007). Translating learning into practice. *Canadian Family Physician, 53*(9), 1477–1485.

Arthur, R., Marfell, J., & Ulrich, S. (2009). Outcomes measurement in nurse-midwifery practice. In R. M. Kleinpell (Ed.), *Outcome assessment in advanced practice nursing* (2nd ed., pp. 229–255). New York, NY: Springer.

Asch, S. M., Baker, D. W., Keesey, J., Broder, M., Schonlau, M., Rosen, M., & Keeler, E. B. (2005). Does the collaborative model improve care for chronic heart failure? *Medical Care, 43*(7), 667–675.

Averis, A., & Pearson, A. (2003). Filling the gaps: Identifying nursing research priorities through the analysis of completed systematic reviews. *JBI Reports, 1*(3), 49–126.

Bailey, D. (2012). *From clinical to academia: The lived experience of the advanced practice nurse's transition to nurse educator* (Unpublished doctoral dissertation). Capella University.

Baker, C. M., Reising, D. L., Johnson, D. R., Stewart, R. L., & Baker, S. D. (1997). Organizational effectiveness: Toward an integrated model for schools of nursing. *Journal of Professional Nursing, 13*(4), 246–255.

Barnes, D. M. (1996). An analysis of the grounded theory method and the concept of culture. *Qualitative Health Research, 6*(3), 429–441.

Batalden, P. B., Nelson, E. C., & Roberts, J. S. (1994). Linking outcome measurements to continual improvement: The serial "V" way of thinking about improving clinical care. *Journal of Quality Improvement, 20*(4), 167–180.

Batalden, P. B., & Stoltz, P. K. (1993). A framework for the continual improvement of healthcare: Building and applying professional and improvement knowledge to test changes in daily work. *Joint Commission Journal of Quality Improvement, 19*(10), 424–447.

Berg, J. A. (2005). Creating a professional poster presentation: Focus on nurse practitioners. *Journal of the American Academy of Nurse Practitioners, 17*(7), 245–248.

Bias. (2003). In *Funk & Wagnall's new international dictionary of the English language* (Comprehensive millennium ed.). Chicago, IL: Ferguson.

Bickerton, J., Procter, S., Johnson, B., & Medina, A. (2011). Socio-phenomenology and conversation analysis: Interpreting video lifeworld healthcare interactions. *Nursing Philosophy, 12*(4), 271–281.

Bischoff, W. R., & Hinjosa, R. H. (2015). A descriptive study of point-of-care reference resource use by advanced practice RNs in Texas. *CIN: Computers, Informatics, Nursing, 33*(Suppl. Topical Collection), TC 23–31.

Boyer, E. L. (1990). Scholarship reconsidered: Priorities of the professoriate. The Carnegie Foundation for the Advancement of Teaching. San Francisco, CA: Jossey-Bass.

Boyer, E. L. (1997). Scholarship reconsidered: Priorities of the professoriate (Rev. ed.). The Carnegie Foundation for the Advancement of Teaching. San Francisco, CA: Jossey-Bass.

Bridges, D. R., Davidson, R. A., Odegard, P. S., Maki, I. V., & Tomkowiak, J. (2011). Interprofessional collaboration: Three best practice models of interprofessional education. *Medical Education Online, 16.* doi:10.3402.meo.v.16i0.6035

Broome, M. E., Riner, M. E., & Allam, E. S. (2013). Scholarly publication practices of doctor of nursing practice-prepared nurses. *Journal of Nursing Education, 52*(8), 429–434.

Brown, S. J. (2005). Direct clinical practice. In A. B. Hamric, J. A. Spross, & C. M. Hanson (Eds.), *Advanced practice nursing: An integrative approach* (3rd ed., pp. 143–185). Philadelphia, PA: W. B. Saunders.

Bundy, E. Y., & Murphy, L. S. (2014). Improving provider compliance in the use of an asthma action plan for patients with asthma in an outpatient setting. *Clinical Scholars Review, 7*(2), 128–142.

Burns, N., & Grove, S. K. (2009). *The practice of nursing research, appraisal, synthesis, and generation of evidence* (6th ed.). St. Louis, MO: Elsevier Saunders.

Burns, S. (2009). Methods of outcome assessment. In R. M. Kleinpell (Ed.), *Outcome assessment in advanced practice nursing* (2nd ed., pp. 73–90). New York, NY: Springer.

Carey, M., Buchan, H., & Sanson-Fisher, R. (2009). The cycle of change: Implementing the best-evidence clinical practice. *International Journal for Quality in Health Care, 21*(1), 37–43. Retrieved from http:www//medscape.com/viewarticle/587379

Carnegie Foundation for the Advancement of Teaching. (1996). *Ernest L. Boyer.* 91st annual report of the Carnegie Foundation for the Advancement of Teaching. Princeton, NJ: Author.

Celik, H., Lagro-Janssen, T. A., Widdershoven, G. G., & Abma, T. A. (2011). Bringing gender sensitivity into healthcare practice: A systematic review. *Patient Education and Counseling, 84*(2), 143–149.

Cochrane Collaboration. (2004). *Cochrane reviewers' handbook.* London, England: The Cochrane Group.

Coe, R. (2002, September). *It's the effect size, stupid: What effect size is and why it is so important.* Paper presented at the annual conference of the British Educational Research Association, University of Exeter, England.

Collins, P. M., Golembeski, S. M., Selgas, M., Sparger, K., Burke, N., & Vaughn, B. B. (2008, January 25). Clinical excellence through evidence-based practice: A model to guide practice changes. *Topics in Advanced Practice E-Journal.* Retrieved from http://www.medscape.com

Conger, M. M., & Plager, K. A. (2008). Advanced nursing practice in rural areas: Connectedness versus disconnectedness. *Online Journal of Rural Nursing and Healthcare, 8*(1), 24–38.

Cooke, L., Smith-Idell, C., Dean, G., Gemmill, R., Steingass, S., Sun, V., . . . Borneman, T. (2004). "Research to practice": A practical program to enhance the use of evidence-based practice at the unit level. *Oncology Nursing Forum, 31*(4), 825–832.

Craft-Rosenburg, M., Krajicek, M. J., & Shin, D. (2002). Report of the American Academy of Nursing Child-Family Expert Panel: Identification of quality and outcome indicators for maternal child nursing. *Nursing Outlook, 50*(2), 57–60.

Crotty, M. (1996). *Phenomenology and nursing research.* Melbourne, Australia: Churchill Livingstone.

D'Amour, D., Ferrada-Videla, M., San Martin-Rodriguez, L., & Beaulieu, M. D. (2005). The conceptual basis for interprofessional collaboration: Core concepts and theoretical frameworks. *Journal of Interprofessional Care, 19*(Suppl. 1), 116–131.

Dearholt, S., & Dang, D. (2012). *Johns Hopkins Nursing evidence-based practice: Model and guidelines.* Honor Society of Nursing, Sigma Theta Tau. Nursing Knowledge International RNL. Retrieved from http://www.reflectionsonnurs ingleadearship.org

Decker, S., & Iphofen, R. (2005). Developing the profession of radiography: Making uses of oral history. *Radiography, 11*(4), 262–271.

Deming, E. W. (1986). *Out of crisis.* Cambridge, MA: MIT Press.

DePalma, J. A., & McGuire, D. B. (2005). Research. In A. B. Hamric, J. A. Spross, & C. Mittenson (Eds.), *Advanced nursing practice: An integrative approach* (3rd ed., pp. 217–249). Philadelphia, PA: Elsevier Saunders.

Diaz-Granados, N., Pitzul, K. B., Dorado, L. M., Wang, F., McDermott, S., Rondon, M. B., & Stewart, D. E. (2011). Monitoring gender equity in health using gender-sensitive indicators: A cross-national study. *Journal of Women's Health, 20*(1), 145–153.

DiCenso, A., Cullum, N., & Ciliska, D. (1998). Implementing evidence-based nursing: Some misconceptions. *Evidence-Based Nursing, 1*(2), 38–39.

Doran, D. M., & Sidani, S. (2007). Outcomes-focused knowledge translation: A framework for knowledge translation and patient outcomes improvement. *Worldviews on Evidence-Based Nursing, 4*(1), 3–13.

Dorn, K. (2004). Caring-healing inquiry for holistic nursing practice: Model for research and evidence based practice. *Topics in Advanced Practice Nursing E-Journal, 4*(4). Retrieved from http://www.medscape.com/viewarticle /496363

Doumitt, G., Gattelliari, M., Grimshaw, J., & O'Brien, M. A. (2007). Local opinion leaders: Effects on professional practice and healthcare outcomes. *Cochrane Database Systematic Review, 4,* Art. No. CD000125. doi:10.1002/14651858. CD000125.pub3

Dreher, M. (1999). Clinical scholarship: Nursing practice as an intellectual endeavor. In Sigma Theta Tau International Clinical Scholarship Task Force, *Clinical scholarship resource paper* (pp. 26–33). Retrieved from http://www. nursingsociety.org/aboutus/PositionPapers/Documents/clinical_scholarship_paper.pdf

Duignan, P. (2006). *Outcomes model standards for systematic outcome analysis.* Retrieved from http://www.parkerduignan.com/oiiwa/toolkit/standards1.html

Dunlop, W. L., & Beauchamp, M. R. (2011). En-gendering choice: Preferences for exercising in gender-integrated and gender-segregated groups and consideration of overweight status. *International Journal of Behavioral Medicine, 18,* 216–220. doi:10.1007/s12529-010-9125-6

Durieux, P., Nizard, R., Ravaud, P., Mounier, N., & Lepage, E. (2000). A clinical decision support system for prevention of venous thromboembolism: Effect on physician behavior. *Journal of the American Medical Association, 283*(21), 2816–2821.

Edwards, S. D. (2001). *Philosophy of nursing: An introduction.* New York, NY: Palgrave.

Fackler, C. A., Chambers, A. N., & Bourbonniere, M. (2015). Hospital nurses' lived experience of power. *Journal of Nursing Scholarship, 47*(3), 267–274.

Fain, J. A. (2009). *Reading, understanding, and applying nursing research* (3rd ed.). Philadelphia, PA: F. A. Davis.

Fain, J. A. (2013). *Reading, understanding, and applying nursing research* (4th ed.). Philadelphia, PA: F. A. Davis.

Fairman, J. (2008). Context and contingency in the history of post-World War II scholarship in the United States. *Journal of Nursing Scholarship, 40*(1), 4–11.

Fawcett, J., & Garrity, J. (2009). *Evaluating research for evidence-based nursing practice.* Philadelphia, PA: F. A. Davis.

Fawcett, J., Watson, J., Neuman, B., Hinton Walker, P., & Fitzpatrick, J. (2001). On nursing theories and evidence. *Journal of Nursing Scholarship, 33*(2), 115–119.

Fishbein, I., & Ajzen, M. (1980). *Understanding attitudes and predicting social behavior.* Englewood Cliffs, NJ: Prentice Hall.

Fitzpatrick, M. L., & Munhall, P. L. (2001). Historical research: The method. In P. L. Munhall (Ed.), *Nursing research: A qualitative perspective* (3rd ed., pp. 403–416). Sudbury, MA: Jones and Bartlett.

French, P. (1999). The development of evidence-based nursing. *Journal of Advanced Nursing, 29*(1), 72–78.

Freshman, B., Rubino, L., & Chassiakos, Y. R. (2010). *Collaboration across the disciplines in health care.* Sudbury, MA: Jones and Bartlett.

Gagan, M., & Hewitt-Taylor, J. (2004). The issues involved in implementing evidence based practice. *British Journal of Nursing, 13*(20), 1216–1220.

Gallagher, R. M. (2009). Participation of the advanced practice nurse in managed care and quality initiatives. In L. A. Joel (Ed.), *Advanced practice nursing: Essentials of role development* (2nd ed., pp. 172–190). Philadelphia, PA: F. A. Davis.

Garrett, B., & Klein, G. (2008). Value of wireless personal digital assistants for practice: Perceptions of advanced practice nurses. *Journal of Clinical Nursing, 17*, 2146–2154.

Gelb, K., Pederson, A., & Greaves, L. (2011). How have health promotion frameworks considered gender? *Health Promotion International, 27*(4), 445–452.

Giddens, A. (1982). *Profiles and critiques in social theory.* London, England: Macmillan.

Gifford, W., Davies, B., Edwards, N., Griffin, P., & Lybanon, V. (2007). Managerial leadership for nurses' use of research evidence: An integrative review of the literature. *World Views on Evidence Based Practice, 4*(3), 126–145.

Giorgi, A. (2000). Concerning the application of phenomenology to caring research. *Scandinavian Journal of Caring Science, 14*(1), 11–15.

Glanville, I., Schirm, V., & Wineman, N. M. (2000). Using evidence-based practice for managing clinical outcomes in advanced practice nursing. *Journal of Nursing Care Quality, 15*(1), 1–11.

Glaser, B. G., & Strauss, A. (1967). *The discovery of grounded theory.* Chicago, IL: Aldine.

Goolsby, M. J., Klardie, K. A., Johnson, J., McNaughton, M. A., & Meyers, W. (2004). Integrating the principles of evidence-based practice into clinical practice. *Journal of the American Academy of Nurse Practitioners, 16*(3), 98–105.

Goolsby, M. J., Meyers, W. C., Johnson, J. A., Klardie, K., & McNaughton, M. A. (2004). Integrating the principles of evidence-based practice: Prognosis and the metabolic syndrome. *Journal of the American Academy of Nurse Practitioners, 16*(5), 178–186.

Graham, W. A., Graham, I. D., & Davies, B. L. (2013). Multi-level barriers to promote guideline based nursing care: A leadership strategy for home health care. *Journal of Nursing Management, 21,* 762–770.

Graling, P. R. (2011). Designing an applied model of perioperative patient safety. *Clinical Scholars Review, 4*(2), 104–114. http://dx.doi.org/10-1891/1939-2095.4.2.104

Griffieon, M., & Halsey, N. (2014). Gender differences in immediate hypersensitivity reactions to vaccines: A review of the literature. *Public Health Nursing, 31*(3), 206–214.

Griffin-Sobel, J. P. (2003). Evaluating an instrument for research. *Gastroenterology Nursing, 26*(3), 135–136.

Grol, R., Dalhuijsen, J., Thomas, S., Veld, C., Rutten, G., & Mokkink, H. (1998). Attributes of clinical guidelines that influence use of guidelines in general practice: Observational study. *British Medical Journal, 317*(7162), 858–861.

Grove, S. K., Burns, N., & Gray, J. R. (2013). *The practice of nursing research: Appraisal, synthesis, and generation of evidence* (7th ed.). St. Louis, MO: Elsevier Saunders.

Gumei, M. K., Tiedje, L. B., & Oweis, A. (2007). Vaginal or cesarean birth: Toward evidence based practice. *American Journal of Maternal Child Nursing, 32*(6), 388.

Hallett, C. (1995). Understanding the phenomenological approach to research. *Nurse Researcher, 3*(2), 55–56.

Halligan, P. (2005). Poster perfect. *World of Irish Nursing and Midwifery, 13*(8), 49.

Hammersley, M. (1989). *The dilemma of qualitative method.* London, England: Routledge.

Hande, K. A. (2013). Measuring endoscopic performance for colorectal cancer prevention: Quality improvement in a gastroenterology practice. *Nursing Clinics of North America, 49,* 15–27. doi:10.1014.j.c.nur

Handley, M., MacGregor, K., Schillinger, D., Sharifi, C., Wong, S., & Bodenheimer, T. (2006). Using action plans to help primary care patients adopt healthy behaviors: A descriptive study. *Journal of the American Board of Family Medicine, 19*(3), 224–231.

Hardicre, J., Devitt, P., & Coad, J. (2007). Ten steps to successful poster presentation. *British Journal of Nursing, 16*(7), 398–401.

Hawkins, R. C., & Clement, P. F. (1984). Binge eating: Measurement problems and a conceptual model. In R. E. Hawkins, W. J. Fremouw, & P. F. Clement (Eds.), *The binge-purge syndrome: Diagnosis, treatment, and research* (pp. 229–251). New York, NY: Springer.

Hess, G., Tosney, K., & Liegel, L. (2013). *Creating effective poster presentations.* Retrieved from http://www.ncsu.edu/project/posters/

Hinkel, J. M., Vandergift, J. L., Perkel, S. J., Waldinger, M. B., Levy, W., & Stewart, F. M. (2010). Practices and productivity of physician assistants and nurse practitioners in outpatient oncology clinics at national comprehensive cancer network institutions. *Journal of Oncology Practice, 6*(4), 182–187.

Hodge, M. B., Asch, S. M., Olson, V. A., Kravitz, R. L., & Sauve, M. J. (2002). Developing indicators of nursing quality to evaluate nurse staffing ratios. *Journal of Nursing Administration, 32*(6), 338–345.

Holleman, G., Eliens, A., van Vliet, M., & van Acterburg, T. (2006). Promotion of evidence based practice by professional nursing associations: Literature review. *Journal of Advanced Nursing, 53*(6), 702–709.

Horsely, J. A., Crane, J., & Bingle, J. D. (1978). Research utilization as an organizational process. *Journal of Nursing Administration, 8*(7), 4–6.

Imberg, W. C. (2008). *The meaning of U.S. childbirth for Mexican immigrant women* (Doctoral dissertation). Available from ProQuest Dissertations and Theses database. (UMI No. 3318193)

Ingersoll, G. (2005). Generating evidence through outcomes management. In B. M. Melnyk & E. Fineout-Overholt (Eds.), *Evidence-based practice in nursing and healthcare: A guide to best practice* (pp. 299–332). Philadelphia, PA: Lippincott Williams & Wilkins.

Ingersoll, G. L., McIntosh, E., & Williams, M. (2000). Nurse sensitive outcomes of advanced practice. *Journal of Advanced Nursing, 32*(5), 1272–1281.

Institute of Medicine. (2001). *Crossing the quality chasm: A new health system for the 21st century.* Washington, DC: National Academies Press.

Institute of Medicine. (2003). *Health professions education: A bridge to quality.* Washington, DC: National Academies Press.

International Development Research Center. (2009). *Confounding.* Retrieved from http://www.idrc.ca/EN/Resources/Publications/Pages/default.aspx

Israni, R. K. (2007). Guide to biostatistics. *MedPage Today.* Retrieved from http://www.medpagetoday.com/lib/content/Medpage-Guide-to-Biostatistics.pdf

Jackson, K. I., & Sheldon, J. M. (1998). Poster presentation: How to tell a story. *Pediatric Nurse, 10*(9), 36–37.

Jamtvedt, G., Young, J. M., Kristofferson, D. T., O'Brien, M. A., & Oxman, A. D. (2006). Audit and feedback: Effects on professional practice and healthcare outcomes. *Cochrane Database of Systematic Reviews, 2,* CD000259.

Johns Hopkins Center for Health Services and Outcomes Research. (2012). Retrieved from http://www.jhsph.edu

The Joint Commission. (2009). *Universal protocol.* Retrieved from http://www.jointcommission.org/standards_information/up.aspx

Kelly, D. R., Cunningham, D. E., McCalister, P., Cassidy, J., & MacVicar, R. (2007). Applying evidence in practice through small group learning: A qualitative exploration of success. *Quality in Primary Care, 15*(2), 93–99.

Kirchoff, K., & Beck, S. (1995). Using the journal club as a component of the research utilization process. *Heart and Lung: The Journal of Acute and Critical Care, 24*(3), 246–250.

Kitson, A., Harvey, G., & McCormack, B. (1998). Enabling the implementation of evidence-based practice: A conceptual framework. *Quality in Healthcare, 7*(3), 149–158.

Kitson, A., Rycroft-Malone, T., Harvey, G., McCormack, B., Seers, K., & Titchen, A. (2008). Evaluating the successful implementation of evidence into practice using the PARIHS framework: Theoretical and practical challenges. *Implementation Science, 3*(1), 1–21.

Kleinpell, R. M. (2007). APNs: Invisible champions? *Nursing Management, 38*(5), 18–22.

Kleinpell, R. M. (2009). Measuring outcomes in advanced nursing practice. In R. M. Kleinpell (Ed.), *Outcome assessment in advanced nursing practice* (2nd ed., pp. 1–63). New York, NY: Springer.

Kleinpell, R. M. (2013). *Outcome assessment in advanced practice nursing* (3rd ed.). New York, NY: Springer.

Kohn, L. T., Corrigan, J. M., & Donaldson, M. S. (2000). *To err is human: Building a safer health system.* A report of the Committee on Quality of Health Care in America, Institute of Medicine. Washington, DC: National Academies Press.

Kovarsky, D. (2008). Representing voices from the life-world in evidence-based practice. *International Journal of Language and Communication Disorders, 43*(S1), 47–57.

Krebbeks, V. P., & Cunningham, V. M. (2013). A DNP managed hepatitis C clinic: Improving quality of life for those in a rural area. *Online Journal of Rural Nursing and Health, 13*(1). Retrieved from http://rnojournal.binghamton.edu

Lambert, M. J., & Burlingame, G. M. (2009). Measuring outcomes in the state of Utah: Practice based evidence. *Behavioral Healthcare, 27*, 16–20. Retrieved from http://www.behavioral.net

Lanthier, E. (2002). *Correlation samples.* Retrieved from http://www.nvcc.edu/home/elanthier/methods/correlation-samples.htm

Lauffenburger, J. C., Robinson, J. G., Oramasionwu, C., & Fang, G. (2014). Racial/ethnic gender gaps in the use of and adherence to evidence-based preventive therapies among elderly Medicare Part D beneficiaries after acute myocardial infarction. *Circulation, 129*(7), 754–763.

Leedy, P. D., & Ormrod, J. E. (2010). *Practical research: Planning and design.* Boston, MA: Pearson.

Library of Congress. (n.d.). *American memory collection.* Retrieved from http://memory.loc.gov/ammem/index.html

Libster, M. M., & McNeil, B. A. (2009). *Enlightened charity.* Farmville, NC: Golden Apple.

Long, C. O. (2015). Weighing in on the evidence. In N. A. Schmidt & J. M. Brown (Eds.), *Evidence-based practice for nurses: Appraisal and application of research* (3rd ed., pp. 417–432). Burlington, MA: Jones & Bartlett Learning.

Lopez-Bushnell, K. (2002). Get research-ready. *Nursing Management, 33*(11), 41–44.

Lowell, J. R. (n.d.). *Scholarship.* Retrieved from http://quotationsbook.com/quote/22196

Lyder, C., & Fain, J. A. (2009). Interpreting and reporting research findings. In J. A. Fain (Ed.), *Reading, understanding, and applying research* (3rd ed., pp. 233–250). Philadelphia, PA: F. A. Davis.

Maggs-Rapport, F. (2001). "Best research practice": In pursuit of methodological rigour. *Journal of Advanced Nursing, 35*(3), 373–383.

Marineau, M. L. (2005). *Exploring the lived experience of individuals with acute infections transitioning in the home with support by an advanced practice nurse using telehealth* (Unpublished doctoral dissertation). University of Hawaii at Manoa. (UMI Order No. AA13198369)

Marinopoulos, S. S., Dorman, T., Ratanawongsa, N., Wilson, L. M., Ashar, B. H., Magaziner, J. L., . . . Bass, E. B. (2007). Effectiveness of continuing medical education. *Evidence Reports in Technology Assessment, 14*, 1–69.

Mark, S., Scott, G., Donviel, D., Leveton, L., Charles, J., Siegel, B., & Mahoney, E. (2014). New NASA and NSBRI report on sex and gender differences in adaptation to space flight. *Journal of Women's Health.* Retrieved from http://onlineliebertpub.com/toc./jwh/23/11

May, C. (2013). Towards a general theory of implementation. *Implementation Science, 8*, 18.

McCaughan, D., Thompson, C., Cullum, N., Sheldon, T. A., & Thompson, D. R. (2002). Acute care nurses' perceptions of barriers to using research information in clinical decision-making. *Journal of Advanced Nursing, 39*(1), 46–60.

McEwen, M., & Wills, E. M. (2014). *Theoretical basis for nursing* (4th ed.). Philadelphia, PA: Wolters Kluwer Health/Lippincott Williams & Wilkins.

McQueen, J., Miller, C., Nivison, C., & Husband, V. (2006). An investigation into the use of a journal club for evidence-based practice. *International Journal of Therapy and Rehabilitation, 13*(7), 311–316.

McSherry, R. (2002). *Evidence informed nursing: A guide for clinical nurses.* London, England: Routledge.

Melnyk, B., & Cole, R. (2011). Generating evidence through quantitative research. In B. Melnyk & E. Fineout-Overholt (Eds.), *Evidence-based practice in nursing and healthcare* (pp. 239–281). Philadelphia, PA: Lippincott Williams & Wilkins.

Melnyk, B., & Fineout-Overholt, E. (2002). Putting research into practice. Rochester ARCC. *Reflections on Nursing Leadership, 28*(2), 22–25.

Melnyk, B., & Fineout-Overholt, E. (2011). *Evidence-based practice in nursing and healthcare: A guide to best practice* (2nd ed.). Philadelphia, PA: Lippincott Williams & Wilkins.

Melnyk, B., & Fineout-Overholt, E. (2015). *Evidence-based practice in nursing and healthcare: A guide to best practice* (3rd ed.). Philadelphia, PA: Lippincott Williams & Williams, Wolters Kluwer Health.

Merryfeather, L., & Bruce, A. (2014). The invisibility of gender diversity: Understanding transgender and transsexuality in nursing literature. *Nursing Forum, 49*(2), 110–123.

Minnick, A. (2009). General design and implementation challenges in outcomes assessment. In R. M. Kleinpell (Ed.), *Outcomes assessment in advanced practice nursing* (2nd ed., pp. 107–119). New York, NY: Springer.

Miracle, V. (2008). Effective poster presentations. *Dimensions of Critical Care Nursing, 27*(3), 122–124.

Mitchell, P. H., Ferketich, S., & Jennings, B. M. (1998). Quality health outcomes model. *Image: Journal of Nursing Scholarship, 30*(1), 43–36.

Monico, E. P., Moore, C. L., & Calise, A. (2005). The impact of evidence-based medicine and evolving technology on the standard of care in emergency medicine. *The Internet Journal of Law, Healthcare and Ethics, 3*(2).

Munhall, P. (1994). *In women's experience.* New York, NY: National League for Nursing.

Munhall, P. (2007). A phenomenological method. In P. L. Munhall (Ed.), *Nursing research: A qualitative perspective* (4th ed., pp. 145–210). Sudbury, MA: Jones and Bartlett.

National Organization of Nurse Practitioner Faculties. (2007). *Nurse practitioner faculty practice: An expectation of professionalism.* Retrieved from http://www.nonpf.com/displaycommon.cfm?an=1&subarticlenbr=13

Newhouse, R., Bobay, K., Dykes, P. C., Stevens, K. R., & Titler, M. (2013). Methodology issues in implementation science. *Medical Care, 51,* 532–540.

Newhouse, R. P., Dearholt, S. L., Poe, S. S., Pugh, L., & White, K. M. (2008). *Johns Hopkins nursing evidence-based practice model and guidelines: Instructor's guide.* Indianapolis, IN: Sigma Theta Tau International.

Nolan, M. (2005). Reconciling tensions between research, evidence-based practice and user participation: Time for nursing to take the lead. *International Journal of Nursing Studies, 42*(5), 503–505.

O'Grady, E. T. (2008). Advanced practice registered nurses: The impact on patient safety and quality. In *Patient safety and quality: An evidence-based handbook for nurses.* Retrieved from http://www.ahrq.gov/qual/nurseshdbk/

Oliver, J. S., Martin, M. Y., Richardson, L., Kim, Y., & Pisu, M. (2013). Gender differences in colon cancer treatment. *Journal of Women's Health, 22*(4), 344–351. doi:10-1089/jwh.2012.3988

Oman, K. S., Duran, C., & Fink, R. (2008). Evidence-based policy and procedures: An algorithm for success. *Journal of Nursing Administration, 38*(1), 47–51.

O'Mathuna, D. P., DiCenso, A., Fineout-Overholt, E., & Johnston, L. (2011). Critically appraising quantitative evidence for clinical decision-making. In *Evidence-based practice in nursing and healthcare: A guide to best practice* (2nd ed., 81–134). Philadelphia, PA: Lippincott Williams & Wilkins.

Patient Protection and Affordable Care Act. (2010). Retrieved from http://www.dpc.senate.gov/healthreformbill/healthbill04.pdf

Patton, M. Q. (1990). *Qualitative evaluation and research methods* (2nd ed.). Newbury Park, CA: Sage.

Pesut, B., & Johnson, J. (2007). Reinstating the "Queen": Understanding philosophical inquiry in nursing. *Journal of Advanced Nursing, 61*(1), 115–121.

Peterson, L. A., Woodward, L. D., Urech, T., Daw, C., & Sookanan, S. (2006). Does pay-for-performance improve the quality of health care? *Annals of Internal Medicine, 145*(4), 265–272.

Polit, D. F., & Beck, C. T. (2008). Is there gender bias in nursing research? *Research in Nursing and Health, 31*(5), 417–427.

Polit, D. F., & Beck, C. T. (2013). Is there still gender bias in nursing research? An update. *Research in Nursing and Health, 36,* 75–83.

Polit, D. F., & Hungler, B. P. (1997). *Essentials of nursing research: Methods, appraisal, and utilization* (4th ed.). Philadelphia, PA: Lippincott-Raven.

Porter, S. (1996). Qualitative research. In D. F. S. Cormack (Ed.), *The research process in nursing* (3rd ed., pp. 113–122). Oxford, England: Blackwell Science.

Prochaska, J. O., & DiClemente, C. C. (1986). Toward a comprehensive model of change. In W. R. Miller & N. Heather (Eds.), *Treating addictive behaviors: Processes of change* (pp. 3–27). New York, NY: Plenum Press.

Prosser, H., Almond, S., & Walley, T. (2003). Influences on GP's decision to prescribe new drugs: The importance of who says what. *Family Practice, 20*(1), 61–68.

Raines, C. F. (2010, March). *The doctor of nursing practice: A report on progress.* Presentation at the annual meeting of the American Association of Colleges of Nursing. Retrieved from http://www.aacn.nche.edu/leading-initiatives/dnp/DNPForum3-10.pdf

Reavy, K., & Tavernier, S. (2008). Nurses reclaiming ownership of their practice: Implementation of an evidence-based model and process. *Journal of Continuing Education in Nursing, 39*(4), 166–172.

Rich, K. A. (2015). Evaluating outcomes of innovations. In N. A. Schmidt & J. M. Brown (Eds.), *Evidence-based practice for nurses: Appraisal and application of research* (3rd ed., pp. 487–504). Burlington, MA: Jones & Bartlett Learning.

Rosenstock, I. M. (1966). Why people use health services. *Milbank Fund Quarterly, 44,* 94–127.

Rosswurm, M. A., & Larrabee, J. (1999). A model for change to evidence based practice. *Image: Journal of Nursing Scholarship, 31*(4), 317–322.

Russell, C., & Gregory, D. (2003). Evaluation of qualitative research studies. *Evidence-Based Nursing, 6*(2), 36–40.

Rutledge, D. N., & Bookbinder, M. (2002). Processes and outcomes of evidence-based practice. *Seminars in Oncology Nursing, 18*(1), 3–10.

Rycroft-Malone, J., Kitson, A., Harvey, G., McCormack, B., Seers, K., Titchen, A., & Estabrooks, C. (2002). Ingredients for change: Revisiting a conceptual framework. *Quality and Safety in Health Care, 11*(2), 174–180.

Rycroft-Malone, J., Seers, K., Titchen, A., Harvey, G., Kitson, A., & McCormack, B. (2004). What counts as evidence in evidence-based practice? *Journal of Advanced Nursing, 47*(1), 81–90.

Sackett, D. L., Richardson, W. S., Rosenberg, W. T., & Haynes, R. B. (1997). *Evidence-based medicine: How to practice and teach evidence-based medicine.* New York, NY: Churchill Livingstone.

Samson, L. (2006). *Building capacity for health disparities research.* Grant 1P20MD001816-01 from the National Center on Minority Health and Health Disparities, National Institutes of Health, Bethesda, MD.

Santucci, S. (2011). A system change: Expansion of primary and secondary prevention services in a marginalized community. *Clinical Scholars Review, 4*(2), 98–103.

Schmidt, N., & Brown, J. M. (2015). Sharing the insights with others. In N. Schmidt & J. M. Brown, *Evidence-based practice for nurses: Appraisal and application of research* (5th ed., pp. 505–529). Burlington, MA: Jones & Bartlett Learning.

Scott-Findley, S., & Pollack, C. (2004). Evidence, research and knowledge: A call for conceptual clarity. *Worldviews on Evidence Based Nursing, 1*(2), 92–97.

Sheratt, C. (2005). The journal club: A method for occupational therapists to bridge the theory-practice gap. *British Journal of Occupational Therapy, 68*(7), 301–306.

Sigma Theta Tau International Clinical Scholarship Task Force. (1999). *Clinical scholarship resource paper.* Retrieved from http://www.nursingsociety.org/aboutus/PositionPapers/Documents/clinical_scholarship_paper.pdf

Simmons-Mackie, N. N., & Damico, J. S. (2001). Intervention outcomes: Clinical applications of qualitative methods. *Topics in Language Disorders, 21*(4), 21–36.

Singleton, J., & Levin, R. (2008). Strategies for learning evidence-based practice: Critically appraising clinical practice guidelines. *Journal of Nursing Education, 47*(8), 380–383.

Soumerai, S. B., McLaughlin, T. J., Gurwitz, J. H., Guadagnoli, E., Hauptman, P. J., Borbas, C., . . . Gobel, F. (1998). Effect of local medical opinion leaders on quality of care for acute myocardial infarction. *Journal of the American Medical Association, 279*(17), 1358–1363.

Spitzer, R. L., Devlin, M., Walsh, B. T., Hasin, D., Wing, R., Marcus, M., & Nonas, C. (1992). Binge eating disorder: A multi-site field trial of the diagnostic criteria. *International Journal of Eating Disorders, 11*(3), 191–203.

Stetler, C. B. (1994). Refinement of the Stetler/Marram model for application of research findings to practice. *Nursing Outlook, 42*(1), 15–25.

Stetler, C. B., & Marram, G. (1976). Evaluating research findings for applicability in practice. *Nursing Outlook, 24*(9), 559–563.

Stevens, K. R. (2011). Critically appraising knowledge for clinical decision-making. In B. Melnyk & E. Fineout-Overholt (Eds.), *Evidence-based practice in nursing and healthcare: A guide to best practice* (2nd ed.). Philadelphia, PA: Lippincott Williams & Wilkins.

Stoekel, P. (2010). Leadership and management role of the doctor of nursing practice in the care of older persons in the USA. *Journal of Clinical Nursing, 19*(Suppl. 1), 145–146.

Strauss, A., & Corbin, J. (1994). *Basics of qualitative research: Grounded theory procedures and techniques.* Newbury Park, CA: Sage.

Strauss, A., & Corbin, J. (1998). *Basics of qualitative research: Techniques and procedures for developing grounded theory.* Thousand Oaks, CA: Sage.

Stroud, S. D., Erkel, E. A., & Smith, C. A. (2005). The use of personal digital assistants by nurse practitioner students and faculty. *Journal of the American Academy of Nurse Practitioners, 17*(2), 67–75.

Stull, A., & Lanz, C. (2005). An innovative model for nursing scholarship. *Journal of Nursing Education, 44*(11), 493–497.

Tanyi, R. A., McKenzie, M., & Chapek, C. (2009). How family practice physicians, nurse practitioners, and physicians assistants incorporate spiritual care in practice. *Journal of the American Academy of Nurse Practitioners, 21*, 690–697.

Timmerman, G. M. (1999). Using a women's health perspective to guide decisions made in quantitative research. *Journal of Advanced Nursing, 30*(3), 640–645.

Titler, M. G. (2002). Use of research in practice. In G. LoBiondo & J. Haber (Eds.), *Nursing research methods: Critical appraisal and utilization* (5th ed., pp. 410–431). St. Louis, MO: Mosby.

Titler, M. G., Klieber, C., Steelman, V., Goode, C., Rakel, B., Barry-Walker, J., . . . Buckwalter, K. (1994). Infusing research into practice to promote quality care. *Nursing Research, 43*(5), 307–313.

Trim, S. (2008). Journal club offers new opportunities. *Kai Tiaki Nursing New Zealand, 14*(11), 23.

Tropello, P. G. D. (2000). *Origins of the nurse practitioner movement: An oral history* (Doctoral dissertation). Rutgers, State University of New Jersey–New Brunswick, and University of Medicine and Dentistry of New Jersey. (UMI Order No. AAI9970979)

Tymkow, C., Shen, J. J., & MacMullen, N. (2006). Project 2: Emergency room usage among uninsured patients with access to a primary care provider. In L. Samson (Ed.), *Building capacity for health disparities research*. Grant 1P20MD001816-01 from the National Center on Minority Health and Health Disparities, National Institutes of Health, Bethesda, MD.

van Manen, M. (1990). *Researching lived experiences: Human science for an action sensitive pedagogy*. Albany, NY: State University of New York Press.

Volker, D. L., & Limerick, M. (2007). Interpretative phenomenological analysis of patient experiences of low back pain. *Clinical Nurse Specialist, 21*(5), 241–249.

Wall, B. M., Edwards, N. E., & Porter, M. L. (2007). Textual analysis of retired nurses' oral histories. *Nursing Inquiry, 14*(4), 279–288.

Watkins, C., Harvey, I., Langley, C., Gray, S., & Faulkner, A. (1999). General practitioners' use of guidelines in the consultation and their attitudes to them. *British Journal of General Practice, 49*(438), 11–15.

Yuh-Min, C., Yueh-Ping, L., & Min-Ling, Y. (2015). Gender differences in the predictors of physical activity among assisted living residents. *Journal of Nursing Scholarship, 47*(3), 211–218.

Zadvinskis, I. M., & Grudell, B. A. (2010). Clinical practice guideline appraisal using the AGREE instrument: Renal Screening. *Clinical Nurse Specialist, 24*(4), 209–214.

Zeeman, L., Aranda, K., & Grant, A. (2014). Queer challenges to evidence-based practice. *Nursing Inquiry, 21*(2), 101–111.

Zuzelo, P. R. (2007). Evidence-based nursing and qualitative research: A partnership imperative for real-world practice. In P. L. Munhall (Ed.), *Nursing research: A qualitative perspective* (4th ed., pp. 481–499). Sudbury, MA: Jones and Bartlett.

Chapter 4

Information Systems/ Technology and Patient Care Technology for the Improvement and Transformation of Health Care

Susan F. Burkart-Jayez

Introduction

The American Association of Colleges of Nursing (AACN) *Essentials of Doctoral Education for Advanced Nursing Practice* (2006) identified "foundational outcome competencies deemed essential for all graduates of a Doctorate of Nursing Practice (DNP) program regardless of specialty or functional focus." This chapter addresses Essential IV in preparing DNP graduates to "utilize information systems to evaluate programs of care, outcomes of care, and care systems" and to "provide leadership within healthcare systems and/or academic settings related to the use of information systems." In a personal communication (September 2011), Bonnie Westra noted that nursing (informatics) competencies need to emphasize patient care and outcomes and that advanced practice nurses (APNs) are in key positions to engage consumers (patients) and transform health care. For the full AACN recommendation, see **Figure 4-1**.

DNP graduates are distinguished by their abilities to use information systems/ technology to support and improve patient care and healthcare systems and provide leadership within healthcare systems and/or academic settings.

Knowledge and skills related to information systems/technology and patient care technology prepare the DNP graduate to apply new knowledge, manage individual- and aggregate-level information, and assess the efficacy of patient care technology appropriate to a specialized area of practice. DNP graduates also design, select, and use information systems/technology to evaluate programs of care, outcomes of care, and care systems. Information systems/technology provide a mechanism to apply budget and productivity tools, practice information systems and decision supports, and web-based learning or intervention tools to support and improve patient care.

DNP graduates must also be proficient in the use of information systems/ technology resources to implement quality improvement initiatives and support practice and administrative decision making. Graduates must demonstrate knowledge of standards and principles for selecting and evaluating information systems and patient care technology, and related ethical, regulatory, and legal issues.

The DNP program prepares the graduate to:

1. Design, select, use, and evaluate programs that evaluate and monitor outcomes of care, care systems, and quality improvement, including consumer use of health care information systems.
2. Analyze and communicate critical elements necessary to the selection, use, and evaluation of healthcare information systems and patient care technology.
3. Demonstrate the conceptual ability and technical skills to develop and execute an evaluation plan involving data extraction from practice information systems and databases.
4. Provide leadership in the evaluation and resolution of ethical and legal issues within healthcare systems relating to the use of information, information technology, communication networks, and patient care technology.
5. Evaluate consumer health information sources for accuracy, timeliness, and appropriateness.

Figure 4-1 Essential IV: Information Systems/Technology and Patient Care Technology for the Improvement and Transformation of Health Care
American Association of Colleges of Nursing. (2006). *The essentials of doctoral education for advanced nursing practice.* Retrieved from http://www.aacn.nche.edu/DNP/Essentials.pdf. Reprinted with permission.

According to Kingsley and Kingsley (2009), "There is a substantial generation gap between college professors and their students . . . students are more comfortable in a *technology* rich environment, but that doesn't equate to knowledge (and/or) critical thinking skills needed to locate, filter, and evaluate information found on line. A core competency for operating in an electronic environment is information literacy . . . (the ability) to apply new knowledge, manage individual and aggregate level information, and assess the efficacy of patient care technology" (p. 7).

Given the nature of this topic, the most efficient use of the material presented is as a guide to building the knowledge, skills, abilities, and toolkits needed to achieve the outcomes recommended by the AACN. Topic background is presented to underscore the saliency of the author's suggestions, but the benefit of this chapter is best realized by performing the tasks as they are presented.

Information Systems/Technology

Computer Literacy/Competency

When faced with novel subspecialty information, it is important to learn the language of the domain. A brief glossary can be found in **Appendix 4-2**, and terms used in this chapter that appear in the glossary are italicized in the text. Because *informatics* is an evolving field, concepts related to it are rapidly changing; therefore, the terms of today continue to expand and evolve as national efforts toward consensus continue. The most exciting aspect of the information to follow is that it brings the reader to the plan developed for *healthcare information technology (HIT)*. The target date for national implementation of competencies in *computer literacy, information technology (IT)*, and *healthcare informatics* was 2014 (Kolbasuk McGee, 2009). Following publication of the 2009 information, the target date was moved to 2015.

Over the years, multiple studies have looked at the *computer competency* of nursing students and staff nurses. Koivunen, Valimaki, Jakobsson, and Pitkanen (2008) "identified different ways of learning computer use and barriers to use; evaluating computer skills; performing a literature search; reflecting findings against the literature search on the most effective teaching and learning computer skills" (p. 302). Although the psychiatric nursing population was the domain of interest, the findings can be generalized to all nursing practice sites. The work identified learning methods and barriers to learning computer skills and the evaluation of the individual nurse's level of skill. This was the basis for developing more effective methods for achieving computer facility.

Nurses' computer skills were evaluated using the European Computer Driving License/International Computer Driving License test (ECDL/ICDL). Readers may review the ECDL at www.ecdl.com.

Building Internet Resources

Table 4-1 consists of a nonexhaustive list of IT *websites* used in preparing this section that should be useful in DNP-level practice.

Table 4-1 Information Technology–Related Websites	
Nursing Informatics Working Group—NIWG	www.amia.org/programs/working-groups/nursing-informatics
American Medical Informatics Association	www.amia.org
Alliance for Nursing Informatics	ANI and the TIGER Initiative: www.allianceni.org
Nelson: Patient Care Technology and Safety	www.ncbi.nlm.nih.gov/books/NBK2686/?report=printable
American Library Association	www.ala.org/aasl/standards-guidelines
Centers for Disease Control and Prevention	www.cdc.gov
National Guideline Clearinghouse	Clinical guidelines: www.ngc.gov
Nursing Informatics: competencies	www.nursing-informatics.com/niassess/index.html
European Computer Driving License	www.ecdl.com
Agency for Healthcare Research and Quality	Government agency for quality: www.ahrq.gov
Health Information Technology	www.healthit.gov
Health Information Technology Scholars Program	www.hits-colab.org
American Library Association	www.ala.org
National Academies Press	Institute of Medicine Collection of Work on Healthcare Quality Improvement Issues: www.nap.edu
The Joint Commission	www.jointcommission.org
National League for Nursing	http://www.nln.org/docs/default-source/professional-development-programs/preparing-the-next-generation-of-nurses.pdf?sfvrsn=6

Table 4-1 Information Technology–Related Websites *(continued)*

Agency for Healthcare Research and Quality	Patient safety work by AHRQ: www.psnet.ahrq.gov
Presidential Message	Presidential call for Electronic Health Records by 2014, Executive order 13,410 at www.whitehouse.gov
	Search "electronic health records"
Healthcare Quality	Private agency for quality: www.leapfroggroup.org
Healthcare Quality	Private agency for quality: www.qualityforum.org
Healthcare Quality	Private agency for quality: www.ihi.org
Healthcare Quality	Quality and safety issues in nursing: www.qsen.org
National Institutes of Health–Nursing Research	www.ninr.nih.gov/Training/OnlineDevelopingNurseScientists/
	www.ninr.nih.gov/Recovery/Home.htm
Office of the National Coordinator	http://search.hhs.gov/search?q=office+of+the+national+coordinator+for+health+information+technology&site=HHS&entqr=3&ud=1&sort=date%3AD%3AL%3Ad1&output=xml_no_dtd&ie=UTF-8&oe=UTF-8&lr=lang_en&client=HHS&proxystylesheet=HHS
Robert Wood Johnson Foundation	www.rwjf.org/en/search-results.html?u=&k=healthcare+technology+projects
Healthcare Quality	www.ihi.org/resources/Pages/Publications/SafePracticesforBetterHealthcare2006Table1.aspx
TIGER	http://thetigerinitiative.org
Tech Terms Dictionary	www.oasismanagement.com/TECHNOLOGY/GLOSSARY
University of Minnesota	www.nursing.umn.edu/icnp

At this juncture, with text in hand, log on to the *Internet* and type in the site information. Select "Favorites" from the toolbar, and "add to" from the drop-down box. Each entry is the address of a website as described. At task completion, the reader will have a beginning collection of places to explore in depth the topics to be discussed in this chapter. Additionally, the list will present the latest in acquiring computer literacy/competency and accessing quality in clinical care standards.

Authors such as Eley, Fallon, Soar, Buikstra, and Hegney (2008) explored nurses' computer competence. The results of the participants' self-assessed computer expertise were as follows: 50% felt that they required more computer/IT training, and 25% felt that their current skill level was a barrier. Those who received on-the-job computer training believed that the training was adequate and timely. These nurses felt that training, though available, was not emphasized as an option and that training interfered with their workload. The group in this study favored a national standard for nursing computer competency.

Computer and Internet skills are necessary for the successful implementation of new IT applications in patient care (Koivunen et al., 2008; TIGER Initiative, 2009; see http://thetigerinitiative.org/docs/ TigerReport_InformaticsCompetencies_000.pdf). Computer literacy is the ability to use computers to perform a variety of tasks. Computer competency is the ability to demonstrate proficiency in use of *software* applications such Microsoft Word, Excel, and PowerPoint, and knowledge in computer use terminology, *hardware* selection, and simple maintenance functions. Literacy is an attribute; competency is the reproducible evaluation of the skills and knowledge related to an attribute. According to Wojner (2001), "Technology is only as good as the skills and knowledge of the clinicians using it . . . the effect of technology varies . . . as a result of the different methods used to prepare and teach the clinicians to use it" (p. 135).

The Technology Informatics Guiding Education Reform (TIGER) Initiative, involving more than 1,100 nursing content experts, completed three years of work in developing a 10-year plan for nursing's path toward computer/information/informatics literacy for patient care as one domain requiring curriculum development. The TIGER Initiative is a large-scale example of *outcomes management (OM)* in methodically unraveling the issue, significance, and outcomes of patient care.

One of the focus areas of the TIGER Initiative is defining the basic technology competency curriculum for nurses (this information is on the TIGER Initiative website). Standardized proficiency in healthcare technology will ensure that the variance in efficacy of technology use will be dampened. The collaborative was funded by federal funds from the National Library of Medicine, the National Institutes of Health (NIH), and the Department of Health and Human Services and by grants from the Robert Wood Johnson Foundation and the Agency for Healthcare Research and Quality (AHRQ). The sponsorship is worth mentioning and indirectly evidences the importance of incorporating

Table 4-2 Sponsors of the TIGER Initiative
Alliance for Nursing Informatics
American Health Information Management Association
American Medical Informatics Association
American Nurses Association
American Nursing Informatics Association
Apptis
Audience Response Systems
Capital Area Roundtable on Informatics in Nursing
Cerner Corporation
Clinical Information Technology Program Office
CliniComp International
CPM Resource Center
Eclipsys
Elsevier
GE Healthcare Systems
Healthcare Information and Management Systems Society
IBM
Independence Foundation
Marion J. Ball
McKesson
MITRE Corporation
Siemens
Sigma Theta Tau International
Tenet Healthcare
Thomson Healthcare
University of Maryland, Baltimore County

computers and technology into nursing's educational base. Each of these entities has its own website. For further background, the reader is invited to type each organization's name into the Internet search box and *browse* areas of interest. See **Table 4-2**.

A second task is to visit and interact with the TIGER summit website (now in your Favorites list). This presents the proposed curriculum content changes that will be introduced into all levels of nursing education over the next 10 years.

The third task is to learn about the ECDL/ICDL through its website, which provides an overview of the ECDL concept. It is recommended that the reader thoroughly explore the site to get a sense of the future nursing curriculum changes that need to occur for the profession to embrace computer competency. How is it that the ECDL/ICDL is identified as core to computer and *information literacy* and competency? In addition to the recommendations of the TIGER summit (2009), other nursing scholars have identified the utility of this toolkit. According to Jones (2005), the ECDL is currently used in teaching basic IT skills to staff in all industries, not just health care. In a survey conducted in the United Kingdom, nurses who had ECDL certification responded that they saved up to 30 minutes a day, which was then available for direct patient care. This study produced information on computer competency's impact on how nurses spend their time following implementation of IT in health care.

Kossman and Scheidenhelm (2008) noted that the recommendations of the Institute of Medicine (IOM) to improve patient safety include the use of IT to automate medication delivery systems, collect patient clinical *data*, and provide clinical decision support. In addition, time burden studies that examined the impact of the *electronic health record (EHR)* use on nurses' time using a variety of methodologies—including time-motion studies, work sampling, and self-report—had varied results: increased/decreased and neutral time burdens with EHRs.

Doctorally prepared advanced practice registered nurses (APRNs) must be competent in computers, IT, and informatics to be able to transform data into the information used in executive decision making; standardized competency is the first step. Because the experts in various nursing and healthcare information organizations proposing computer competency curriculum recommend the ECDL/ICDL as foundational, the reader is encouraged to achieve ECDL/ICDL certification regardless of level of educational preparation (Jones, 2005; TIGER Initiative, 2009).

In the literature, many subscribe to the core requirement of computer literacy for nurses. In "Curriculum Strategies to Improve Baccalaureate Nursing Information Technology Outcomes," Fetter (2009) identified "enhancing information technology (IT) competence as one of nursing's most significant and urgent priorities" (p. 4), and one that has vast potential to reduce health errors and improve care quality, access, and cost-effectiveness. The strategy, outlined in the February 2009 article, includes policy-based incentives for networking nursing programs, clinical agencies, vendors, and accrediting bodies to introduce standard IT and information literacy and competency into nursing education and practice. Examples of Veterans Affairs (VA) healthcare technology are presented in the patient care technology section of this chapter.

Information Literacy

The framework for the steps and skills needed for providing the best patient care in a technology-rich environment includes the ability to use critical thinking and assessment skills to determine what information is needed. The reader should find the information based on all available resources, including colleagues, policies, and literature in various formats; evaluate the information through critical thinking and determining the validity of the source; put the information into practice; and evaluate whether use of the information resulted in improved patient care. Doctoral-level nurses need to be experts in critically evaluating the available information using multiple sources.

In 1991, Berwick, Roessner, and Godfrey noted that more time spent on training in the use of basic tools translates into more rapid gains. Berwick gave examples of information literacy found in everyday practice: Pareto diagrams (representing largest to smallest frequency), line graphs/run charts (identifying trends over time), pie charts (showing relative parts of a whole), bar graphs (comparing categorical data), histograms (showing frequency distribution of continuous data like time, weight, size, temperature), and control charts (determining if a process can be considered stable/thus predictable or unstable/thus unpredictable). Such information presentation is common, yet not all viewers are fully knowledgeable as to what the concepts behind these graphics are, much less when to use which type. As one becomes information literate, one gains the ability to generate data and to transform the data into information for executive decision making. McNeil et al. (2003), in surveying nurses exiting their education program regarding IT skills, found that "e-mail use, bibliographic retrieval via library-based resources or the Internet, use of the Internet and *World Wide Web*, and use of presentation graphics software were most frequently cited as computer competency skills acquired. Information technology tools such as remote monitoring devices, online consumer health tools, and hand-held computers were examples given by the group studied as examples of information literacy skills." This indicated the need for nursing curricula to include information management (literacy) as found in daily nursing practice. The American Library Association (ALA) website (www.ala.org) has the "25 best teaching and learning sites" for information management, literacy, and technology-based tools.

Informatics

Thede, Allen, and Pierce (2003) considered that Scholes and Barber first used the term "informatics" in 1980 in an address to MEDINFO and that nursing informatics (NI) is "the use of computer technology in all endeavors: services, education and research." Thede et al. further stated that "informatics offers many benefits for health care: the ability to create and use aggregated data, to prevent errors, and to provide better medical records" (p. 6). The National Center for Nursing Research (1993) proposed seven areas for NI: "using data, information, and knowledge for patient care; defining data in nursing care; acquiring and delivering knowledge about patient care; creating new tools for patient care from new technologies; applying patient care ergonomics to patient-nurse-machine interaction; integrating systems; and evaluating the effects of nursing systems" (p. 192). Twenty-two years later, nursing education still struggles with the core curriculum to ensure that students and graduates are able to achieve competency in these areas.

Ornes and Gassert (2007) emphasized that "nursing programs must integrate informatics content into their curricula to prepare nurses to use information technology" (p. 75) and cited Staggers, Gassert, and Curran (2002), who noted that nurses need "fundamental information management and computer technology skills" so they can "use existing information systems and available information to manage their practice" (p. 386).

The National League for Nursing (NLN, 2008) position statement on preparing the next generation of nurses for practice addressed incorporating informatics competencies into nursing education, noting that informatics is one of the IOM's five quality and safety competencies. The other quality and safety competencies are patient-centered care, teamwork and collaboration, evidence-based practice, quality improvement and safety. The NLN further recommended forming partnerships between clinicians and informatics people at the agency level to "help faculty and students develop competence in informatics, and to ensure that all faculty members have competence in computer literacy, information literacy, and informatics" (NLN, 2008). The full document can be found at the NLN website (www.nln.org).

One often cited master list of competencies was developed by Staggers and Gassert (Staggers et al., 2002). This study, reported by Page (2004), had as its focus the production of a research-based master list of informatics competencies differentiated by level of nursing practice. Informatics knowledge is the theory; informatics skills are the methods, tools, and techniques; and computer literacy is learning how to manipulate computer technology.

Lin, Lin, Jiang, and Lee (2007) defined informatics competency as the knowledge and skills necessary to use computers and IT in nursing practice. One of their suggested competencies was in basic programming skills using software such as Microsoft Excel. In their report, Lin et al. stated that the conceptual framework for NI competency includes "hardware, software and network concepts; computer application principles; computer use skills; programming design; computer limitations; personal and social issues; and attitudes toward computers" (p. 54). Charles (2008) presented informatics, in the context of *evidence-based medicine (EBM)*, as using tested, objectively measurable care guidelines and following best practices to reduce variability in care outcomes. Reviewing the content of the AHRQ website provides information on EBM and the informatics available for incorporating guidelines into practice for the DNP.

Kirkley (2004) explained how the use of clinical IT in bedside nursing mirrors Magnet-level qualities. She described a *computer information system (CIS)* introduced within a healthcare agency in 1998 as having an online decision support system (DSS), clinical documentation, care planning, and *computerized physician order entry (CPOE)*. The core nursing functions included results reporting, clinical documentation, medication charting, patient assessments, and performance reports, thus giving nurses the knowledge they need to make informed decisions at the point of care. At the facility studied, all educational materials, policies, and procedures were consolidated online for open access to all staff, and nurses completed competency training by computer. This supported the Magnet aspect that nurses are accountable for their own practice as well as the coordination of care.

Patient Care Technology

What is patient care technology? According to Audrey Nelson, in *Patient Safety and Quality: An Evidence-Based Handbook for Nurses*, "Patient care technologies can be classified in many ways . . . direct nursing care delivery technology, indirect nursing care delivery technology, communication technology, patient and nurse protective devices, nurse protective devices, patient assessment, monitoring and surveillance, patient assistive devices, remote monitoring, continued learning, and pattern identification. Well-designed technology allows nurses to focus on care-giving functions and promoting the health of patients" (Powell-Cope, Nelson, & Patterson, 2008, pp. 2–3). The fourth task is to access Nelson's patient safety information using the website provided in Table 4-1. Current APRN practice includes the "hospitalist" role, that is, providing oversight of the care provided to the inpatient population in various settings. Doctorally prepared APRNs need to be familiar, if not highly experienced, with each of the patient care technology types because they both oversee and provide direct patient care.

The Joint Commission (2008) reported that *adverse events* related to healthcare IT arise from several sources, including lack of inclusion of frontline staff in developing and implementing new technologies, poor human–machine interfaces, absence of use of best practices information, and poor resources for maintaining technologies once implemented. Recommendations to avoid unintended and/or adverse outcomes include involving end users in examining care processes for potential risks before implementing technological changes. Training programs are also recommended for all levels of clinicians and staff involved in the use of technology. The disconnect between available technology and clinical utility was identified early on by Wojner (2001), who viewed technology as "only as good as the skills and knowledge of the clinicians using it" (p. 135), adding that "the effect of technology varies between hospitals as a result of the different methods used to prepare and teach the clinicians to use it . . . particularly patient monitoring technologies" (p. 135). Wojner described a common disconnect between the specific use of technology and the availability of devices, using pulse oximetry as an example. In collecting data on critically ill patients, one measure commonly collected is the pulse oximetry reading, without consideration for the utility of the information rendered. Patients treated for gastrointestinal bleeds or myocardial infarction in the emergency department are as likely to have pulse oximetry readings as the patient with chronic obstructive pulmonary disease, pneumonia, or pulmonary embolism. However, using the information obtained is crucial for the latter group, less so for the former. An analogy is monitoring body temperature in the suspected septic patient versus the patient with an acute orthopedic injury: a task is performed because the technology is available, and data are obtained and recorded but not necessarily essential in evaluating the presumed condition. The utility of the measurement is for supplemental oxygen and other pulmonary-related interventions, yet the information is collected regardless of diagnosis as part of a routine task. Wojner cautioned us that "the use of technology in healthcare must be tempered by education, training, and appropriate application in order to be of optimal benefit to patient outcomes" (p. 135). That is, development of technology-based patient care solutions in provision of direct care must have saliency; whether one is measuring vital signs, utilization of clinical pathways, readmission rates, or clinical performance/outcome measures, the task and tools must make sense.

Conversely, Nelson noted, "Given that 5,000 types of medical devices are used by millions of health care providers around the world, device related problems are inevitable" (Powell-Cope et al., 2008, p. 1). The common pitfalls include poor design, poor design interface with the intended application (patient centered), poor planning for technology-driven practice changes, and poor technology maintenance after implementation. This has led to the concept of "yet-to-be errors"—adverse events caused by unforeseen outcomes of using new technology. According to Simpson (2009, p. 302), the best way to eliminate human-induced errors is to improve human behavior, and for nurses, better behavior results in better care. Standard competency assessment for using technology is one facet of improving behavior. Performance management and monitoring patient care indicators can also improve nursing behaviors by helping nurses map outcomes to practice through objective feedback on an individual's efficacy in providing care. Nurses have incredible knowledge and influence on healthcare outcomes, yet there is often variation in the quality of nursing care and in nurse-sensitive outcomes. According to Delaney (personal communication, October 1, 2009), "all technology will change practice as will practice influence technology."

In work completed by Lee (2007, p. 109), patients' perceptions of nurses' behavior in the use of information in health care was found to fall into three categories: increased work efficiency (providing everyday care information: more time on patient care, less on documentation); privacy and confidentiality issues (because of easy data access); and satisfaction of relationships (patients did not care about personal digital assistant use as long as they received the care they needed and did not see a difference in care). The use of technology-based tools by nurses was found to be of no concern to patients, as long as the tools did not interfere with direct patient care.

Transformation of Health Care

Quality

Between the health care we have and the care we could have lies not just a gap, but a chasm. Failing to use available science is costly and harmful: it leads to overuse of unhelpful care, underuse of effective care and errors in execution. Simple innovations spread faster than complicated ones.

—Berwick (2003, p. 1969)

Although the need for curriculum changes to integrate technology into nursing education has been discussed in the literature for nearly 30 years, the complexities of the innovations are a barrier. Until now, there has been little in policy and funding at the national level to encourage the changes required. However, the $21 billion for health IT programs in the U.S. economic stimulus bill will create career opportunities and fuel educational programs for professionals to acquire a mix of technology and clinical expertise (IT) (Kolbasuk McGee, 2009). In the first year of incentives, hospitals could receive up to $1.5 million for effectively using *electronic medical record (EMR)* systems, and doctor practices can eventually earn around $40,000. It is estimated that only 20% of hospitals currently have fully functional HIT/EMR systems. With hospitals and other clinical practice sites making the leap to computerized patient records, the nursing education system will need to respond rapidly with appropriate classroom and practical training.

Technology impacts safety (order entry [OE] decreased prescribing errors), effectiveness (clinical reminders), enhancement of patient-centered care (increases clinical knowledge through Web resources), timeliness (e-health), and efficiency, all domains of interest for DNP clinical care and professional education.

According to a report by Clancy (2005), better quality health care using IT means making patient information available at the point of care at any time and to all team members in order to provide the right treatment, without delay, using best practice guidelines, while preventing medical errors. An EMR coordinates patient care by "giving multiple providers access to the same, accurate and current information, extending medical resources to underserved populations through telehealth, measuring performance for comparing providers by linking front end processes (DSS to assist in providing treatment) and back end feed-back systems to show outcomes."

Goldstein and Blumenthal (2008, pp. 709–710) concurred that HIT "facilitates the transparency and sharing of information that already exists—essential for improving the quality of care, reducing costs and reducing health care disparities." The IOM is an advocate of HIT/EMR as a component fundamental to patient safety. Goldstein and Blumenthal described four essential components: a fully functional EMR with the ability to collect and store patient data electronically; an EMR capable of making information available to providers on request; CPOE; and the ability to access computerized decision support. A minimally functional EMR has limited CPOE and limited DSS. Recommendations by the National Quality Forum (NQF) are found on its website (www.qualityforum.org).

Outcomes Management

In Wojner's (2001) work *Outcomes Management: Applications to Clinical Practice,* there is a self-instruction module introducing OM and use of technology in health care. If OM is not part of the student's current course of study, the text will serve to initiate the reader in understanding concepts of OM and how computer competency is core to building OM plans.

One of this chapter author's research projects in OM was to measure the impact of technology on bedside acute care and intensive care nurses' time in rendering patient care. The project, *Research Protocol: Research Collaborative: Examining the Connection Between Patient Care, Nursing Sensitive Adverse Events, and Environment of Care Intensity* (Burkart-Jayez & Spath, 2008; see Appendix 4-1), funded by a seed grant from the American Organization of Nurse Executives, was a small-scale OM evaluation built on computer literacy, technology literacy, information literacy, and informatics competency. The method used was nurses' self-report. The two objectives of the research/quality improvement study were: (1) to measure the distribution of nursing time constraints for direct, indirect, unit-support, and standby activities (with a subset of computer usage tasks for medication administration and all documentation) on a nursing care unit basis, and (2) to analyze known adverse events, in the context of the derived intensity factor (IF), in order to evaluate for the existence of a relationship not yet described in nursing literature. Competencies required by the researcher, acquired over the course of completing the study, included all the basics recommended as core computer competencies for all nurses and others in health care. Weak competencies in technology selection, software selection, and advanced information literacy were barriers in the course of conducting the study and illustrate the need for the curricula of doctorally prepared APRNs to include standard competencies as proposed by the TIGER II Initiative. The study illustrates how technology impacts the provision of patient care and services as a function of time required when introducing meaningful use of HIT.

According to Houston (1996), the utility of OM in health care is in the use of aggregate variance data to change a system of healthcare practices, where variance is any event that alters patient progress toward the expected outcome. Sources of variance include practitioner behavior (competency), the severity of illness, as with high-risk patients, and practice patterns that either expedite care or inhibit delivery of care. Although technology has the potential for vast improvements in the provision of health care, without competency in the end user and adequate training and resources for continued maintenance of equipment and user performance, technology can be the source of "yet-to-be" errors. It is incumbent on nurse educators and nurse clinicians to be fully aware of the intent of use of each technological innovation, and on nurse scientists, at both the bedside and the podium, to have the requisite knowledge, skills, and abilities to function in the coming conversion to an electronic environment.

Translational Science

The goal of translational science is to incorporate scientific, patient-centered research into health gains. Toward this end, the NIH developed a "road map for medical research," charged with finding new approaches in biologic research, reducing artificial barriers to research, and cultivating patient-oriented research by "re-engineering the clinical research enterprise" (Zerhouni, 2005). The website for the NIH division of nursing research can be found in Table 4-1.

Translational science means taking research-based concepts—whether medications, medical devices, or technology—and moving the research into practice. This requires the interface of multiple disciplines in developing the practical applications. A simple example would be advances in wireless technology being incorporated into how nurses administer medications at the bedside. It requires the knowledge base of multiple professions to operationalize: computer engineers to develop hardware and software to capture the tasks required by end users; pharmacists, clinicians, and nurses to address the process requirements of each domain; quality management professionals to ensure compliance with clinical standards; and informatics nurses to support the education, training, and troubleshooting for the end users.

The American Medical Informatics Association (AMIA) website defines informatics researchers as those who develop methods in areas such as data mining, text processing, human interface design, decision support, *databases*, and other tools for data analysis. The work of informatics is interdisciplinary and aims to develop new solutions using IT. In 2009, the International Medical Informatics Association (IMIA) Special Interest group on Nursing Informatics defined NI as "the science and practice that integrates nursing, its information and knowledge, with management of information and communication technologies to promote the health of people, families and communities." The reader should view the AMIA website (www.amia.org), search "nursing informatics," and read the core areas of the work of NI. Expert clinical nurses, as "translational scientists," are integral to the translation of nursing and clinical informatics into the practice of nursing. This is one of the areas identified by the Office of the National Coordinator (ONC, 2011) as necessary for the rapid preparation of a workforce capable of implementing EHRs. One of the university-based training sites, as part of the HIT for Economic and Clinical Health (HITECH) Act, is the University of Minnesota University Partnership for Health Informatics (UP-HI) (www.uphi.umn.edu) (Westra, 2011). This program addresses the goals described in the next section.

Meaningful Use

The preceding section is a brief overview of the literature on information systems/technology (computer literacy/competency, information literacy, informatics), patient care technology, and quality and OM—topics embedded in the concept of "meaningful use." But what is meaningful use?

The American Recovery and Reinvestment Act of 2009 allocated billions of dollars in funding for the transformation of healthcare system IT. The agenda for the transformation is the HITECH Act. In 2010, the Affordable Care Act (Health Care and Education Reconciliation Act of 2010) built on the HITECH Act for health IT. The federal entity for accomplishing the work of HIT is the Office of the National Coordinator (ONC). The ONC has a strategic plan with five goals (2011):

1. Achieve adoption and information exchange through *meaningful use* of HIT.
2. Improve care, improve population health, and reduce healthcare costs through the use of HIT.
3. Inspire confidence and trust in HIT.
4. Empower individuals with HIT to improve their health and the healthcare system.
5. Achieve rapid learning and technological advancement.

The reader is advised to view the ONC website for information on each of the goals (see Table 4-1).

The document is a road map to facilitate Health Information Exchange (IIIE) adaptation. Meaningful use is geared to accelerate the use of EHRs, to support information exchange, and to use HIT for public health and population-based needs. This includes recording patient data, use of decision support software, transmitting prescriptions through electronic order entry, all while maintaining security and confidentiality. Funding will be provided for the purchase of tools and education of necessary IT professionals through the HITECH program. Meaningful use will also require integration of its concepts into clinical education programs, alignment among federal agencies, and interoperability.

Stage 1 of the ONC Strategic Plan is well under way across public and private healthcare practices, as evidenced by electronic prescriptions and recording of patient demographics, vital signs, and laboratory and imaging results. Funding is available to all practices, including rural, underserved areas. For those who do not adopt meaningful use by 2015, Medicare payment/reimbursements will be reduced.

The APRN's Role in Informatics

NI is computer literacy/competency, information literacy/competency, and the science of informatics on a platform of nursing science/expertise. This specialty role continues to evolve as the field of HIT expands. Sensmeier (2007) described the demand for NI in terms of developing and implementing health information systems. Factors cited as driving the field were the need to increase efficiency, promote safety, and improve patient care (e.g., meaningful use). These responsibilities for the NI role were identified in surveys conducted in 2004 and 2007. Identified barriers to the required activities were financial and technological (i.e., interoperability of systems). Sensmeier's recommendations for the future role include utilizing NI in implementing HIT software, EHR systems, and hardware selection. Of note is that Sensmeier identified the need for the NI to have both patient care expertise and informatics skills.

One example of how technology can support APRN workflow has been documented by Ridge (2011). Telehealth, specifically telemergency care, is used by nurse practitioners (NPs) who practice with an emergency medicine group, with physicians available by teleconference. This technology has enabled the NPs to successfully treat ~60% of patients presenting to the emergency department, while ensuring immediate access to physician input. Zytowski (2003) described the APRN role as both liaison/interpreter between nursing practice and IT innovation, and end user reliant on technology for patient care information access, reimbursement, and evidence-based practice. If NI is being introduced into your organization, Struk and Moss (2009) recommend starting small and focusing on changing attitudes and gaining organization commitment. This means initiating a limited demonstration project, such as instructing nurses in Internet use as it applies to evidence-based practice changes, using informatics content experts as consultants to attract early adopters, and gearing activities toward the organizational strategic plan to gain leadership commitment in order to keep NI "on the radar."

The American Nurses Association (ANA) updated *Nursing Informatics: Scope and Standards of Practice* in 2008. Information on these is available on the ANA website (www.nursingworld.org). The standards address concepts salient to meaningful use and translational science (i.e., how NI impacts health teaching, promotion, and education; quality of practice; research; and resource utilization).

Opportunities for the DNP-APRN exist in many domains of informatics. A few that are readily apparent:

1. Information/systems/technology—educating staff in computer literacy/competency, information literacy, and patient care technology.
2. Consulting as content experts for development of patient care documentation software congruent with nurses' workflow and the nursing process; translational scientist.
3. Transformation of health care:
   a. Quality—software development of documentation tools that are derived from evidence-based practice guidelines; use of clinical decision support tools.
   b. Outcomes management—use of performance data that are population based to compare patients' outcomes in order to identify opportunities for improvement.
   c. Meaningful use—lead change as advocates for adoption of HIT; conduct implementation projects in practices at the beginning of incorporation of EMRs; engage and educate patients in their electronic personal health information; apply for funding to support small and rural practices' achievement of technology capability.
   d. Research on all aspects of HIT and patient-centered technology. The author of this chapter believes that paramount is the need to understand how the integration of HIT and patient care technology impacts the amount of time the professional nurse has for direct care of each patient. Few, if any, of the technological advances within the nursing care of patients are intended as time- or labor-saving devices; they are meant to lead to safe patient care.

Conclusion

What is the emerging image of the nurse clinician? He or she will be certified competent in computer, information, and informatics technology. The nurse clinician's day will begin with an electronic overview of each patient's treatment plan. In a technology-rich environment, nurses will have wireless communication devices for instant contact with other members of the healthcare team. For bedside nurses, portable computer stations will be situated within steps of their patients, supplemented by laptop computers on rolling stands, and they will be used for documentation, data collection on patient outcomes, and dispensing of medications using bar-coding technology. Supplies for the patients' care (dressings, linen, etc.) will be stored in closets that open to the room and the corridor; assistive personnel will stock these "nurse-servers" and track inventory with hand-held bar-coding devices. Each day will bring the capacity for face-to-face follow-up with patients in their homes using *telehealth* networks, as well as live and Web-based educational opportunities. Moving patients safely will involve such devices as inflatable transfer mats placed under patients as they travel from their unit, to x-ray, and to procedures, which will replace the multiple-staff manual lift. For example, after hip surgery, patients will begin near immediate rehabilitation using ceiling-based lifts with walking slings, eliminating the fear of falling and the pain that initial weight-bearing brings. The work area will be less noisy as phones and call-bell systems give way to wireless devices. In addition, wireless tools will transmit vital signs and other monitoring modalities directly into the computer-based medical record, eliminating the need for transcription of data and the potential errors associated with redundant and/or manual documentation. Throughout each nurse's shift, workload and staffing data will be monitored and staffing levels adjusted accordingly. Throughout the day, as a result of careful resourcing and maintenance of the tools used and ongoing education of end users, nurses will have more time for direct patient care, thus decreasing the possibility for *nursing-sensitive adverse events*.

For APRNs, many of the same tools will augment their provision of services; faced with challenging patient care issues, the DNP-APRN can access the DSS for clinical pathways and best practices and collect outcomes data for improving patient care. All of this is available now, with the goal of widespread adaptation by 2015. APRNs must be familiar with all forms of patient care technology because the APRN both oversees and provides direct patient care. For the APRN working within the VA, all aspects of meaningful use are part of everyday practice. **Figure 4-2** shows the first screen that the NP sees once he or she is logged on to the secure EMR site and selects a patient.

Across the top of the screen, the NP has options for File, Edit, View, Tools, and Help. Under Tools, the NP can do such things as access medication information, view actual x-rays, access clinical references, and develop graphs of lab results, to note a few options. On the next band,

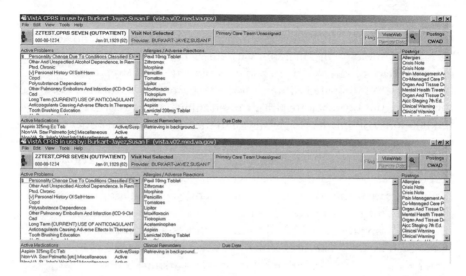

Figure 4-2 Opening Screen of a Patient Record in the Department of Veterans Affairs Computerized Patient Record-Keeping System
U.S. Department of Veterans Affairs.

the NP can access the patient demographics, add "flags" to the chart for acute health conditions, add allergy information, access other VA systems for remote data, and look at "clinical reminders"—primary-care-based interventions due at the time of the patient's visit (e.g., preventive health screenings, immunizations, and so on). The next bar shows the problem list (to expedite finding primary documentation, clicking on the problem shows when the diagnosis was first made and by whom), a list of documented allergies, and a list of flags. The next bar shows the medication list for reconciliation, and the clinical reminders due. The next bar shows the most recent lab work ordered, the most recent vital signs, and a list of clinical appointments. By clicking on the individual vital sign, the NP can view a graph over time for trends. Next are the chart tabs, where the content is stored and where documentation occurs. All services are entered and recorded electronically.

On the bottom of the screen, the NP can access the VA intranet, which has direct links to library references, literature search engines, clinical guidelines/pathways, and clinical data (for nurses, this includes veterans affairs nursing outcome data [VANOD]-VA).

How, then, to prepare for this impending future? The NP should achieve basic computer literacy with such products as the ECDL/ICDL, basic information competency using such resources as the American Library Association website, and basic informatics competency through any distance learning website, and begin exploring the use of OM in daily processes. All of these can be obtained through self-study while awaiting the redesign of nursing curriculum. Early training and adaption to technology, although not without risk, will improve each patient's receipt of safe, efficient, and effective care.

For the DNP-prepared APRN, information, computer, and technological literacy and competency are already essential in daily practice. The quality and quantity of information available to the healthcare consumer and provider continue to expand. Knowing how to provide the right care, the right way, with the right outcome is no longer sufficient. Patients are no longer apt to be passive recipients of healthcare services. The DNP must be able to communicate with these patients using technology and information-based platforms, including telehealth, e-mail, Web-based health education, and EBM. As hospitalists, DNP-APRNs must understand the time burdens associated with patient care technology when implementing plans of care and balance innovation with insight into the nursing process.

References

American Association of Colleges of Nursing. (2006, October). *The essentials of doctoral education for advanced nursing practice.* Washington, DC: Author. Retrieved from http://www.aacn.nche.edu/DNP/pdf/Essentials.pdf

American Nurses Association. (2008). *Nursing informatics: Scope and standards of practice.* Silver Spring, MD: Springhouse.

Berwick, D. (2003). Disseminating innovations in health care. *Journal of the American Medical Association, 289*(15), 1969–1975.

Berwick, D., Roessner, J., & Godfrey, A. B. (1991). *Curing health care: New strategies for quality improvement.* San Francisco, CA: Jossey-Bass.

Burkart-Jayez, S., & Spath, D. (2008). *Research protocol: Research collaborative: Examining the connection between patient care, nursing sensitive adverse events, and environment of care intensity.* AONE seed grant.

Charles, R. (2008, December). Making the most of EBM: Evidence-based medicine moves forward with clinical decision support (Decision Support/EBM). *Health Management Technology, 29*(12), 22–23.

Clancy, C. M. (2005, September 9). *Health information technology and the "quality movement."* Second Health IT Summit. Washington, DC: Agency for Healthcare Research and Quality. Retrieved from http://archive.ahrq.gov/news/sp090905

Eley, R., Fallon, T., Soar, J., Buikstra, E., & Hegney, D. (2008, October). The status of training and education in information and computer technology of Australian nurses: A national survey. *Journal of Clinical Nursing, 2758*(10), 17–20.

Fetter, M. S. (2009). Curriculum strategies to improve baccalaureate nursing information technology outcomes. *Journal of Nursing Education, 48*(2), 78–85.

Goldstein, M. M., & Blumenthal, D. (2008). Building an information technology infrastructure. *Journal of Law, Medicine & Ethics, 36*(4), 709–715.

Houston, S. (1996). Getting started in outcomes research. *AACN Clinical Issues, 7*(1), 146–153.

International Medical Informatics Association. (2009). *Special interest group on nursing informatics.* Retrieved from http://www.amia.org

The Joint Commission. (2008, December 11). *Safely implementing health information and converging technologies* (Issue Brief No. 42, p. 1). Retrieved from http://www.jointcommission.org/assets/1/18/SEA_42.PDF

Jones, J. R. (2005, November 16). Driving the information highway: The NHS IT strategy is an opportunity for nurses to get ahead of the game. *Nursing Standard, 70*(2), 70.

Kingsley, K. V., & Kingsley, K. (2009). A case study for teaching information literacy skills. *BMC Medical Education, 9*, 7.

Kirkley, D. (2004, June). Clinical IT: Powering up data analysis for the nurse executive [Data analysis to inform executive decision making: EMRs and other CIS functionality provide the hard data needed to guide these types of high-level decisions]. *Nursing Economic$, 22*(3), 147–156.

Koivunen, M., Valimaki, M., Jakobsson, T., & Pitkanen, A. (2008, September). Developing an evidence-based curriculum designed to help psychiatric nurses learn to use computers and the Internet. *Journal of Professional Nursing, 24*(5), 302–314.

Kolbasuk McGee, M. (2009, February 11). Stimulus bill will stimulate health IT adoption, jobs. *Information Week, 1.* Retrieved from http://www.information week.com/healthcare/stimulus-bill-will-stimulate-health-it-adoption-jobs/d/d-id/1076541

Kossman, S. P., & Scheidenhelm, S. L. (2008, March/April). Nurses' perceptions of the impact of electronic health records on work and patient outcomes. *CIN: Computers, Informatics, Nursing, 26*(2), 69–77.

Lee, T. T. (2007, March/April). Patients' perceptions of nurses' bedside use of PDAs. *CIN: Computers, Informatics, Nursing, 25*(2), 106–111.

Lin, J. S., Lin, K. C., Jiang, W. W., & Lee, T. T. (2007). An exploration of nursing informatics competency and satisfaction related to network education. *Journal of Nursing Research, 15*(1), 54–65.

McNeil, B. J., Elfrink, V. L., Bickford, C. J., Pierce, S. T., Beyea, S. C., Averill, C., & Klappenbach, C. (2003, August). Nursing information technology knowledge, skills, and preparation of student nurses, nursing faculty, and clinicians: A U.S. survey. *Journal of Nursing Education, 42*(8), 341–349.

National Center for Nursing Research. (1993). Report by Pillar and Golumbic: Secondary citation in Thede work, p. 192.

National League for Nursing. (2008, May 9). *Preparing the next generation of nurses to practice in a technology-rich environment: An informatics agenda* (Position statement). Retrieved from http://www.nln.org/docs/default-source/professional-development-programs/preparing-the-next-generation-of-nurses.pdf?sfvrsn=6

Office of the National Coordinator for Health Information Technology. (2011). *Federal health information technology strategic plan* (pp. 4–18). Retrieved from http://www.DHHS.gov

Ornes, L. L., & Gassert, C. (2007, February). Computer competencies in a BSN program. *Journal of Nursing Education, 46*(2), 75–78.

Page, A. (Ed.). (2004). *Keeping patients safe. Transforming the work environment of nurses.* Washington, DC: National Academies Press.

Powell-Cope, G., Nelson, A. L., & Patterson, E. S. (2008, March). Patient care technology and safety. In R. G. Hughes (Ed.), *Patient safety and quality: An evidence-based handbook for nurses* (Prepared with support from the Robert Wood Johnson Foundation). AHRQ Publication No. 08-0043. Rockville, MD: Agency for Healthcare Research and Quality.

Ridge, R. (2011, June). Future of nursing special: Practicing to potential. *Nursing Management, 42*(6), 32–37.

Sensmeier, J. (2007, May/June). Survey demonstrates importance of nurse informaticist role in health information technology design and implementation. *CIN: Computers, Informatics, Nursing, 25*(3), 180–182.

Simpson, R. L. (2009, March). The softer side of technology: How IT helps nursing care. *Nursing Administration Quarterly, 28*(4), 302–305.

Staggers, N., Gassert, C. A., & Curran, C. (2002, November/December). A Delphi study to determine informatics competencies for nurses at four levels of practice. *Nursing Research, 51*(6), 383–390.

Struk, C., & Moss, J. (2009, May/June). Focus on technology: What can you do to move the vision forward? *CIN: Computers, Informatics, Nursing, 27*(3), 192–194.

Thede, L. Q., Allen, M., & Pierce, S. T. (2003). *Informatics and nursing: Opportunities and challenges* (2nd ed.). Philadelphia, PA: Lippincott Williams & Wilkins.

The TIGER Initiative. (2009). *Technology Informatics Guiding Education Reform.* Retrieved from http://thetigerinitiative.org/docs/TigerReport_Informatics Competencies_000.pdf

Westra, B. (2011, June). HITECH University-based training. *CIN: Computers, Informatics, Nursing, 29*(4), 263–264.

Wojner, A. W. (2001). *Outcomes management: Applications to clinical practice.* St. Louis, MO: Mosby.

Zerhouni, E. (2005). Translational and clinical science—Time for a new vision. *New England Journal of Medicine, 353,* 1621–1623.

Zytowski, M. (2003, August). Nursing informatics: The key to unlocking contemporary nursing practice. *Advanced Practice in Acute and Critical Care, 14*(3), 271–281.

Research Protocol: Research Collaborative: Examining the Connection Between Patient Care, Nursing-Sensitive Adverse Events, and Environment of Care Intensity*

Susan F. Burkart-Jayez and Deborah Spath

The facility in which the project occurred experienced the nursing-sensitive adverse events (NSAE) common to all healthcare facilities: medication errors, falls, decubitus, and unanticipated deaths.

An intensity factor (IF) of the nursing units' workload was calibrated for each unit, based on historical workload data, as a measure of activity within a patient care unit as a whole (see **Table A-1**). Initially developed by others as a tool for calculating gaps in staffing strength, an earlier project by the principal investigator used this factor: findings from the project held promise for being used to forecast and avert work environment conditions conducive to NSAE.

The project objectives were:

1. To measure the distribution of nursing time constraints for direct, indirect, unit-support, and standby activities (with a subset of computer usage tasks for medication administration and all documentation) on a nursing care unit basis, and
2. To analyze known adverse events in the context of the derived IF in order to evaluate for the existence of a relationship not yet described in nursing literature.

*The material presented does not represent the Department of Veterans Affairs, Veterans Health Administration, or the Samuel S. Stratton Veterans Administration Medical Center. The project was funded by the American Organization of Nurse Executives (AONE) through the support of the Albany Research Institute.

Table A-1 Calculation of Unit- and Facility-Specific Intensity Factors

Unit	Benchmark Range of ADT/Month*	Range of ADT for 24 Months by Nursing Unit	Average ADT for 24 Months by Nursing Unit	Low 1	Average 2	High 3	Critical 4	Average Intensity Factor (IF) for Project Interval	Average Nominal Value for Project Interval
Intensive care	85–98	81–143	112	23–71	72–119	120–167	>168	1.59	3
Acute care—7B	50–55	206–238	238	14–42	43–71	72–101	>101	1.45	4
Acute care—8B	50–55	158–259	104	14–42	43–71	72–101	>101	1.38	4

ADC = average daily census
ADT (per 24 hour period) = admissions + discharges + transfers
IF = intensity factor = ADT + ADC/ADC
Low-Average-High-Critical: unit values using industry standard as pivot point for quartile averages
*After Couvaras, 2001

Developed in collaboration with Kate Toms, PhD. For inclusion in Burkart-Jayez, S. (2004). *Nursing competency assessment and outcomes management* (Unpublished doctoral dissertation). Rush College of Nursing, Chicago, IL.

Significance of the Project

Healthcare quality research supports that 27% of nursing time spent in direct care is the lower limit necessary to positively impact NSAE. In linking processes and outcomes, such as workflow and NSAE, we can identify what needs to change and how, and what happens as a result of factor modification. This protocol is an example of outcomes management (OM): data pertaining to workload, nurses' time obligations in the direct care setting, and NSAE were analyzed for opportunities in improving patient outcomes, using both qualitative and quantitative data. Currently, the institution uses the root cause analysis (RCA) methodology to look at events with serious patient care impact. The teams are clinically based, can range from three to eight members, and take 49 to more than 100 hours cumulatively. The average salary at the institution for nursing was $37/hour at the time of calculation (the first three-quarters of fiscal year 2003). Given the diverse composition of the teams, this figure is a fair estimate of hourly costs. All figures are estimates, based on existent data, and represent the cost of the least possible scenario (Burkart-Jayez, 2004). The sample cost of current activities for monitoring/managing NSAE is shown in **Table A-2** and represents a potential for cost avoidance should an early warning be developed for adverse patient outcomes. Simply put, the figures calculated for the monitoring events without OM can be viewed as "the cost of doing nothing," because monitoring never ends. One intended outcome of this project is the derivation of a mathematical portent of adverse events for evaluation against other, more complex structure issues (such as staff mix, staff education level, and staff expertise) that can be readily analyzed in subsequent studies.

Background

As Buerhaus et al. (1997) proposed, as nurses, we must know what needs to be done or not done, we must know that what requires clinical expertise is occurring, and we must know why we are doing what we are doing. Thus, by defining time utilization at the bedside—using categories of direct care, indirect care, unit support, and "other" activities—the first step toward understanding the facility-specific work environment was taken. This process engaged the bedside nurses in the research process from its inception and fostered ever essential participation in the activities and results that follow.

Perkins, Connerney, and Hastings (2000) described OM as relying on clinical resource management, quantitative and qualitative analyses,

Table A-2 Approximate Cost of Risk Management of Nursing-Sensitive Adverse Events, FY 2003	
Activity	
RCA	$35,834.50
ADE	$88,882.20
Case reviews	$9,800.00
Total estimated review costs	$134,096.70

RCA = root cause analysis: team-based adverse events reviews, calculated from number of staff hours/salary rates in participating on each RCA for FY 2003.
ADE = number of medication errors × % of errors likely to cause harm × recovery cost of harm, FY 2003.
Case reviews = number of patient care charts reviewed by an RN × 2 hours average review time × average facility salary for RN, FY 2003.

From Burkart-Jayez, S. (2004). *Nursing competency assessment and outcomes management* (Unpublished doctoral dissertation). Rush College of Nursing, Chicago, IL.

and indicators that are patient, provider, or organizationally focused. In linking processes and outcomes, such as workflow and NSAE, we can identify what needs to change and how, and what happens because of factor modification. This pilot is an example of OM: inspection of data pertaining to workload, nurses' time obligations in the direct care setting, and NSAE will be analyzed for opportunities in improving patient outcomes, using both qualitative and quantitative data.

Aiken, Sochalski, and Lake (1997); Laschinger, Almost, and Tuer-Hoedes (2003); and Perkins et al. (2000), among others, articulated the linkage between processes and outcomes, organizational attributes and outcomes, and working conditions and outcomes. Aiken et al. suggested that unraveling this linkage between factors and outcomes will create a new understanding of ways to improve quality of patient care and patient-centered outcomes.

Common indicators of NSAE identified in nursing literature include medication errors, intravenous-device-associated infections, and transfusion error rates per thousand bed days of care (BDOC). The National Quality Forum also identified skin breakdown, hospital-acquired urinary tract infections, pneumonia and upper gastrointestinal bleeds, cardiac arrest, falls, length of stay, adverse drug events, patient and family complaints, and surgical wound infections as issues responsive or sensitive to nursing care (see www.qualityforum.org). Factors initially proposed to be analyzed in this project included falls, medication errors, nosocomial infections, decubitus, and mortality. Nosocomial infections are analyzed as a facility annual rate and are compared with annual average IF, BDOC, nursing task, and NSAE rates per thousand BDOC. The additional indicator calculated for this project as a potential risk adjustment is an IF—the "busy"-ness of the nurses' work environment. BDOC captures one patient's journey through the system. An IF shows intensity of the work environment based on each patient's journey; that is, each patient has one BDOC but may have been treated on several nursing care units within one 24-hour interval. For example, a patient with heart disease may be admitted to the emergency department, transferred to the intensive care unit (ICU) for stabilization/observation, transferred to the operating/recovery room for stent placement, and transferred back to the ICU. Once stable, the patient could then be transferred to an acute care nursing ward. In theory, up to five different nursing teams would have provided care to this patient, but the patient would be counted only once in the average daily census (ADC), which is based on the patient's location at midnight. By demonstrating the actual number of patients served in a 24-hour period as a percentage of the ADC on which staffing methods are based, nurse leaders will have an additional tool for illustrating nurse staffing requirements (see Table A-1).

Goals of OM include increasing quality of care and decreasing adverse events. Quality is the degree to which patient care services increase the probability of positive outcomes and reduce the probability of negative outcomes. Care process components of technical, interpersonal, and professional skills contribute to variation in outcome and recognize the provider skill in delivery of care (Houston, 1996).

As noted by Woods (2002), as healthcare professionals, we will be called on more and more to communicate what we are doing to ensure patient safety. This project set out to reduce adverse events in a population of patients through strengthening workload assessment processes and by enumerating core responsibilities for the nursing staff. Inherent in this project was the need to collect, analyze, and interpret data for communication of safety issues to leadership and frontline staff.

Flood (1994) noted that evidence from organizational theory on evaluation suggests that voluntary internal monitoring is most effective in change management because people respond to information about their performance; thus, a self-reporting methodology was used. These processes are related to better quality of care. The nursing leaders at the project's facility want the culture to be one of nursing excellence. They agree with Aiken and colleagues' (1997) position that unraveling the linkage between organization attributes/culture and outcomes can provide significant understanding of ways to improve quality of care and patient outcomes. These leaders supported the proposed project as a tool in linking processes and outcomes: The co-Principal Investigator is the facility associate director for patient and nursing services (nurse executive).

Outcome indicators for patient care efficacy align with organizational features such as nursing surveillance, nurse–clinician communication and collaboration, and the quality of the work environment. Adverse events may be an even more sensitive marker of organizational quality than other types of performance measures such as cost, length of stay, and patient satisfaction. For example, mortality rates are associated with organizational processes such as communication. The greater the degree of reciprocal interdependence (exchange of time, expertise, and resources), the greater the effect on outcomes (Mitchell & Shortell, 1997). Some of the factors that Mitchell and Shortell cited include technology, RN-to-patient ratio (nurse staffing intensity), professional expertise (competency, skill mix), professional influences (autonomy), and collaboration and coordination of care—all facets of nursing's domain (Mitchell & Shortell, 1997).

A subset of mortality data, failure to rescue (FTR), described in Agency for Healthcare Research and Quality (AHRQ) (2003) "as preventable death related to complications of hospitalization" and "the key indicator of quality of professional care," was collected through the PI's review of charts of patients who died during the interval studied. FTR has limitations as an indicator of quality. One limitation is the variation in definition of FTR. Dr. Lucian Leape of the Harvard School of Public Health proposed conservatively that 1 in 25 patients (4%) are harmed by errors and that an overall increase in deaths comes almost entirely from adding FTR (AHRQ, 2003). Dr. Leape described FTR as a delay in recognizing and intervening on behalf of a patient who becomes suddenly ill. As part of the second objective, examination of all NSAE identified to date and mortality data, coupled with analysis of workload, may produce tools for continued event avoidance.

Project

Following expedited review and approval of the proposal by the facility's institutional review board (IRB), the PI met with nursing staff on each unit to explain the project. Common activities specific to a unit's provision of nursing care and services were identified and determined to be one of four categories, based on nursing literature: direct care, indirect care, unit support, and standby time. The nursing staff self-assessed/recorded their activities for aggregation using a paper workload collection tool (see **Figure A-1**). In the cases in which a staff nurse was more comfortable being assessed by an observer logging his or her activities, the staff nurse was observed by the PI. As the project continued, nurses initially committed to data collection found that participation was an additional time constraint; therefore, it was necessary for the PI to capture data to complete the baseline. Data were collected three times for each shift for all acute care units—two medical-surgical units and the ICU. The data were anonymously aggregated into direct care, indirect care, unit support, and "other" categories, and a subset of computer-based tasks, producing a profile of the patient care environment in real time. Concurrently, data collected from multiple databases of workload proxies included:

1. ADC: measured as the number of patients present within a facility at midnight, by unit.
2. Mortality data were retrieved from the Automated Medical Information System (AMIS) and converted to a rate per thousand BDOC.
3. Nosocomial events (infections, decubitus formation) were to be extracted from secondary diagnoses at discharge as a function of date and location only; because of coder-staffing limitations, the only readily accessible information was for skin ulcer and infection rates.

Data for the latter were examined for fiscal year (FY) 2005 through FY 2006 (October 1, 2004, through September 30, 2006) as a baseline. All the data were received as an anonymous aggregate from primary sources.

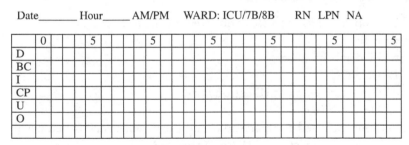

Date_____ Hour_____ AM/PM   WARD: ICU/7B/8B   RN LPN NA

NB: Actual tool has 12 5-minute marks across face, and is double sided=2 hours of time
D= Direct: Admission, assessment, VS, crisis, IV care, transfusions, ADL care, discharge, skills requiring scope of practice/competency assessment, teaching (family/patient), procedures
BC= BCMA
I= Indirect: Report, MD rounds, documentation, patient classification, care plan, narcotic counts
CP= CPRS/any computer use
U= Unit-Support: Transport, supplies, audits, empty/stock lined, wait, food trays, "down time," errands off of unit
O= Other: Committee/staff meetings, personal time, breaks, personal phone calls

Figure A-1 Workload Collection Tool
From Burkart-Jayez, S. (2004). *Nursing competency assessment and outcomes management* (Unpublished doctoral dissertation). Rush College of Nursing, Chicago, IL.

Neither individual patients nor individual employees were identifiable from the data sets used because the sole purpose was to identify trends.

The admission-discharge-transfer (ADT) factor was used to calculate an IF and was also transformed into a nominal/quantitative set of low, average, high, and critical levels. This manipulation has been used in the prior work of the PI and yields information reflecting the intensity of the environment in which nurses work (see Table A-1).

The invasion of privacy of individual patients and employees was assessed as being of minimal risk. Data received by the PI had no patient identifiers, only anonymous aggregate numbers by category of occurrence, date, and patient care location. Only the PI and co-PI had access to data collected for the study prior to analysis. The physical security of all information was safeguarded. Computer access codes were not shared, and the workstation for data storage was locked when not in use and located in a locked office. Data were backed up on floppy discs and stored in a locking file cabinet within the PI's locked office.

The project took place at a tertiary care facility with 53 acute care (10 ICU), 50 long-term care, and 10 acute behavioral care beds. The scope of the project initially included all inpatient units but was reduced to examining the acute care units in order to facilitate project progress and completion.

Data Collection Activities

1. Pearson correlations were conducted for the following:
   a. Falls
   b. Medication errors
   c. Ulcers
   d. Operator-related medication errors
   e. Deaths/FTRs

Manipulations included comparison of indicators with each other, with BDOC, and with the calculated IF (see **Table A-3**).

2. Nursing time obligations were collected for:
   a. Direct care
   b. Indirect care
   c. Unit support
   d. Other
      i. Computerized Patient Record System (CPRS)/all computer time except *bar coding medication administration (BCMA)*, and
      ii. BCMA use

These are demonstrated in **Table A-4**.

Table A-3 Pearson Correlation of Indicators Evaluated for Nursing-Sensitive Adverse Events and Novel Intensity Factor Calculated as a Function of Average Daily Census Plus Average Daily Admissions, Discharges, and Transfers

Correlations

		ADC+TO/A	Total Med Error Rate/ Thousand BDOC	Rate of Reported Falls/ Thousand BDOC	Rate of All Reported Skin Ulcers/ Thousand BDOC	FTR/ Thousand BDOC	Rate of Death/ Thousand BDOC
ADC+TO/ ADC	Pearson Correlation	1	.099	-.541	.250*	.000	.511**
	Sig. (2-tailed)		.408	.000	.034	.999	.000
	N	72	72	72	72	72	72
Total med error rate/ thousand BDOC	Pearson Correlation	.099	1	-.068	.044	.035	-.035
	Sig. (2-tailed)	.408		.568	.715	.770	.770
	N	72	72	72	72	72	72
Rate of reported falls/ thousand BDOC	Pearson Correlation	-.541	-.068	1	-.182	.050	-.386**
	Sig. (2-tailed)	.000	.568		.125	.678	.001
	N	72	72	72	72	72	72
Rate of all reported skin ulcers/ thousand BDOC	Pearson Correlation	.250*	.044	-.182	1	.291*	.115
	Sig. (2-tailed)	.034	.715	.125		.013	.338
	N	72	72	72	72	72	72

Table A-3 Pearson Correlation of Indicators Evaluated for Nursing-Sensitive Adverse Events and Novel Intensity Factor Calculated as a Function of Average Daily Census Plus Average Daily Admissions, Discharges, and Transfers *(continued)*

Correlations

		ADC+TO/A	Total Med Error Rate/ Thousand BDOC	Rate of Reported Falls/ Thousand BDOC	Rate of All Reported Skin Ulcers/ Thousand BDOC	FTR/ Thousand BDOC	Rate of Death/ Thousand BDOC
FTR/ thousand BDOC	Pearson Correlation	.000	.035	.050	.291*	1	.276*
	Sig. (2-tailed)	.999	.770	.678	.013		.019
	N	72	72	72	72	72	72
Rate of death/ thousand BDOC	Pearson Correlation	.511**	-0.35	-.386**	.115	.276*	1
	Sig. (2-tailed)	.000	.770	.001	.338	.019	
	N	72	72	72	72	72	72

Note: Bed Days of Care (BDOC)
**Correlation is significant at the 0.01 level (2-tailed).
* Correlation is significant at the 0.05 level (2-tailed).

Table A-4 Comparison of Nursing Time-Task Categories in Minutes

Unit	BDMA	Direct	Indirect	Computer	Unit Support	Other	Total
8B	561	1545	811	1160	456	518	5051
	11.11%	30.59%	16.06%	22.97%	9.03%	10.26%	
7B	1293	1602	453	947	787	347	5429
	23.82%	29.51%	8.34%	17.44%	14.50%	6.39%	
ICU	1068	1274	749	1060	92	339	4782
	22.33%	26.64%	15.66%	22.17%	6.11%	7.09%	

From Burkart-Jayez, S. (2004). *Nursing competency assessment and outcomes management* (Unpublished doctoral dissertation). Rush College of Nursing, Chicago, IL.

Findings

Summary of Time Analysis

1. Overall, with the exception of BCMA time, nursing reported times are similar, with near identical graphs as evidenced in the Unit Comparison line graph (see Table 4-6 and **Figure A-2**).
2. Direct patient care time recorded ranged from 26.6% to 30.6%; literature cites 27% as the point at which NSAEs are more likely than not to occur. Nurses' time with their patients is at the near minimum level for uneventful care.
3. The predicted "down time" (other) is 10.4% (based on contract-defined rest breaks), yet nurses report only 7.9% other (breaks, lunch periods, in-services). Nurses invested more time each shift and still could not exceed 30% direct patient care time.
4. Time spent on technology-based tasks approached 39.9%. This is significant in that staffing models are based on patient acuity and volume and do not take into account the time dedicated to technological adaptations for standard nursing tasks (medication administration and documentation within an electronic medical record). Thus, nurse-to-patient staffing ratios are underestimated by up to 39.9%.
5. Unit support time (activities requiring no nursing education/licensure) averaged 10.1%. Delegation of such activities would thus return 10.1% of nursing time to patient-centered activities.

Evaluation of Time Analysis

1. A more precise method of analyzing nursing time spent on technology-based activities would support the reported time. One method would involve running file reports for both BCMA and CPRS use time. The total staffing available for each shift reported could then be used to calculate the exact amount of available nursing time spent on these tasks.
2. Identification of recurring nonnursing tasks would lend itself to shifting such work to alternate staff resources.
3. Although initially proposed as a time study, it will be useful to analyze the time totals in comparison with adverse event rates at the unit/shift level.

Unit Comparisons-Nursing Time

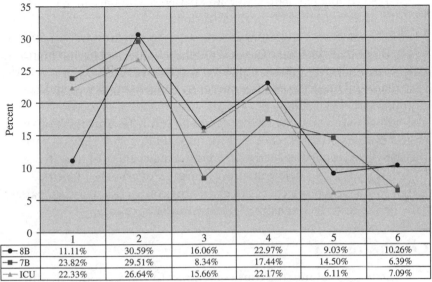

	1	2	3	4	5	6
●— 8B	11.11%	30.59%	16.06%	22.97%	9.03%	10.26%
■— 7B	23.82%	29.51%	8.34%	17.44%	14.50%	6.39%
▲— ICU	22.33%	26.64%	15.66%	22.17%	6.11%	7.09%

1=BCMA 2=Direct 3=Indirect 4=Computer 5=Unit Support 6=Other

Figure A-2 Comparison of Three Acute Patient Care Units for Self-Reported Time-Task Commitments Showing Similar Distribution Across Diverse Patient Care Populations: Medical/Medical-Surgical and Intensive Care Units
From Burkart-Jayez, S. (2004). *Nursing competency assessment and outcomes management* (Unpublished doctoral dissertation). Rush College of Nursing, Chicago, IL.

Summary of the Connection Between NSAE and IF

These findings suggest that calculation of a unit's IF based on "real time" unit activity could contribute to quality patient care through informing nursing leadership as to current patient activity and nursing unit workload in development of an overarching nurse staffing model. For example, end-of-shift census and acuity of care as a basis for the number of nursing staff required for the next shift capture one moment in the 8-hour work shift (the total number of patients and their needs "category" at the end of the tour). The acuity of care level is based on 20-plus-year-old measures, in a time of open-ended lengths of stay. Twenty years later, patients whom we would categorize as 1 and perhaps 2 on a 5-point scale would not necessarily meet current admission and length-of-stay criteria. The IF, on the other hand, calculates the actual number of patients served in the same period, taking into account the patients who have been admitted into, transferred into and out of, and discharged from a particular unit, and patients who have met a much more complex standard for hospitalization.

The calculation of an IF may serve as an early warning system: that is, as the IF reaches the high to critical range, patients may be at a higher risk for skin ulcer formation and adverse events contributing to unanticipated death. Quality assurance and/or nursing research would further illuminate these findings.

For now, for one facility's acute care unit and ICUs, information on time, demands on direct care, and the impact of patient flow on patient care have been identified. This information may be useful in staffing level/bed availability determinations. Future work on the identified trends by nursing researchers can clarify the connection between patient care, NSAE, and the intensity of the environment of care.

Conclusion

The distribution of nursing time constraints for direct, indirect, unit-support, and standby activities was calculated for two acute medical-surgical nursing units and one ICU. A "hidden" time commitment, the technology used for documentation and administration of medications, accounted for up to 41% of nurses' time. Nurses continue to provide services that do not require a nurse's education/licensure for up to 11% of their workday. The latter provides an opportunity to shift workload to appropriate ancillary staff, resulting in a relative "professional nurse staffing increase" of 11%. An in-depth analysis of nursing-computer time, using time reports from each computer application, would yield more precise data that are illustrative of the impact of technology on nursing resources allocated for direct care.

As examined in previous work (Burkart-Jayez, 2004), nursing OM requires attention to and intervention focused on the indicators identified in the literature as reflective of quality nursing care: medication errors, infections, transfusion errors, skin breakdown, hospital-acquired urinary tract infections, pneumonia and upper gastrointestinal bleeds, cardiac arrest, falls, length of stay, adverse drug events, patient and family complaints, and surgical wound infection rates per thousand BDOC. The addition of an "outcomes manager"—a nursing clinician dedicated to monitoring all NSAE—would be valuable in examining the occurrence of, and contributing factors to, such events, followed by an intervention/ prevention plan. Such a clinician would be in the position of providing evidence-based guidance to nursing staff. This guidance would enhance the patient care environment and improve access to quality care.

References

Agency for Healthcare Research and Quality. (2003). *Morbidity and mortality rounds on the Web: Current cases and commentaries: Nursing.* Retrieved from http://www.qualityindicators.ahrq.gov

Aiken, L. H., Sochalski, J., & Lake, E. T. (1997). Studying outcomes of organizational change in health services. *Medical Care, 35*(11), NS6–NS18.

Buerhaus, P. I., Clifford, J., Erickson, J. I., Fay, M. S., Miller, J. R., Sporing, E. M., & Weissman, G. K. (1997). Effective nursing leadership: Summary of the Harvard Nursing Research Institute's follow-up conference. *Journal of Nursing Administration, 27*(4), 12–20.

Burkart-Jayez, S. (2004). *Nursing competency assessment and outcomes management* (Unpublished doctoral dissertation). Rush College of Nursing, Chicago, IL.

Couvaras, C. (2001, January). *The impact of admissions, transfers, and discharge on budgeting and scheduling.* Paper presented at the meeting of the Forum on Healthcare Leadership, Philadelphia, PA.

Flood, A. B. (1994). The impact of organizational and managerial factors on the quality of care in health care organizations. *Medical Care Review, 51*(4), 381–428.

Laschinger, H. K., Almost, J., & Tuer-Hoedes, D. (2003). Workplace empowerment and magnet hospital characteristics. *Journal of Nursing Administration, 33*(7–8), 410–422.

Mitchell, P. H., & Shortell, S. M. (1997). Adverse outcomes and variations in organization of care delivery. *Medical Care, 35*(Suppl. 11), NS19–NS32.

Perkins, S. B., Connerney, I., & Hastings, C. E. (2000). Outcomes management: From concepts to application. *AACN Clinical Issues, 11*(3), 339–350.

Woods, D. K. (2002). Realizing your market influence, Part 1. Meeting patient needs through collaboration. *Journal of Nursing Administration, 32*(4), 189–195.

Glossary

Adverse events: Injuries caused by healthcare worker interventions, not due to the patients' healthcare condition: often due to an individual or system error (doing the right thing the wrong way, doing the wrong thing the right way).

Bar coding medication administration (BCMA): Use of a scanner to identify medication to be administered to a patient and ordered in an electronic medical record.

Browse: (1) In database systems, to browse means to view data. Many database systems support a special browse mode, in which you can flip through fields and records quickly. Usually you cannot modify data while you are in browse mode. (2) In object-oriented programming languages, to browse means to examine data structures. (3) To view formatted documents. For example, you look at Web pages with a *Web browser.* "Browse" is often used interchangeably with "surf."

Computer competency: The ability to demonstrate proficiency in use of software applications such as Microsoft Word, Excel, and PowerPoint, and knowledge in computer terminology, hardware selection, and simple maintenance functions.

Computer information system (CIS): A computer system that usually includes an online decision support system, clinical documentation, care planning, and computerized physician order entry. The core nursing functions of such systems include results reporting, clinical documentation, medication charting, patient assessments, and performance reports.

Computer literacy: The level of expertise and familiarity someone has with computers. Computer literacy generally refers to the ability to use applications rather than to program. Individuals who are very computer literate are sometimes called power users.

Computerized physician order entry (CPOE): Use of a software application for the ordering of medications, laboratory/radiology testing, consultation, and referral requests. The CPOE is the electronic replacement for paper prescriptions and written/verbal orders in both the inpatient and outpatient setting and is cited as an important tool in avoidance of medical errors and provision of patient safety.

Data: (1) Distinct pieces of information, usually formatted in a special way. All software is divided into two general categories: data and programs. Programs are collections of instructions for manipulating data. (2) The term *data* is often used to distinguish binary machine-readable information from textual human-readable information. For example, some applications make a distinction between data files (files that contain binary data) and text files (files that contain ASCII data).

Database: An organized collection of information that is easy to maintain, sort, and search (Burke & Weill, 2005).

Electronic health record (EHR): An EHR is a type of healthcare information technology, which is the digital version of the patient's medical file. A fully functional EHR allows recording of patient information and demographics, results viewing and management, order entry management (including e-prescribing), and clinical decision support. A minimally functional EHR lacks full order entry capabilities and clinical decision support. Also known as an electronic medical record (EMR).

Electronic medical record (EMR): See *electronic health record (EHR)*.

Evidence-based medicine (EBM) (see also evidence-based practice): Integration of the best available evidence from the scientific literature with clinical judgment and expertise in making healthcare decisions for the individual patient.

Hardware: An object or objects that you can actually touch, such as disks, disk drives, display screens, keyboards, printers, boards, and chips. In contrast, software is untouchable. Software exists as ideas, concepts, and symbols, but it has no substance. Books provide a useful analogy. The pages and the ink are the hardware, whereas the words, sentences, paragraphs, and the overall meaning are the software. A computer without software is like a book full of blank pages—you need software to make the computer useful, just as you need words to make a book meaningful.

Healthcare information technology (HIT): Use of computer hardware and software for the processing, storage, and retrieval of healthcare-related information, including all clinical components of care and administrative data. An example of HIT is the EHR.

Healthcare informatics: The integration of computer science, information science, and health care. Examples of tools in healthcare informatics include clinical guidelines, EHRs, patient care technology devices, and databases of healthcare outcomes.

Informatics: The integration of information and information management with electronic processing and communication technology.

Information literacy: Information literacy is the ability to identify information needed for a specific purpose; to locate pertinent information, evaluate the information, and apply it correctly (Englebardt & Nelson, 2002).

Information technology (IT): The broad subject concerned with all aspects of managing and processing information, especially within a large organization or company. Because computers are central to information management, computer departments within companies and universities are often called IT departments. Some companies refer to this department as IS (information services) or MIS (management information services).

Internet: A global network connecting millions of computers. More than 100 countries are linked into exchanges of data, news, and opinions. Unlike online services, which are centrally controlled, the Internet is decentralized by design. Each Internet computer, called a host, is independent. Its operators can choose which Internet services to use and which local services to make available to the global Internet community. Remarkably, this anarchy by design works exceedingly well.

Nursing-sensitive adverse events (NSAE): Failure to rescue, nosocomial infections, pressure ulcers, falls, medication errors, transfusion errors.

Outcomes management (OM): The use of aggregate variance data to change a system of healthcare practices, where variance is any event that alters patient progress toward the expected outcome. Sources of variance include practitioner behavior (competency), the severity of illness (as with high-risk patients), and practice patterns that either expedite care or inhibit delivery of care (Houston, 1996).

Software: Anything that can be stored electronically. Software is often divided into two categories: systems software, which includes the *operating system* and all the utilities that enable the computer to function, and applications software, which includes programs that do real work for users, such as word processors, spreadsheets, and *database management systems*.

Technology: (1) (a) The application of science, especially to industrial or commercial objectives. (b) The scientific method and material used to achieve a commercial or industrial objective. (2) Electronic or digital products and systems considered as a group. (3) Anthropology. The body of knowledge available to a society that is of use in fashioning implements, practicing manual arts and skills, and extracting or collecting materials.

Telehealth: Telemedicine and other health-related activities using telecommunication lines and computers, including education, research, public health, and administration of health services (Burke & Weill, 2005).

Web browser: See *browse*.

Websites: Files in which information on the Web is stored (Burke & Weill, 2005).

World Wide Web (Web or WWW): The part of the Internet that is most accessible and easiest to navigate, organized as sites with hyperlinks to one another (Burke & Weill, 2005).

References

Burke, L., & Weill, B. (2005). *Information technology for the health professions* (2nd ed.). Upper Saddle River, NJ: Pearson/Prentice Hall.

Englebardt, E. P., & Nelson, R. (2002). *Health care informatics: An interdisciplinary approach.* St. Louis, MO: Mosby.

Chapter 5

Healthcare Policy for Advocacy in Health Care

Angela Mund

> *There are three critical ingredients to democratic renewal and progressive change in America: good public policy, grassroots organizing and electoral politics.*
>
> —Paul Wellstone

Introduction

In 2001, the Institute of Medicine (IOM) challenged all healthcare professionals to improve the quality of patient care, with an emphasis on increasing its safety, effectiveness, efficiency, equitability, timeliness, and patient centeredness (IOM, 2001). With the release of the IOM report, "The Future of Nursing: Leading Change, Advancing Health" (IOM, 2011), nurses are tasked with being active partners in this transformation of health care. However, advanced practice registered nurses (APRNs) continue to be encumbered by scope of practice restrictions and challenges to obtaining parity in reimbursement. These barriers can be removed through political advocacy. In addition, to create widespread change in the delivery of health care and in the structure of America's health systems, policies supporting quality improvement must be researched, developed, funded, and implemented. The complexity of today's healthcare environment and the increase in volume of scientific knowledge demand the involvement of nurses educated in the legislative process and prepared to influence policy on the local, state, and national levels.

APRNs have the advantage of an appreciation of the patient care experience and the challenges of working within complex healthcare systems. According to Lyttle (2011), "Nurses in political office are also likely to do exactly what they've been doing in health care settings for years: adjust and adapt to ever-changing situations; listen carefully; gather facts; and discern, decide, and deal thoughtfully with unexpected outcomes and turns of events" (p. 19).

However, those unique experiences must be combined with an education in the intricacies of policy and politics in order to create true and effective change. Policy activism translates into patient advocacy. In 1992, Ham described five basic elements critical to understanding the inherent complexity of policy. These elements are just as relevant today and include the following concepts:

1. Reviewing policies includes studying formal decisions and actions.
2. A policy may include a network of interacting decisions rather than a single decision.
3. Policies change over time.
4. Policies that were not acted on should also be included when reviewing policymaking.
5. It is important to identify the policies that were created out of clear decision-making and to use that information to develop an effective process of policy making. (Hewison, 1999, p. 1378)

During the creation of the American Association of Colleges of Nursing's (AACN) *Essentials of Doctoral Education for Advanced Nursing Practice*, the AACN recognized and supported the integral relationship between policy and practice. Therefore, the AACN included the curricular requirement of instruction in "health care policy for advocacy in health care" in the *Essentials* (AACN, 2006). According to the AACN, doctorally educated nurses will have the tools to engage in and serve as leaders in the development and implementation of healthcare policy that affects financing, *regulation*, quality improvement, and equitable access to health care.

In 2000, Rains and Carroll asserted that there has never been a greater need for nurses to be involved in the political process in order to ensure the best use of shrinking resources, to provide affordable health care for all, and to advocate for changes in healthcare policy. Although nurses are increasingly being recognized as leaders in U.S. regulatory agencies, from Marilyn Tavenner, former administrator of the Centers for Medicare and Medicaid Services (CMS), to Mary Wakefield, current administrator of the Health Resources and Services Administration (HRSA), nurses continue to be underrepresented in the legislative arena. In the 114th United States Congress, nurses make up less than 1% of the total members.

The ability to effectively engage in influencing policy can be created by obtaining an understanding of the foundations of nursing policy, the elements of the political process, and the relationship between leadership and policy making. APRNs can be at the forefront of changing the system of healthcare delivery in the United States by shaping local and legislative decision-making processes.

History of the Relationship Between Nursing and Policy Making

The integration of nursing and policy is not a new concept. During the Crimean War, Florence Nightingale recognized the connection between policies made by Parliament and the British soldiers' poor living conditions (Ennen, 2001). Nurses' policy involvement has waxed and waned since the 19th century, when Nightingale exerted influence on the public policies of sanitation and infection control practices. There was a lack of political interest and influence in the early 20th century (Milstead, 2008, p. 2). After a few decades of silence, individual nurse leaders such as Lillian Wald and Lavina Dock spoke up and publically supported suffrage, women's rights, nursing licensure, and the right to health care (Rubotzky, 2000). Nursing as a collective field, however, did not speak out on the issues. In 1985, Huston described several factors explaining nurses' lack of political involvement, including the "socialization to view power and politics negatively and the invisibility of nurses in the media" (Rains & Carroll, 2000, p. 37). From the 1970s through the 1990s, nurses were gaining in the areas of nursing science and education, use of technological knowledge and clinical skills, and in the creation of a new paradigm of advanced practice nursing. APRNs were now confronted with understanding the political and practice implications of state and national legislation and with creating policies that supported the continued advancement of the profession.

During the 1970s, the Department of Health, Education, and Welfare created the Committee to Study Extended Roles for Nurses. This committee recommended further studies on cost-benefit analysis and attitudes toward the use of APRNs and recommended increased federal funding for nurse practitioners (NPs) (Hamric, Spross, & Hanson, 2000). The 1970s also brought battles over prescriptive authority, the right for APRNs to use the word "diagnose," and the right to directly bill Medicare for nurse anesthesia services (Hamric et al., 2000). The 1980s brought the concepts of cost containment and diagnosis-related groups and the associated legislation that would have an impact on APRN practice. NPs and nurse anesthetists encouraged lawmakers and the Health Care Financing Administration, currently the CMS, to create policies and pass legislation concerning reimbursement procedures that would support the profession of advanced practice nursing. In 1989, nurse anesthetists became the first APRN group allowed to obtain direct reimbursement from Medicare for anesthesia services. The passage of this legislation is considered "one of the greatest lobbying achievements not only of the American Association of Nurse Anesthetists (AANA) but of the whole of nursing" (Bankart, 1993, p. 167).

Throughout the 20th century, nursing organizations were created and led by nurses who acknowledged the need for involvement in the policy arena, the necessity of professional leadership, and the importance of strong grassroots efforts by their nurse members. The 1990s were a decade of growth in the numbers of APRNs and of both NP and nurse anesthetist programs. Comprehending the increased complexity of patients and of healthcare systems, APRN educational programs transitioned to requiring a master's-level education for entry to practice. APRN organizations continued to develop a voice, while the American Nurses Association (ANA), realizing the need for access to legislators, moved its headquarters to Washington, D.C. (Hamric et al., 2000; Milstead, 2008).

As we move into the 21st century, nurses and nursing organizations have demonstrated a continued and growing presence in Washington, D.C., in the offices and chambers of Congress and in the meeting rooms of the regulatory agencies. Conflicts over physician supervision, prescriptive authority, scope of practice, equal access to healthcare providers, and the quality, safety, and cost-effectiveness of health care are still being waged at the state and federal levels. These challenges will continue to support the need to educate all nurses in how to become influential in the policy arena. The incorporation of policy into the APRN role and the doctor of nursing practice (DNP) degree requirements is leading to a resurgence of interest in the responsibility of influencing healthcare reform, the promotion of global health, and the protection of the profession.

Influencing the Health Policy Agenda

Public policy is created by governmental legislation and involves laws and regulations. It has been defined as "the purposeful, general plan of action developed to respond to a problem that includes authoritative guidelines" (Sudduth, 2008, p. 171). According to Mason, Leavitt, and Chafee (2002), "Public policy often reflects the value, beliefs and attitudes of those designing the policy" (p. 8). Public policy can be further divided into social policy, which concerns communities, and then into health policy, which focuses on the health of the individual (Mason et al., 2002). The word *politics* has both positive and negative connotations. On one hand, it brings to mind images of corruption, misbehavior, and "politics as usual." However, politics should also have positive undertones as the decision-making process whereby APRNs can influence the development of legislation and the allocation of resources. As APRNs are increasingly becoming empowered to engage in the process of transforming health care, they must be actively engaged in influencing the health policy agenda. A potential avenue to effect change in health policy is for APRNs to author a policy brief. Nurses have the public's trust as well as the education and healthcare expertise to provide credible information to legislators and regulatory agencies. The purpose of a health policy brief is to provide background and to propose a solution to an issue facing a person or a group that does not have a background in health care. A policy brief can be defined as a brief report that addresses the interests and needs of policy makers though application of best evidence in an effort to produce a solution to a problem (DeMarco & Tufts, 2014). See **Table 5-1** for considerations on developing a policy brief.

DNP graduates are well positioned to influence the content and quality of healthcare legislation. Along with their extensive clinical

---

Table 5-1 Considerations for the Development of a Policy Brief

- Make it brief and understandable for a non–healthcare provider audience.
  - Know your audience and what problem they are interested in solving.
  - The brief should be no longer than 4 pages.
- A typical format consists of four sections: an executive summary; background and significance; statement of the author's position; and a reputable reference list.
- Determine the most efficacious timing for submitting the brief.
  - A sense of urgency is a powerful motivator in seeking solutions.
- Provide a convincing argument through a systematic review of the literature.
  - Advocate for a desired solution based on the information.
  - Provide data that refute objections to the solution proposed within the brief.
- Demonstrate credibility and expertise in the area of concern.

Modified from DeMarco, R., & Tufts, K. A. (2014). The mechanics of writing a policy brief. *Nursing Outlook, 62,* 219–224.

background and a well-developed comprehension of the issues, APRNs must have a working knowledge of the language of legislation and regulation.

The Process of Legislation

The legislative process is rarely the very linear, rational process described in textbooks. Instead, it is a process whereby competing interests attempt to influence policy making by creating bargains, trading votes, and using rhetoric to convince legislators that their policy agenda is the best. APRNs have the opportunity and responsibility to educate lawmakers as legislation moves through the legislative bodies and government agencies. **Figure 5-1** notes the basic steps of moving a bill through the state or federal process. In the federal policy arena, proposed legislation is called a bill until it is passed by both houses of Congress and signed into law by the president. At the state level, a bill moves via a similar process and is passed by the state legislature and signed into law by the governor.

Although APRNs can draft legislation, it is more common to partner with an interested and supportive legislator in either the state or federal House of Representatives or the Senate. The drafting process may include only a small number of persons or may involve a significant number of interested parties. It will be beneficial at this stage to allow any stakeholder nursing groups to review the language of the proposed legislation. Why is this important? Not all language is viewed the same by all groups, and what may be good for one APRN group may be detrimental to another. The time to find this discrepancy is not during the *hearing*

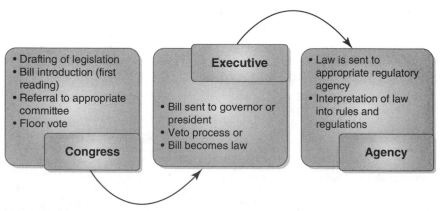

Figure 5-1 Movement of a Bill

phase, when the ability to influence legislation may be limited by time constraints and lack of coalition support.

The greater the political power of the sponsoring legislator, the greater the probability of successfully passing a piece of legislation. The likelihood of successful passing of legislation will also improve if supportive legislators introduce the bill to both chambers of Congress at the same time. Bipartisan support from both Republican and Democratic sponsors further increases the likelihood of successful movement of legislation through Congress. Following the drafting of the legislation, the senator or representative will introduce the proposed legislation to the chamber; the legislation will then be referred to the proper committee, typically based on the recommendation of the sponsoring legislator. The bill is given a number corresponding to the chamber in which it was introduced (e.g., S.252). The details of each bill can be found at www.thomas.gov. The selection of the "proper" committee is based primarily on the appropriateness of the committee but can also be a political decision based on whether members of the committee support or oppose the proposed legislation. In theory, members usually author bills that will be referred to the committees where they have *jurisdiction*. While the legislation is in committee, interested parties and stakeholders may be invited to submit written or oral testimony either supporting or refuting the legislation. The legislation then undergoes a process called *markup* in which the committee debates the legislation, discusses the flaws, and amends the legislation as necessary.

During this process, APRNs should be prepared to serve as content experts while advocating for the profession of nursing and shaping the healthcare agenda. It is imperative at this point to know the "enemies" of your legislation and be able to generate a strategy for managing controversy. Well-prepared testimony includes a description of who is doing the testifying (e.g., a family NP in a rural practice), the background of the issue, and why the legislation is supportive or detrimental in resolving the issue. Effective testimony must also include what the APRN testifying would like the committee to do. Submitting oral testimony may be a stressful situation, but the key to presenting a logical, persuasive report is to prepare in advance. When preparing testimony, it is very important to be able to discuss the issue in great detail, know the influential legislators on the committee, and include the potential impact on patient care.

Once the committee agrees on the content and language of the bill, it is then moved to the Senate or House floor and voted on by the members. The submitting committee must create a report to accompany the bill. The report includes such information as the intent of the legislation, the potential financial implications, dissenting opinions, and amendments to the initial bill. The bill may be referred back to committee, approved, or voted down. Meanwhile, "companion legislation" is introduced in the other chamber of Congress, typically with similar wording; however, rarely is the wording exactly the same. The passage of the original legislation in one chamber encourages the forward movement of the companion legislation in the other chamber. Following the passage of both companion bills, one in the Senate and one in the House, the bill may be moved to a conference committee to work out any differences. The conference committee is composed of both senators and representatives. Both chambers must concur and approve their respective bills prior to the bill passing out of Congress and moving to the executive branch. If the bill does not come out of committee before the end of the legislative session, the bill is dead and must be reintroduced during the following session.

An important role for APRNs during this phase is to contact their representatives or senators and to build coalitions with other professional associations. The importance of creating these relationships prior to the introduction of any legislation will become evident as the bill moves through Congress. Nurses must not wait until the proposed legislation is being voted on—this is too late! Instead, nurses must be involved during the very early stages. Although the emphasis of influencing legislation often lies within the Congress, at the federal level, the executive branch has the power to either veto the legislation or sign it. Again, a similar process occurs at the state level. Another important factor to consider is the power of the office of governor or president in supporting or blocking the legislative effort.

The Process of Regulation

An equally important but maybe more complex segment of policy is regulation. Regulation is the implementation process of legislation and occurs at both the state and federal levels. After a bill is passed through Congress and signed into law by the president, it is sent to a regulatory agency within the government, which then interprets the law and creates the rules and regulations that shape the way the new law is executed. Congress rarely includes explicit directions for implementation within the legislation and in fact may be purposefully vague. Again, stakeholders are invited to comment on the proposed draft of the rules and regulations. It is important not to overlook this phase because a hard-fought battle to produce legislation favorable for nursing may become something completely different during the regulatory process. Conversely, if policy cannot be changed in the legislative arena, APRNs may be able to persuade the regulatory agency to publish rules that are favorable to nursing. This may be a dangerous game to play, because regulations must be consistent with the enabling *statute*. In the event that the regulation is inconsistent with the law, the law supersedes the regulation.

Federal agencies of interest to APRNs include the Department of Health and Human Services, the CMS, the Department of Veterans Affairs, the Indian Health Service, and the armed forces. CMS is the primary agency regulating reimbursement for APRN services, including supervision requirements. Before a regulation is put into effect, two steps must occur. First, the proposed rule is published in the *Federal Register*, and information is included on how the public can participate in the process by providing comment and attending the meetings (Loversidge, 2008). The second step involves the agency considering all the information and deciding on a course of action. The final regulation is then published in the *Federal Register* and becomes effective after 30 days. The *Federal Register* is a daily journal of the government of the United States that contains the public notices of all the government agencies, executive orders, and presidential proclamations. All the information from the *Federal Register* is in the public domain and can be accessed by any APRN at https://www.federalregister.gov/. Many professional organizations have paid staff to monitor the *Federal Register* for regulations that may have an impact on APRNs.

Boards of nursing, medicine, and pharmacy are examples of state regulatory agencies that may create rules and regulations that affect nurses and the delivery of health care within states. These agencies have the power to control entry into the profession, monitor and discipline licensees, and ensure continued competency of licensees (Loversidge, 2008). State agencies obtain their rule-making authority through enabling laws. An enabling law is "one in which the state legislature delegates to an administrative agency the authority to adopt regulations to implement the law's purposes" (Tobin, 2001, p. 113). In essence, enabling laws give regulatory agencies the power to create rules and regulations. APRNs should assist in maintaining a collegial relationship between their state professional organizations and the board of nursing. Most appointments to state boards are made by the governor and necessitate the support of legislators and professional organizations. APRNs must be represented on boards of nursing to monitor the actions of the board and offer recommendations related to advanced nursing practice.

Boards of medicine may attempt to regulate nursing practice through language concerning supervision and collaboration. Therefore, it is advisable for APRNs to be aware of the regulatory agenda of all state boards that may have an interest in limiting APRNs' scope of practice and patient access. This involvement may include having an APRN presence at the board meetings of nursing and nonnursing state boards. When reviewing proposed regulations, it is important to understand the intent of the regulation and evaluate the language of the regulation for possible limits to APRN scope of practice and reimbursement. Other possible avenues to influence the regulatory process include seeking appointment to CMS panels, providing testimony at regulatory hearings, obtaining a position on advisory panels to the National Council of State Boards of Nursing (NCSBN), and agreeing to serve as an APRN expert during drafting of regulatory policy.

The NCSBN is a coalition of state boards of nursing that provides an avenue for state boards to examine regulatory issues and "counsel together on matters of common interest and concern affecting public health safety and welfare," including performing policy analysis, licensure, and research (NCSBN, n.d.). In 2008, the NCSBN partnered with the APRN Consensus Work Group and created the Consensus Model for APRN Regulation. The Consensus Model grew out of a concern that because each state determines the legal scope of practice and the criteria for entry to practice and competence through certification examinations, the ability of APRNs to move between states is limited, and access to health care for patients may decrease. The Consensus Model promotes a uniform regulatory process based on nationally accepted standards for certification, licensure, and practice. All APRN stakeholder professional associations were invited to comment on the proposed Consensus Model. It was essential throughout this process that all APRN groups had a place at the table and were able to discuss concerns with the regulatory language, create a coalition of a wide variety of nursing groups, and generate a model that all the nursing stakeholders could support.

The APRN Model Act on Rules and Regulations was approved by the NCSBN in August 2008 and has slowly gained a foothold in state legislative and regulatory processes. During 2014, states increasingly became in line with adoption of parts or the whole of the Consensus Model. States have passed laws and regulations that recognize all four clinical specialties as APRNs; that allow for NPs to order home health; and that have provider-neutral language. Additional work is being done to address

issues of lack of claim payment, enhanced reimbursement
of primary care services, and widened authorization for prescriptive authority (Phillips, 2015). As of January 2015, 14 states have full practice
authority for NPs, and an additional 6 states have full authority following a postlicensure/postcertification period.

The IOM (2011) has supported the NCSBN Model for Nurse Practice Act
and has recommended that Congress "limit federal funding for nursing
education programs to only those programs in states that have adopted
this model" (p. 278). Although the intent of the IOM is to remove scope of
practice barriers through consistent education and regulation, these statements could have a profound and unexpected effect on APRN practice.
Therefore, as language from the Consensus Model continues to appear in
proposed state legislation, it is imperative that APRNs monitor the legislative language to ensure that the intent of the model is correctly displayed
in the legislation at both the state and federal levels.

Therefore, in policy making, it is important to consider all phases and
potential areas for influence throughout the entire process. Although
similarities exist between states, APRNs should also understand the
peculiarities of their state of licensure and the differences between federal and state legislation and regulation. APRNs can influence policy by
providing proactive solutions to the problems facing health care rather
than lamenting the problems. The solutions should contain information
on practicality, feasibility, financial implications, and the benefits for the
profession of nursing and for overall health care. Armed with an understanding of the background of policy making, the APRN will be able to
build coalitions, foster *grassroots lobbying* efforts, and cultivate effective
lobbying skills.

Professional Organizations, Grassroots Lobbying, and Coalition Building

The powerful combination of a united political voice through professional organizations and the grassroots efforts of APRNs has the power
to influence the healthcare agenda. Through membership dues and
other revenue sources, professional organizations have the resources
to create a network of federal government lobbyists, state government
political affairs directors, and political action committees (PACs).

Strength in numbers and coalition building are an important part of creating political influence. Membership in a professional organization is the
responsibility of all APRNs. **Table 5-2** lists examples of APRN professional
organizations. Professional organizations all have healthcare advocacy on

Table 5-2 APRN Professional Organizations
American Academy of Nurse Practitioners (AANP)
American Association of Colleges of Nursing (AACN)
American Association of Nurse Anesthetists (AANA)
American College of Nurse-Midwives (ACNM)
American Nurses Association (ANA)

their agenda, but their approach to influencing policy varies. The yearly legislative agenda for each professional organization is based on the current policy climate, the presence of pronursing members of Congress on important committees, and the current needs of the profession. Some organizations have offices based in Washington, D.C., with paid office staff, professional lobbyists, and PACs. Others operate primarily on a grassroots-type scale, with members providing the majority of the legislative work. Regardless of the organizational makeup, all members should maintain a two-way channel of communication to facilitate the flow of policy information and generate a network of involved members for grassroots lobbying efforts.

It is important to remember that political decisions are not made in the Senate or House chamber on the day of the vote but in offices throughout the legislative session. Decisions may be based on external pressures from other legislators, constituents, friends, and professional groups. A potentially powerful grassroots approach to influencing policy is to become involved in the election campaign of an official running for public office. Involvement may range from knocking on doors to discuss the campaigner's stance on the issue of access to health care to hosting a fundraising event. Visibility is critical. When elected, the legislator will remember the supporters who were involved in the early stages of his or her run for a position in the local, state, or federal government. An indication of effective involvement can be when a legislator introduces an APRN to another legislator with the words "the APRNs were with me from the beginning." This early involvement translates into an open-door policy with the legislator for members of the organization.

Lobbying is not a dirty word but an important part of the legislative process bound by ethical rules of conduct. Lobbyists are registered, educated professionals hired by both state and federal organizations to influence decisions made by legislators. One approach to influence legislation is to ensure that the legislators have all the pertinent information before making a decision on a certain piece of legislation. For example, in the recent healthcare bill, a legislator who has a reputation of being

"CRNA friendly" proposed an amendment for reimbursement for pain management services. However, the wording covered only physician services. After a discussion with the AANA lobbyist, the amendment was changed.

Because healthcare professional organizations are composed of members with full-time careers in the clinical arena, lobbyists are an integral part of influencing the healthcare agenda. Lobbyists are able to be continuously available during the legislative process. The lobbyists have cultivated relationships with legislative staff and understand the inner workings of Congress. Professional lobbying activities performed on behalf of an organization can include monitoring ongoing and proposed legislation, developing an agenda of legislative goals, advising on distribution of PAC funds, communicating with the membership, and educating members during grassroots lobbying efforts. Lobbyists often assist in creating a voice for the professional organization in developing oral and written testimony. Professional lobbyists do not create the message. APRNs have the message; the lobbyist just knows how to get the message to the right people and in the correct manner.

Legislators are more likely to listen to the concerns of their constituents and to support the efforts of a group of constituents. APRNs must take on the professional responsibility of advocating for nursing and healthcare reform by contacting their representatives and senators in Congress. APRNs have the ability to tell the story of their patients who cannot afford preventive health care, or the small-town hospital that is closing because of budget cuts, or the patient who does not have access to health care because of lack of providers. Personal stories told by a clinician in one of the most respected and trusted professions can be a powerful tool for influencing legislation. Also, storytelling can be the least intimidating entry into the world of grassroots lobbying. When APRN DNP students share their personal difficulties in obtaining funding for education and research, it creates a more lasting impression than when a nonstudent discusses the challenges of financing education. APRN students can also share the real risk of a decline in the number of providers because of the high cost of education, especially at a time when the healthcare system may see a large influx of patients as a result of healthcare reform measures.

Professional organizations play a significant role in preparing the membership and alleviating some of the fears of grassroots lobbying. For example, the AANA's Federal Government Affairs Office creates "Action Alerts" to encourage members to contact their representatives or senators. A portion of the AANA website contains the information that members who are certified registered nurse anesthetists (CRNAs) can use to contact their legislators. At a yearly assembly held in Washington, D.C., the staff at the AANA's D.C. office educates CRNAs on the legislative process as a whole, on the current issues facing health care and healthcare reform, and on the issues specific to CRNAs. A portion of the assembly is spent practicing for lobbying, including the dos and don'ts of presenting the issues and very specific details on the agenda for lobbying visits to Capitol Hill. Attending these professional meetings can be a very empowering experience, creating an understanding of what one individual, as part of a larger organization, can do to advocate for the profession of nursing and for the health of the nation. **Table 5-3** lists examples of effective lobbying techniques.

Table 5-3 Effective Lobbying

- Lobby in person or on paper.
  - Send letters to your member of Congress when necessary.
  - Obtain face time with legislators early on and throughout their term(s).
  - Make an appointment rather than just drop by (not just in Washington but at home too).
  - Be professional in appearance and demeanor.
  - Be punctual.
- Understand how the policy-making process works.
  - Attend educational "boot camps."
  - Maintain two-way communication with your professional organization regarding the organization's legislative agenda.
- Use your professional organization's lobbyist.
- Cultivate relationships with key legislative staff.
  - Take the time and opportunity to educate staff on nursing issues.
- Research your issues.
  - Be knowledgeable, confident, and articulate.
  - Know the number and status of the bill you are supporting or opposing (www.thomas.gov).
- Research the legislator you will be lobbying.
  - Build legislative profiles.
  - Is there a healthcare provider in the legislator's family?
  - Is the legislator on a committee with jurisdiction over healthcare issues? Is he or she the chair of the committee or a ranking member?
  - Drive the discussion.
  - Tell your story.

Table 5-3 Effective Lobbying (*continued*)

- Provide credible, "at the bedside" information about the impact of policies on health care.
- Discuss the impact of proposed legislation on the individual in his or her district—on constituents, the healthcare consumer, and the overall health of the United States.
- Never bash or speak poorly of your adversaries' position on the legislation.
- If applicable, ask the legislator to sign on to cosponsor a bill you are supporting.
- Stay in touch.
  - Send a handwritten thank you note as follow-up.
  - Include your business card and how to contact you for questions or assistance.
  - Flaunt your credentials!
- Exemplify professionalism.
  - Focus on advocacy, trust, knowledge, and competency.
  - Focus on the unique role, skills, and pivotal position of APRNs in the health-care system

Another essential aspect of lobbying is appreciating the roles and responsibilities of congressional staff. Each member of Congress has a chief of staff, also called an administrative assistant (AA), who is responsible for overseeing the overall management of the office, including managing the media and public relations and serving as a political advisor. Legislative directors are responsible for the "day-to-day legislative activities and may have more policy expertise" (Wakefield, 2008, p. 70). *Legislative assistants (LAs)*, often postcollege interns or fellows participating in a fellowship program, have the most contact with *special interest groups* such as nursing professional organizations. LAs can be very influential because they advise the member of Congress on health policy issues. They control what information is presented to the member of Congress and what groups get face time with the senator or representative. LAs are assigned to a specific issue, such as health or veterans' affairs; this does not mean that the LA is an expert in that area, however! When meeting with an LA for the first time, it is crucial to determine what he or she knows about advanced practice nursing and nursing's stance on healthcare issues. It is important to spend time educating the LA, in a nondefensive, noncondescending manner, regarding APRN practice and the professional organization's legislative agenda. Even if the exact goal of the lobbying visit was not met, the LA will have obtained a greater understanding of APRNs, including those with doctoral education, which may increase the probability that a DNP may be sought out for advice on proposed legislation. An established relationship with the member of Congress's health LA will serve as a communication conduit for information regarding upcoming legislation and committee hearings.

Although the blend of money and politics may not always appear to be a good combination, a strong PAC will increase access to and gain the attention of members of Congress. A PAC is a "group that is formed by an industry or an issue oriented organization to raise and contribute money to the campaign of political candidates who likely can advance their issue" (Twedell & Webb, 2007, p. 279). PACs have been involved in the campaign process over the last 60 years. Two types of PAC exist: separate segregated funds (SSFs) and nonconnected committees. SSFs are established and administered by organizations, whereas nonconnected committees are not sponsored by any organization (Federal Election Commission, 2009). Nursing PACs collect funds from their membership, pool the money, research the candidates, and distribute the money to legislators who are more likely to support the agenda of the nursing organization. PACs may contribute primarily to Democratic or Republican candidates, but often the PAC may be nonpartisan, supporting the candidate with similar priorities or the candidate who is influential on healthcare issues. Nurse anesthetists (NAs), NPs, clinical nurse specialists (CNSs), and certified nurse midwives (CNMs) have APRN-specific PACs. The ANA's PAC also contributes to candidates that support APRN issues.

As Congress addresses campaign reform, PACs have come under increased scrutiny and have been required to increase transparency in regard to sources of funding, donation amounts to candidates, and relationships with Congress. The Federal Election Campaign Act of 1971 prohibited organizations from using their general funds and membership dues to fund campaign contributions, and the Bipartisan Campaign Reform Act of 2002 placed further limits on contributions (Twedell & Webb, 2007). However, in 2010, Citizens United, a conservative nonprofit organization, successfully used the First Amendment's prohibition on the government placing limits on political spending by corporations or unions as a mechanism to allow for financing political expenditures through a corporation's general treasury. This ruling by the United States Supreme Court allows for the creation of a "SuperPAC" with access to significant amounts of money to spend on media campaigns for or against a certain candidate. All PACs must continue to be transparent, as required from previous legislation related to campaign reform (Summary of Citizens United v. Federal Election Commission, 2010).

Physician groups and pharmaceutical companies continue to have the top-spending PACs in health care, which often translates into greater political influence. During the 2008 election cycle, the only nursing PAC to break into the top 10 PACs was that of the AANA. Interestingly, the American Society of Anesthesiologists led PAC contributions from specialty physician groups (Center for Responsive Politics, 2009). According to the U.S. Department of Health and Human Services, in 2008, there were 250,527 APRNs (Health Resources and Services Administration, 2010). If each APRN donated $50 to his or her PAC, the resultant $12.5 million could move APRN PACs toward the top of the list of influential healthcare PACs. Information regarding individual PACs, including where the money comes from, how it is spent, and the overall worth of each PAC, can be found at www.opensecrets.org/index.php. With nursing's positive public image and a well-funded PAC, imagine the possibilities to influence legislation and advocate for improved quality and access to health care.

Coalition building is an effective approach to obtaining legislative and regulatory approval for an organization's policy agenda. Coalitions may last for the short term or long term, with the objective of combining resources to achieve a common goal. Nursing organizations can form coalitions either with other healthcare organizations or between APRN groups. For example, a coalition of over 30 nursing organizations created the Nursing Community Consensus Document (2008) requesting improved funding for doctoral education and calling for the removal of the rule that limits traineeship grants for doctoral education. Although the emphasis is on increasing nursing faculty, the importance of removing the cap on doctoral grants for entry-level doctoral students should not go unnoticed. According to Rice (2002, p. 122), the essential ingredients for strong coalitions include "leadership, membership, and serendipity." As in all organizations, it is important to have a leader who can organize the work of the coalition and motivate the group to stay on target (Rice, 2002). This could be an important venue for a DNP. Membership is essential to increase the productivity and the visibility of the organization. Coalitions may be formed by unforeseen opportunities. For example, proposed state legislation to remove the collaboration requirement for prescriptive authority may bring together the state nursing association and the state APRN organizations. The North Dakota Nurse Practitioner Association recognized the need to create a coalition of varied stakeholders before seeking a sponsor for a bill to change their nurse practice act (NPA). A dedicated group of NPs approached the North Dakota Board of Nursing for support and then obtained additional support from select North Dakota hospitals, county commissioner boards, the North Dakota Association of Nurses, individual physicians, and others (Madler, Kalanek, & Rising, 2014).

Just as there are benefits for organizations in coming together, there are also potential pitfalls and challenges to effective functioning of the group. When forming a coalition, it is essential to have all the right people: members who will work hard and people with a stake in the common goal (Rice, 2002). One of the challenges of working in a group of differing organizations is the presence of varying perspectives. Although the group may have one common goal, each member organization may have contradictory perspectives on other goals. When this occurs, it is essential to have a leader, potentially one with a DNP degree, who will seek out diverse opinions, allow members to agree to disagree, and "work toward achieving decisions which members can live with" (Rice, 2002, p. 128). Although opposing organizations may not agree on all topics, it is important to handle conflict effectively in order to maintain a working relationship if the need for collaboration does occur.

Coalitions may be created for the purpose of countering a threat to the ability of member organizations to practice to the full scope of their professional licensure. The Coalition for Patients' Rights (CPR) is composed of 35 organizations representing a variety of licensed healthcare professionals. CPR, with strength in numbers and a diverse group of providers, aims to offset the efforts of the American Medical Association's Scope of Practice Partnership (SOPP) initiative, which is designed to limit patients' choice of healthcare providers and ultimately patient access to health care (CPR, n.d.). Some coalitions may be formed without the express purpose of policy making. However, the data obtained by these nursing groups can be used to give a statistical significance to a proposed legislative agenda item. The Interagency Collaborative on Nursing Statistics (ICONS) "promotes the generation and utilization of data, information, and research about nurses, nursing education, and the nursing workforce" (ICONS, 2006).

Coalitions of like-minded organizations may join forces to ensure a seat at the table while the details of the composition of healthcare reform legislation are debated. The Patients' Access to Responsible Care Alliance (PARCA) is a coalition of nonphysician organizations that "aims to provide federal policymakers with access to information from all areas of the healthcare community . . . and is committed to quality cost-effective care and ensuring patients have options in the delivery of such care" (PARCA, n.d.). The inclusion of nondiscriminatory language for reimbursement for services provided by a nonphysician is critical for the future of APRNs and for equitable access to health care for all. This coalition was successful in getting nondiscrimination language included in the Patient Protection and Affordable Care Act (ACA) of 2010. PARCA is composed of nursing APRN organizations, the American Academy of Audiology, the American Chiropractic Association, the American Optometric Association, the National Association of Social Workers, and others. As evidenced by the composition of PARCA, an important aspect to consider when building effective coalitions is the significance of connecting diverse groups, including both depth and breadth of professions.

Healthcare Reform

Because of increasing healthcare costs, "the insecurity resulting from basing healthcare insurance on employment," and the significant number of uninsured, the American public grew increasingly dissatisfied with the state of health care in the United States throughout the 1990s (Schroeder, 1993, p. 945). In 1993, the Clinton administration attempted to reform health care in the United States. The proposed national Health Security Act (HSA) of 1993 included guaranteed comprehensive benefits, limitations on health insurance premiums, and increased emphasis on quality, and it mandated employers to provide insurance coverage through regulated health maintenance organizations (National Health Security Plan, 1993). The proposed plan, spearheaded by then first lady Hillary Clinton, had significant opposition from conservatives, small business owners, and the health insurance industry because of its cost and complexity, significant government oversight and control, and the potential to limit patient healthcare choices. In the end, legislation for healthcare reform was not passed.

Because of the difficulty in creating a coalition for support and the appearance of political shenanigans, the American public's interest in healthcare reform declined during the time that the HSA legislation was drafted. For the first time, nursing, the largest group of healthcare providers, had a significant presence during the debate over how to reform the U.S. healthcare system. This presence was due to the work of a small group of nurses who understood the importance of creating legislative relationships and of suggesting solutions to the problem and who demonstrated a "willingness to compromise in the present to secure the greater gain in the future" (Milstead, 2008, p. 20).

In advance of the presidential and legislative impetus to restructure the healthcare system, the ANA created a task force in 1989 to begin work on an agenda to reform health care. Nursing's Agenda for Healthcare Reform, published in 1992, focused on the contribution that reforming health systems would make in improving access to care while controlling costs and improving outcomes. The agenda called for a "federal standard of uniform basic benefits package for all U.S. citizens and residents financed through public-private partnerships using a variety of healthcare providers including provisions for community health and quality measurement" (Trotter Betts, 1996, p. 4). Despite the failure of the HSA, the activism during this period allowed nurses to obtain increased visibility in the policy arena and develop skills in policy making. Nursing and the ANA came out better informed, with greater access to legislators, and better armed for the next legislative challenge (Rubotzky, 2000; Trotter Betts, 1996).

Blendon and Benson, in a 2001 review regarding American opinions on health policy over the last 50 years, found that "Americans may have expressed dissatisfaction with private health insurance and managed care but most don't trust the federal government to take over as a single-payer provider or are satisfied enough with their current medical payment arrangements" (cited in Jamelske, Johs-Artisensi, Taft, & German, 2009, p. 17). However, given the 2008 downturn in the economy, Americans and Congress are again concerned with enacting some variety of healthcare reform. With the rising cost of healthcare premiums and the increase in the number of Americans who are uninsured or underinsured, Americans have begun to realize that the potential to lose coverage in the future does exist. Policy lessons learned during the previous attempts at healthcare reform have set the stage for organized nursing to influence policy that will ensure improved health care for all Americans. An incremental healthcare reform policy would begin with small changes, allowing for the addressing of political dynamics at each stage. Influential policy makers exist on both sides of the plan for reform: creation of an immediate, all-encompassing change versus making small adjustments at regular intervals.

In March 2010, President Barack Obama signed the ACA into law despite a lack of bipartisan support. The impetus for the passage of the ACA was the recognition that the United States spends more per capita on health care than any other country and is the one developed country that does not provide coverage to all its citizens (Hall & Lord, 2014). The ACA's wide-ranging provisions address many of the issues that were facing health care in the prior decades including outmoded approaches to reimbursement, provider discrimination, lack of access to healthcare insurance at a reasonable cost, disparities in health care among all citizens, and rampant healthcare costs. Although many of the supporters of healthcare reform may have preferred a sweeping movement to publicly provided health care for all, many in Congress remembered the failures of the Clinton Administration and supported incremental, narrower calculated initiatives. The ACA was a middle-of-the-road approach that mandated individual health insurance but continued to preserve many aspects of the existing health insurance systems (Gable, 2011, p. 343). It expands Medicare coverage and provides for increased federal support for the Children's Health Insurance Program. An important achievement of the ACA is universal insurability, which precludes insurers from refusing to cover preexisting conditions (Hall & Lord, 2014). Of particular interest for APRNs is that it encourages the creation of new patient care models—accountable care organizations (ACOs)—and provider non-discrimination language in reimbursement for service. Other diverse components include linking of Medicare payments to quality indicators, increased access to preventive care, and increased federal financial support for careers in nursing.

In this author's opinion, it remains to be seen whether the ACA will result in broad healthcare reform as it moves through the U.S. judiciary, regulatory agencies, and state government. According to Gable (2011), "the ultimate effects and significance of the ACA remain uncertain" (p. 340), and the same obstacles exist, including political opposition, concerns over constitutionality of mandates, and overall implementation of the legislation. The critics of the ACA were further encouraged by the issues with the Department of Health and Human Services rollout of the insurance exchange website. However, once the issues were resolved, the website has successfully enrolled previously uninsured and underinsured Americans.

Political influence developed by the ANA and nursing leaders in the 1980s and 1990s must be sustained throughout the upcoming legislative challenges during the anticipated long road to sustainable healthcare financing reform.

Long-Standing Policy Goals

Before advocating for improvements in health care, it is crucial to understand the issues that have been at the forefront of nursing policy and politics for over four decades and that continue to warrant nursing's legislative and regulatory involvement. According to Malone (2005, p. 139), "it is important to understand the recent history of any policy issue to better understand the obstacles and resources in play."

Nursing Workforce Development

As the demand for health care rises, the demographics of our population change, and the new ACA is being implemented, the nursing profession continues to be challenged with an overall nursing workforce shortage. Although the primary factor behind the nursing workforce shortage changes over time, "consistent factors include unfavorable working conditions, relatively low income potential, more satisfying alternative job opportunities, and lack of nursing faculty" (McHugh, Aiken, Cooper, & Miller, 2008, p. 6). Doctorally prepared APRNs and nursing faculty are drawn from the relatively small pool of baccalaureate-prepared nurses; therefore, deficiencies in the number of registered nurses (RNs) affects APRN vacancy rates and ultimately may limit patient access to care. Vacancy rates change over time relative to the changing economic times and healthcare market. Therefore, when advocating for legislative change concerning workforce development, it is necessary to have updated facts on past and current vacancy rates, the impact of past funding efforts on the shortage of nurses, and the impact of vacancy rates on healthcare delivery. For example, data from the U.S. Bureau of Labor Statistics (BLS) can be used to support the need for additional educational funding due to a projected need for a 31% increase in APRNs between 2012 and 2022 (BLS, 2015). The average rate of growth for all occupations is 11%. Additional information in the 2015 BLS Occupational Outlook Handbook reported that all four APRN specialties—CNS, CRNA, CNM, and NP—will be in "high demand particularly in medically underserved areas," and "relative to physicians, these RNs increasingly serve as lower-cost primary care providers." The BLS handbook also acknowledges the role that changes in state NPAs will play regarding the need for more APRN practitioners as barriers to practice are removed and the public increasingly recognizes the role of APRNs.

According to McHugh et al. (2008), "The nursing shortage is not only of total numbers but also of the level of nursing education" (p. 7). Over the last decade, nursing organizations have continued to lobby for legislative support to increase funding for nursing education at both the baccalaureate and graduate levels. One legislative mechanism for funding is through the Nursing Workforce Development Programs (Title VIII of the Public Health Service Act). Title VIII programs have been the largest source of federal funding for nursing education over the last 45 years. In the 1960s, nursing leaders lobbied Congress to enact legislation that would alleviate the nation's nursing shortage by funding nursing education. In 1964, President Lyndon Johnson signed the Nurse Training Act of 1964. In the years since its inception, Title VIII has expanded to include funding for advanced practice nursing education, for the education of disadvantaged and minority students, for nurse faculty loan programs, and for nurse education, practice, and retention grants (Nursing Community Consensus Document, 2008). Title VIII grants are an essential component for increasing the number of APRN graduates and for ensuring that medically underserved areas receive access to healthcare services. However, the level of funding is not guaranteed, and, despite the increased costs of education and inflation, the relative level of funding has remained unchanged. It is through the continued action of involved nurses that Title VIII funding consistently remains in the national budget and on the legislative agenda.

Along with a greater demand for nurses, the changing complexity of health care and healthcare systems requires that a greater number of APRNs and nursing faculty be prepared at the graduate level. APRNs must continue to monitor and support legislative issues that alleviate the nursing shortage by expanding funding for nursing education, promoting a favorable work environment, and eliminating barriers to practice.

Reimbursement

Although the complexity and changing nature of regulation make a detailed discussion of APRN reimbursement impractical for this venue, it is appropriate to discuss the fundamentals and historical background within the framework of advocating for APRN practice. It is imperative for the APRN provider to understand the challenges in achieving equality and to monitor for threats to APRN practice in the economic healthcare market within public policy. For over three decades, APRN groups have challenged our legislators to remove the financial barriers to practice (Sullivan-Marx, 2008).

For example, until 1989, all direct reimbursement for anesthesia services was limited to anesthesiologists. CRNAs were reimbursed from the money paid to the institution through Part A of Medicare. The disparity in the ability to directly bill for services created an inequality between providers delivering the same care. The Omnibus Budget Reconciliation

Act of 1987 required the federal Medicare program to create a separate payment plan for the anesthesia care delivered by a CRNA, which is now known as Medicare Part B. The change was budget neutral because responsibility for payment was moved from the Medicare Part A division to the Part B division (Broadston, 2001). The regulatory agency responsible for determining Medicare reimbursement was the Health Care Financing Administration (HCFA). When Medicare federal regulation changed, private insurance providers and state public health plans followed suit and opted to directly reimburse CRNAs for services provided (Broadston, 2001). It was essential during this time of legislative and regulatory change that CRNAs at all levels of the profession maintain close contact with Congress and the agencies responsible for transforming Medicare reimbursement.

During the 1970s and 1980s, as the number of NPs grew and diagnosis-related groups (DRGs) were created, nursing leaders in the ANA recognized the need for parity between physician and NP reimbursement. The ANA pressed for a mechanism to change Medicare rules through legislation (Sullivan-Marx, 2008). During this same time period, three policy reports were released supporting the role of NPs and the removal of barriers to reimbursement: the Graduate Medical Education National Advisory Council's (GMENAC) report, the Office of Technology Assessment's report to Congress, and the Physician Payment Review Commission's report (Sullivan-Marx, 2008). The reports cited barriers, including the lack of NP Medicare reimbursement. The GMENAC report concluded that direct reimbursement by Medicare and Medicaid would be necessary to facilitate full use of NPs and CNSs (Sullivan-Marx, 2008, p. 122). Finally, with the passage of the 1990 Omnibus Budget Reconciliation Act, NPs and CNSs in rural health clinics and in nursing homes were allowed to directly bill Medicare at 85% of the physician rate. CNMs were allowed to bill at 65% of the physician rate (Sullivan-Marx, 2008). An additional seven years of encouraging legislators to act was required to include all NPs in direct reimbursement from Medicare. The Balanced Budget Act of 1997 granted NPs and CNSs the ability to bill Medicare in all geographic areas and settings, but still at only 85% of the prevailing physician rate (Abood & Franklin, 2000).

These initial wins for parity in reimbursement demonstrated the importance of the political advocacy role for APRNs in influencing the structure of legislation and regulation that influence finance. The next step has been to remove the artificial barrier of supervision as a requirement for Medicare payment. In 2000, CRNAs lobbied extensively (and won) for a change at the federal level. Initial gains in removing the supervision requirement were lost with the change in presidential administration in 2001. However, the AANA and CRNAs fought to develop a compromise that would lead to the Medicare "opt-out" language that allowed states to decide whether to make physician supervision of CRNAs a requirement for reimbursement. As of January 2015, 17 states have "opted-out" (www.aana.com). Although much of the fight for parity in reimbursement between APRNs and physicians has focused on Medicare/Medicaid, APRNs must stay vigilant to prevent limitations in reimbursement from other insurance providers.

According to Abood and Franklin (2000), the ability to document and bill for APRN services creates transparency regarding which provider is actually performing the patient care. This documentation allows for connecting patient outcomes to healthcare providers and gives APRNs an additional tool to demonstrate their value to both the institution and policy makers. As we move forward with healthcare reform, through the knowledge gained during doctoral education and practice, APRNs can provide the skills necessary to analyze and engage in the discussion of cost-effectiveness, pay for performance, and reimbursement.

State Nurse Practice Acts and Scope of Practice

The first board of nursing and the first NPA were created in 1903 in the state of North Carolina (Loversidge, 2008, p. 96). Initially, NPAs focused on protecting the use of the RN title rather than defining the delivery of nursing care (Tobin, 2001). Following the 1971 report of the Department of Health, Education, and Welfare's Committee to Study Extended Roles for Nurses, state NPAs began to change to include regulations governing APRN practice (Tobin, 2001). The NPA is an example of an enabling law and contains the laws and regulations that credential and govern a profession (Loversidge, 2008). As noted in a previous section, boards of nursing and NPAs were created to protect the well-being of patients by ensuring consistent minimum standards of licensure and qualifications. Each state has a different NPA, which defines the scope of practice for all nurses within that state and delineates the officers, staff, and powers of the state regulatory board (e.g., the board of nursing).

NPAs include language that defines the roles and responsibilities of APRNs, including "accepting referrals from, consulting with, cooperating with, or referring to all other types of health care providers" and "must practice within a health care system that provides for consultation and collaborative management and referral as indicated by the health status of the patient" (Minnesota Board of Nursing, 2008). The evolution of the NPA is evident in the language regarding the roles of nurses. The initial ANA model definition of nursing practice in 1946 included the provision that the scope of practice for nursing is "not deemed to include acts of diagnosis or prescription of therapeutic or corrective measures" (Tobin, 2001). The ANA amended the model definition to allow for nurses to perform specific tasks (diagnosis and treatment) "under emergency or special conditions as are recognized by the medical and nursing professions" (Tobin, 2001). In 1996, the ANA revised the model practice definition to broaden the scope of practice of professional nursing, and a definition of APRN practice was explicitly included. The 2008 APRN Consensus Model grew out of the need for state NPAs to continue to evolve to meet the needs of the profession of nursing and the healthcare needs of the American public. During their successful attempt to grant full practice authority to APRNs in North Dakota, the NPs were able to convince the legislators that the current regulatory language was antiquated, did not meet the changing healthcare needs in the state, and "did not contribute to the advancement of North Dakotans' health" (Madler et al., 2014, p. 115).

State NPAs vary widely in defining the scope of practice of APRNs. Some states have very few restrictions, whereas others limit the ability of the APRN to prescribe medications, independently administer chronic pain injections, admit patients, and conduct a prehospital history and physical. NPAs also include rules on delegation of duties to non-RN providers, continuing education requirements, and the administration of certain medications, such as Propofol, a potent amnestic. NPAs include the rules for prescriptive authority for APRNs. The authorization for APRNs to prescribe with or without a written collaborative agreement with a physician must be expressly written into the agreement. States differ in the authority for APRNs to prescribe controlled substances. CRNAs may be exempt from some of the prescriptive language requiring written collaboration in order to administer anesthetic agents and their adjuncts during the perioperative period.

Historically, APRNs have had to be diligent in monitoring proposed changes to an NPA and to prevent other entities from attempting to supersede the power of the state board of nursing in defining APRN scope of practice. In 2005, the American Medical Association created the SOPP and stated, in the report of the board of trustees, "[AMA] agreed that it was necessary to concentrate the resources of organized medicine to oppose scope of practice expansions by allied health professionals that would threaten the health and safety of the public" (American Medical Association, 2005). The SOPP objective is to fund studies refuting claims that APRNs were necessary to improve access to care in rural states and to create studies comparing the educational, training, and licensure requirements of physician and nonphysician providers. Just as nursing organizations should have no role in defining the practice of medicine, physician groups are in no position to define APRN practice, licensure, certification, or education. According to the CPR, rather than creating division among healthcare professionals, the AMA and the allied health members of CPR should be working together to find solutions to the current healthcare challenges.

Any time a state nurse practice act is opened, whether the intent is to broaden scope of practice or not, the opportunity exists for language to be inserted regarding increasing the need for supervision by a physician or removing prescriptive authority. State nursing organizations may be reluctant to open their NPA for just those reasons. Before any decision to open up a state NPA, nursing organizations should have a well-developed supportive relationship with legislators who serve the committee that is reviewing any proposed changes. APRNs are responsible for remaining knowledgeable of the current status of the NPA in their state and for practicing within the limits of their scope of practice.

DNP graduates will be expected not only to exhibit the skills of advanced clinical practice and systems thinking but also to be accountable for driving the discussion that sustains nursing workforce development, maintains parity in reimbursement, and removes barriers to the full scope of practice for APRNs.

Integration of Policy with Ethics, Research, and Education

Ethics and Policy Making

Just as a vital link exists between policy and practice, so too should the connection between policy and ethics be strong. The 2001 Code of Ethics for Nurses with Interpretive Statements (ANA, 2001) includes the following statement: "The profession of nursing, as represented by associations and their members, is responsible for articulating nursing values, for maintaining the integrity of the profession and its practice, and for shaping social policy."

Policy decisions are ethical decisions on many different levels, from choices made by professional organizations, to prioritizing a legislative or regulatory agenda, to the allocation of scarce resources. A political ethical conflict "occurs when what one is told to do (either covertly or overtly) by those having more power in the organization or what one feels compelled to do by the organization is in conflict with one's ethical belief structure" (Silva, 2002, p. 180). It becomes more of a challenge when the policy initially appears at odds with one's values, but upon further examination, the eventual outcome of policy implementation does support the needs of the profession and public. For example, APRNs may have the ethical dilemma of supporting a legislator through PAC contributions who does not have the same values as organized nursing but sits in a position of power to influence legislation. Kent and Liaschenko (2004) examined the connection between nursing values and ANA PAC donations. They encouraged the ANA PAC to continue to evaluate the donation process for successful outcomes that are important to nursing while maintaining a connection with legislative leadership—Democratic or Republican (Kent & Liaschenko, 2004). As nursing continues to become more influential in the policy arena, it is important to develop partnerships on both sides of the legislative aisle. Regardless of the occasional differences in political viewpoints, it is necessary to ensure equal access when issues important to nursing arise.

Clinical APRNs are often the central decision makers in the allocation of resources, including laboratory and invasive testing, time spent in the delivery of patient care, medical equipment, and referrals for additional interventions (Aroskar, Moldow, & Good, 2004). This array of patient care concerns has the potential for both policy and ethical implications. Aroskar et al. (2004) used focus groups to examine the clinical nurse's perspective on changes in healthcare policy that affect patient care. Changes in legislative policy influence institutional policy, which in turn influences patient care. The most frequently noted themes included the policy implications of cost containment, the effects of policy on quality of care and patient education, and the overall effect on nurses and nursing (Aroskar et al., 2004). Medicare regulations may dictate where patients may receive care and how much care will be reimbursed. Legislation may influence the appropriate allocation of healthcare resources as well as the decision makers who define "appropriate." Regulation regarding APRN licensure may affect quality-of-life and end-of-life matters if patients do not have access to all providers who can provide pain management and palliative care. However, the researchers found that although all the focus groups stressed the importance of nursing having a voice in policy development, the recognized need for "assertiveness does not always translate to advocacy for patients or participation in policy development" (Aroskar et al., 2004, p. 274).

APRNs educated and experienced in policy will have the ability to comprehend the ethical implications of policy development and implementation and be able to integrate both while achieving the ultimate goals of improving health and supporting the profession of nursing. According to Silva (2002), the solution to successful resolution of an ethical conflict between values and politics involves either integration or compromise. Integration includes the incorporation of all points of view into the policy, whereas compromise encourages all parties to forfeit something for the overall common good (Silva, 2002). Just as APRNs have a professional responsibility to be involved in policy, as noted by the ANA's Code of Ethics, they also have an ethical responsibility to the public to be engaged in healthcare policy.

Research and Policy Making

The initial link between nursing policy, practice, and research may have begun in the 1960s as nurse researchers sought federal funding and an equal playing field with medicine for research dollars (Milstead, 2008). Research and policy are connected in two interrelated ways: there is nursing research, and there is policy research. Nursing research is used to supply the data and background information for creating policy. Policy research is the "analysis of a social problem to provide policy makers with alternative recommendations for future initiatives aimed at alleviating problems" (Nagelkerk & Henry, 1991, p. 20). During the process of restructuring health care in the United States, both types of research will be essential for creating an evidence-based plan that includes an examination of the alternatives. Nurse researchers have begun to realize that when using research to create policy, the largest challenge may originate from the inherent potential for ambiguous data to produce different interpretations and then different policies. In these situations, the successful APRN leader must shape the policy agenda such that the issue becomes defined as a problem backed by research requiring legislative or regulatory action. Often nursing research is "published by nurse academicians in the nursing literature but policymakers do not access their work" (Short, 2008, p. 266). APRNs can be the experts who bring the data to the legislator and discuss the outcomes and how they can be applied to public policy. Short (2008) encouraged nurses to submit their research studies to journals outside nursing and to include the potential policy implications of nursing research.

The media can be used to open a window of opportunity on an issue important to nursing. When the media started reporting on the childhood obesity epidemic, nurse researchers were the content experts who used supporting data to influence public policy. Because nurses have a favorable public impression, they are able to convey health-related information in a manner that is considered fact without a particular bias or slant. An institution or organization's public relations staff can be used as a tool to stimulate public and legislator interest in nursing health policy research (Diers, 2002). Because research can be uninteresting or overwhelming to the lay public, the ability to translate research into powerful stories or anecdotes can serve as a catalyst for legislative activity.

Although the value of evidence-based research outcomes is not disputed, the ability of evidence to influence policy in the manner and to the degree expected by the researcher is still debated. Policy decisions are political decisions, and thus the rational, correct decision is not always made; instead, the decision may be a compromise between competing interests. The majority of citizens, who may have competing values at odds with the best policy evidence, must also support policy decisions. The quality of the research or the research design may be less important than an understanding of the current political agenda or the agenda of special interest groups. In that case, the research may even be called into question despite solid methodology, or politicians and healthcare providers may use researched outcomes selectively to back an alternative course of action. APRNs educated in healthcare policy will be able to anticipate political trends, discover areas lacking in data, and design studies to seek out the answers. The Future of Nursing Campaign for Action (CFA) engaged state and national nursing coalitions to support the recommendations of the IOM "Future of Nursing" report. To understand the progress of the implementation, the Robert Wood Johnson Foundation (RWJF) developed metrics, planned for statistical analysis, and developed a dashboard as an approach to graphically demonstrate progress on the recommendations (Spetz et al., 2014).

Evidence-based practice data may be used to influence healthcare financing policy. Rather than focus on "this is the way we do it here," the impetus should instead be to focus on whether "the evidence support[s] the need for a procedure with increased cost without a proven benefit." According to P. R. Orszag (2009), former director of the Congressional Budget Office and of the Office of Management and Budget, when looking at the correlation between cost and quality, "the higher cost providers, the higher cost hospitals, the higher cost regions are not generating better health outcomes than the lower cost, more efficient providers"

(p. 74). Outcome-based research may be assisted by the use of information technology. With the increased emphasis on the use of electronic health records (EHRs), APRNs must be involved in the development of data entry points to support further research of outcomes relative to nursing care, including cost versus quality. Program evaluation is an integral part of policy research. Doctorally prepared APRNs are experts in program evaluation. As experts, APRNs must continue to use feedback to ensure that "old problems are being addressed, new problems are being identified and appropriate solutions are being considered" (Milstead, 2008, p. 21).

The political agenda is often shaped by cost, quality, and access to care. Research designed with that in mind can be used to a professional organization's benefit. In a May 2009 letter to the Senate Finance Committee answering a request for input into financing healthcare reform, Jackie Rowles, past president of AANA, used data from a Government Accountability Office study (2007, p. 15) to communicate the financial incentive for including CRNAs in the blueprint for healthcare financing reform. Then-president Rowles stated, "CRNAs predominate where there are more Medicare patients than average. CRNAs also predominate where private payment is lower than average, which is also where the gap between Medicare and private payment is less. Where anesthesiologists predominate, private payments are higher than average and the gap between Medicare and private payment is greater" (Rowles, 2009). Recognizing that the current anesthesia staffing patterns may become unsustainable in an age of cost containment and healthcare reform, the AANA funded a study conducted by non-CRNA economists who analyzed a variety of staffing approaches. Hogan, Seifert, Moore, and Simonson (2010) were able to use economic modeling to prove that CRNAs working independently were more cost effective to hospitals. These data can prove powerful when discussing implementation of healthcare reform legislation.

The IOM "Future of Nursing" report (2011) stressed the importance of better data collection on workforce planning and transforming the clinical practice environment. Outcomes research data continue to become more important as pressures to reduce cost and improve quality become a critical part of the conversation when APRNs meet with legislators and discuss removing barriers to practice. In recent years, professional nursing organizations and individuals have begun to take a more proactive role in gathering and publishing these important data. For example, Newhouse et al. (2011) conducted an extensive systematic review and found positive patient outcomes when APRNs were involved in the care of a variety of patients. Dulisse and Cromwell (2010) examined the impact of removal of the CRNA Medicare supervision rule on patient outcomes and found that there was no increased risk to patients in states that had opted out. An important facet of the Dulisse-Cromwell research was its inclusion in a nonnursing journal, *Health Affairs.*

Clinical systems research, inherent in the final scholarly or capstone project of the DNP degree, is a useful means to provide an evidence-based approach to making policy changes within local, state, or federal health systems. Challenges within health care can often be traced back to a systems problem. APRNs with the clinical background and the education in evidence-based practice and policy will be able to frame the questions to search for the solutions. Is there a need to create policies that providers must follow to ensure delivery of evidence-based diabetes care or guarantee on-time immunizations? Why are some medical centers more efficient than others, and should their processes be emulated? How do we ensure access to care with a sustainable health policy?

Education, Practice, and Policy Making

According to Malone (2005), too often policy is not consistently emphasized as a part of nursing education even though policy can influence many aspects of patient care. When policy development has been included as part of nursing education, the primary focus has been on identifying and using an institution's policy manual (Malone, 2005). Policy-making skills are an integral part of doctoral education. Just as nurses learn the clinical skills necessary to care for patients, they are also compelled to learn the skills necessary for influencing policy. When new graduates have a sense of competency obtained through education and practical experience, they are more likely to become involved in the process. In the past, there were limited opportunities for formal policy education within nursing. Most skills were learned on the job through mentoring or self-directed education. With the increased complexity of health care and an increased need for nurses to become politically involved, the education process should now include a focused, systematic, consistent approach.

One approach in educating APRNs in how to influence public policy is to apply the nursing process—assess, diagnose, plan, implement, and evaluate. For example, the nursing process can be applied to the challenges in delivering health care in the United States and the current outcome of the ACA of 2010.

Begin with an assessment of the situation. A bipartisan report released by the U.S. Senate Finance Committee on May 18, 2009, noted that "46 million Americans lack health insurance coverage, employer-sponsored health care premiums have increased 117 percent between 1999–2008, and annual health care spending is expected to outpace annual growth in the overall economy by 2.1 percent in the next ten years. Also, in 2009, health spending will increase 5.5 percent while gross domestic product is expected to decrease 0.2 percent" (Senate Finance Committee, 2009). It is important to include both a financial and social perspective, for example, "The United States ranks last among industrialized nations in mortality from conditions preventable with timely and effective care" (Gable, 2011, p. 342).

The next step in the process is to identify or diagnose the problem. Armed with data from government sources, including the Department of Health and Human Services, Centers for Disease Control and Prevention, and the CMS, APRNs can recognize many of the problems in healthcare systems, including a healthcare delivery system that does not provide access to all Americans, the uncontrolled rise in healthcare cost, and the lack of preventive health care.

Following a diagnosis of the problem, the biggest challenge becomes how to plan for resolution of the crisis while anticipating potential obstacles. According to Malone (2005), obstacles to policy intervention include "lack of media attention, ideological opposition from those in decision-making positions, lack of money, advocacy leadership struggles and efforts from those actively opposed" (p. 141). The doctorally prepared APRN will be prepared, informed, and empowered to challenge any Congress or presidential administration to support a healthcare policy that meets the six aims of the IOM: safe, effective, patient centered, timely, efficient, and equitable (IOM, 2001). The search for innovative solutions while using the resources at hand may prove to be more difficult than anticipated, as evidenced by the failure of the Clinton plan. How can the United States ensure equal access to high-quality care for all Americans while controlling cost? Is the U.S. nursing workforce substantial enough to handle the potential influx of patients into the healthcare system? APRNs may be asked to provide expert testimony, serve as content experts, and garner support from legislators during this stage of the process.

While the legislation is being implemented, APRNs must continue their political activism with vigilance and a skeptical eye regarding any drafts, testimony, or regulations that do not support the intent of the reform legislation. The last step of the process—which should actually occur throughout the progression of legislation—is to evaluate whether the legislation works. Formative evaluation of the policy process should occur from the beginning. Did APRNs become involved, and how effective were they? What were the obstacles to policy legislation and implementation? Were the obstacles recognized early in the process? Does the legislation meet the six aims of the IOM? Does the legislation provide for equal access to providers and for patients? How will outcomes be measured, and will they be measured equitably for all providers? Will this plan be sustainable?

Maynard (1999) described a four-dimensional intersecting model for teaching healthcare policy that includes information, commitment, initiative, and involvement. The first step is the responsibility that nurses have to remain informed and up to date about the health policy agenda. The second step is the commitment to act on an issue. Initiative, the third step, is the "power, ability, or instinct to begin or follow through with a plan or task" (p. 193). Although the model is not intended to be linear, the final step is involvement in the process of influencing policy. As the content of policy education is formalized within the curriculum of DNP programs, educators will need to be able to demonstrate the relevance of policy to practice. One approach to accomplish this is to instruct APRNs on how to determine the basis of proposed policy changes.

An awareness of where legislation and regulation originate may be critical to understanding and influencing policy. Taft and Nanna (2008) stressed the importance of educating nurses on the sources of healthcare policies that affect practice, including organizational, public, and professional sources. Examples of organizational sources are consumers of health care (patients), the media, and insurers. Patients who have experienced difficulties in the healthcare system are frequently an impetus for legislative change—for example, changes in insurance coverage for preventive exams. Public sources include the government at all levels and all branches, economic and demographic trends, and special interest groups (Taft & Nanna, 2008). Healthcare disciplines, including nursing, universities, and research-generating organizations, comprise the final type of source: professional sources. Professional APRN associations have played an integral role in proposing legislation that influences health care and have been involved in the regulatory role.

Nursing educators at all levels of entry to nursing practice must serve as mentors by becoming role models for political activism, risk taking, and health policy advocacy. Experienced nurses can successfully communicate the connection between professional commitment and political responsibility. Rather than merely encouraging nurses to be politically involved, nursing faculty should equip students with the knowledge and skills to feel confident in their ability to influence policy. According to

Rains and Carroll (2000), "Health policy education at the graduate level has the potential to increase the political skills, involvement, and competence of nursing's future leaders" (p. 37). It is crucial during doctoral education that APRN students become actively involved in the process by lobbying on Capitol Hill, by serving as student representatives on professional organization committees, and by successfully demonstrating the ability to articulate the legislative and regulatory process. Policy-educated APRN clinicians should serve as role models to the next generations of baccalaureate- and graduate-prepared nurses. APRNs will be able to create a teaching environment that synthesizes didactic knowledge with the practice and work environments (Short, 2008). J. A. Milstead proposed that hospitals consider developing a "health policy/researcher" position to combine advanced clinical skills with the research skills necessary to influence health policy decisions within the organization and on a larger scale (Peters, 2002).

Although all APRNs must participate in healthcare policy at some level, it is unrealistic to assume that all APRNs should become policy experts in addition to their roles providing direct patient care. The extensive commitment of time and energy necessary to effectively perform all the duties of both roles may not be achievable. Instead, the future of advanced practice nursing may include the specialty of health policy APRN. As nurses become more informed about and interested in policy, especially after doctoral education, they may choose to focus their career on influencing legislation and serving as a health policy expert. Nurses can gain practical experience by applying for policy fellowships in Washington, D.C. Perhaps the most well known is the Robert Wood Johnson Foundation (RWJF) Health Policy Fellowship. Historically, nurses have not taken advantage of these opportunities. In the RWJF Fellowship's 37 years, over 230 fellowships have been awarded, but only 27 nurses have been fellows (Robert Wood Johnson Foundation Health Policy Fellowships Program, n.d.). Health policy fellowships offer nurses an opportunity to brief legislators on healthcare issues, develop proposals, and staff conferences and hearings.

Although the relationship between policy and practice has focused on clinical care, nurse executives with a doctoral education foundation can play a critical role in influencing the policies that have a direct impact on patient care. Peters (2002) compared influencing policy to teaching an elephant to dance: difficult to do, but it can be accomplished if approached methodically. Administrators must be "committed to political activism; stay informed through formal and informal channels; challenge the status quo; identify a base of support; and get the issues on the agenda" (pp. 5–7).

Phases of Policy Involvement

All APRNs have the responsibility to their patients to become involved in the political process at some level. Various authors have described levels of political involvement and emphasized that the focus is on finding a level at which the individual can be engaged and that is compatible with where the individual may be in his or her career. Boswell, Cannon, and Miller (2005) identified "three primary levels of commitment: survival, success, and significance" (p. 6). As APRNs become more engaged in the process, they may move through the levels, or they may choose to stay at the level where they are comfortable. At the survival level, the individual takes part in the voting process or may serve on a community board. At the next level, success, the individual "chooses to become influential in the policy arena" by becoming involved on the state or national level (Boswell et al., 2005, p. 6). Significance is the final level of involvement, whereby the individual is intensely involved in all aspects of healthcare policy, assuming leadership positions in influencing legislation at the state and national level.

Hewison (2008) described nursing involvement in policy as a continuum from policy literacy, to policy acumen, to policy competence, and, finally, to policy influence (p. 292). Rather than finding a level of engagement, Hewison (2008) applied the strategy to where individuals are in their careers, from novice to expert. Policy literacy may only involve reviewing the literature, defining the issues, and analyzing health policy research. This early stage provides a framework for the more experienced nurse to develop policy acumen. Policy acumen is "an awareness and understanding distilled from a policy analysis" that allows nurses to influence the manner in which health care is organized and delivered (Hewison, 2008, p. 293). APRNs who have come to understand the issues and can analyze policy that translates into action would be able to persuade policy leaders to make healthcare decisions that are favorable to nursing and to their patient population. They can make the transition from the introspective realm of acumen to the action of competence (Hewison, 2008). The final level of policy influence brings together all the elements of the previous levels. The APRN who has achieved this level integrates the issues with health policy research, formulates the agenda, and influences policy on the national and international scale.

Most authors agree that all nurses have the responsibility of becoming involved in the policy process (Boswell et al., 2005; Hewison, 2008; Peters, 2002). Although it may be an intimidating task for both the novice and the experienced APRN, there are opportunities for involvement at all levels and in all areas of interest to nursing, including legislation and regulation, research, ethics, and practice.

Conclusion

According to Peters (2002), nurses should start to look at policy as not just the legislative process but as a comprehensive method of identifying healthcare issues and then bring those issues to the legislature and the American public. "Nurses will not be effective in politics or policy-making until they value their voices, develop policy agendas that embrace their core values, and learn the skills of policy making and influencing" (Mason et al., 2002, p. 12). Political expertise is essential for success. Nursing practice and health care must no longer be shaped by other dominant interest groups but instead by the inclusion of nurses using their education in policy combined with their unique understanding of the patient perspective.

Nurses must take advantage of positive public opinion and their pivotal position in the healthcare system as the largest group of providers. Patient advocacy should include policy advocacy, with APRNs increasing their knowledge of the issues and increasing political involvement. APRNs can be a crucial part of reforming health care by offering guidance and support to elected leaders. In the United States, APRNs have never been in a better position to influence health care as a whole, but it will require a group of "policy initiators who are willing to work toward eliminating the inequality of healthcare resources" (Peters, 2002, p. 5). This statement has been borne out in the last few years; nurses are increasingly involved at the state and federal level as their expertise is recognized as a crucial part of ensuring that healthcare reform is implemented in a manner that is cost effective, accessible, and based on the evidence.

According to health policy expert Mary Wakefield (2008), "If nurses want to be sought out as health care resources and to have their views reflected in health policy, nurses have to get off the porch to run with the big dogs" (p. 86). It has been argued that clinically engaged APRNs already have a full daily agenda, so how can they take on the additional responsibility of influencing policy? A more vital question should be, how can we not? Political activism provides nurses with the means to promote overall health through passing supportive health policy legislation, using evidence-based policy to transform institutional and national health systems, and employing policy language that prevents discrimination in reimbursement and patient access to providers. The doctorally prepared APRN is in the position to become this political advocate.

Acknowledgments

A special acknowledgment and thank you go out to my policy mentors: Laura Cohen, CRNA, and Brian R. Bullard, MBA, MPH, MA.

References

Abood, S., & Franklin, P. (2000). Why care about Medicare reimbursement? *American Journal of Nursing, 100*(6), 69–70, 72.

American Association of Colleges of Nursing. (2006). *The essentials of doctoral education for advanced nursing practice.* Retrieved from http://www.aacn.nche .edu/DNP/pdf/essentials.pdf

American Medical Association. (2005). *Scope of practice partnership.* Retrieved from http://www.camlawblog.com/articles/health-trends/ama-scope-of-practice-partnership/

American Nurses Association. (2001). *Code of ethics for nurses with interpretive statements.* Retrieved from http://www.nursingworld.org/MainMenuCategories/ EthicsStandards/CodeofEthicsforNurses.aspx

APRN Consensus Work Group & National Council of State Boards of Nursing. (2008, May 7). *Consensus model for APRN regulation: Licensure, accreditation, certification and education.* Retrieved from www.aacn.nche.edu/education-resources/APRNReport.pdf

Aroskar, M. A., Moldow, D. G., & Good, C. M. (2004). Nurses' voices: Policy, practice and ethics. *Nursing Ethics, 11*(3), 266–276.

Bankart, M. (1993). *Watchful care: A history of America's nurse anesthetists.* New York, NY: Continuum.

Boswell, C., Cannon, S., & Miller, J. (2005). Nurses' political involvement: Responsibility versus privilege. *Journal of Professional Nursing, 21*(1), 5–8.

Broadston, L. S. (2001). Reimbursement for anesthesia services. In S. Foster & M. Faut-Callahan (Eds.), *A professional study and resource guide for the CRNA* (pp. 287–311). Park Ridge, IL: AANA Publishing.

Bureau of Labor Statistics. (2015). Nurse anesthetists, nurse midwives, and nurse practitioners. In *Occupational outlook handbook, 2008–09 edition.* Retrieved from http://www.bls.gov/ooh/healthcare/nurse-anesthetists-nurse-midwives-and-nurse-practitioners.htm

Center for Responsive Politics. (2009). *Health professionals' PAC contributions to federal candidates, 2006–2008.* Retrieved from http://www.opensecrets.org/ pacs/industry.php?txt=HO1&cycle2008

Coalition for Patients' Rights. (n.d.). *About us.* Retrieved from http://www .patientsrightscoalition.org/Main-Menu/About-Us

DeMarco, R., & Tufts, K. A. (2014). The mechanics of writing a policy brief. *Nursing Outlook, 62,* 219–224.

Diers, D. (2002). Research as a political and policy tool. In D. J. Mason, J. K. Leavitt, & M. W. Chaffee (Eds.), *Policy and politics in nursing and healthcare* (pp. 141–156). St. Louis, MO: Saunders.

Dulisse, B., & Cromwell, J. (2010). No harm found when nurse anesthetists work without supervision by physicians. *Health Affairs, 29*(8), 1469–1475.

Ennen, K. A. (2001). Shaping the future of practice through political activity: How nurses can influence health care policy. *Journal of the American Association of Occupational Health Nurses, 49*(12), 557–569.

Federal Election Commission. (2009). *Quick answers to PAC questions*. Retrieved from http://www.fec.gov/ans/answers_pac.shtml

Gable, L. (2011). The Patient Protection and Affordable Care Act, public health, and the elusive target of human rights. *Journal of Law, Medicine, and Ethics, 39*(3), 340–354.

Government Accountability Office. (2007, July 27). *Medicare physician payments: Medicare and private payment differences for anesthesia services*. Report to Subcommittee on Health, Committee on Ways and Means, U.S. House of Representatives (GAO Report GAO-07-463). Retrieved from www.gao.gov/new.items/d07463.pdf

Hall, M. A., & Lord, R. (2014). Obamacare: What the Affordable Care Act means for patients and physicians. *British Medical Journal*. Retrieved from http://dx.doi.org/10.1136/bmj.g5376

Hamric, A. B., Spross, J. A., & Hanson, C. M. (2000). *Advanced practice nursing: An integrative approach* (3rd ed.). St. Louis, MO: Elsevier Saunders.

Health Resources and Services Administration. (2010). *The registered nurse population: Findings from the 2008 National Sample Survey of Registered Nurses*. Retrieved from bhpr.hrsa.gov/healthworkforce/rnsurveys/rnsurveyfinal.pdf

Hewison, A. (1999). The new public management and the new nursing: Related by rhetoric? Some reflections on the policy process and nursing. *Journal of Advanced Nursing, 29*(6), 1377–1384.

Hewison, A. (2008). Evidence-based policy: Implications for nursing and policy involvement. *Policy, Politics, and Nursing Practice, 9*(4), 288–298.

Hogan, P. F., Seifert, R. F., Moore, C. S., & Simonson, B. E. (2010). Cost effectiveness analysis of anesthesia providers. *Nursing Economic$, 28*(3), 159–169.

Institute of Medicine. (2001). *Crossing the quality chasm: A new health system for the 21st century*. Washington, DC: National Academies Press.

Institute of Medicine. (2011). *The future of nursing: Leading change, advancing health*. Washington, DC: National Academies Press.

Interagency Collaborative on Nursing Statistics. (2006). Home page. Retrieved from http://www.iconsdata.org

Jamelske, E. M., Johs-Artisensi, J. L., Taft, L. B., & German, K. A. (2009). A descriptive analysis of healthcare coverage and concerns in west central Wisconsin. *Policy, Politics, and Nursing Practice, 10*(1), 16–27.

Kent, R. L., & Liaschenko, J. (2004). Operationalizing professional values through PAC donations. *Policy, Politics, and Nursing Practice, 5*(4), 243–249.

Loversidge, J. M. (2008). Government regulation: Parallel and powerful. In J. A. Milstead (Ed.), *Health policy and politics: A nurse's guide* (pp. 91–127). Sudbury, MA: Jones and Bartlett.

Lyttle, B. (2011). Politics: A natural step for nurses. *American Journal of Nursing, 111*(5), 19–20.

Madler, B. J., Kalanek, C. B., & Rising, C. (2014). Gaining independent prescriptive practice: One state's experience in adoption of the APRN Consensus Model. *Policy, Politics, and Nursing Practice, 15*(3–4), 111–118.

Malone, R. E. (2005). Assessing the policy environment. *Policy, Politics, and Nursing, 6*(2), 135–143.

Mason, D. J., Leavitt, J. K., & Chaffee, M. W. (2002). *Policy and politics in nursing and healthcare* (4th ed.). St. Louis, MO: Saunders.

Maynard, C. A. (1999). Political influence: A model for advanced nursing education. *Clinical Nurse Specialist, 13*(4), 191–195.

McHugh, M. D., Aiken, L. H., Cooper, R. A., & Miller, P. (2008). The U.S. presidential election and health care workforce policy. *Policy, Politics, and Nursing, 9*(1), 6–14.

Milstead, J. A. (2008). *Health policy and politics: A nurse's guide* (3rd ed.). Sudbury, MA: Jones and Bartlett.

Minnesota Board of Nursing. (2008). *Nurse Practice Act.* Retrieved from http://mn.gov/health-licensing-boards/nursing/laws-and-rules/nurse-practice-act/

Nagelkerk, J. M., & Henry, B. (1991). Leadership through policy research. *Journal of Nursing Administration, 21*(5), 20–24.

National Council of State Boards of Nursing. (n.d.). *About NCSBN.* Retrieved from http://www.ncsbn.org/about.htm

National Health Security Plan. (1993). *Table of contents.* Retrieved from www.cbo.gov/sites/default/files/cbofiles/ftpdocs/79xx/...Orhttp://r.search.yahoo.com/_ylt=A0LEV71Do.RVIFoA.BonnIlQ;_ylu=X3oDMTBybGY3bmpvBGNvbG8DY mYxBHBvcwMyBHZ0aWQDBHNlYwNzcg--/RV=2/RE=1441076164/RO=10/RU=http%3a%2f%2fwww.cbo.gov%2fsites%2fdefault%2ffiles%2fcbofiles %2fftpdocs%2f79xx%2fdoc7945%2f93doc08b.pdf/RK=0/RS=o4IRvW1pXq .N1rnDDcVAd.QK0ho-

Newhouse, R. P., Bass, E. B., Steinwachs, D. M., Stanik-Hutt, J., Zangaro, G., Heindel, L., . . . Fountain, L. (2011). Advanced practice nurse outcomes 1990–2008: A systematic review. *Nursing Economic$, 29*(5), 1–21.

Nursing Community Consensus Document. (2008). Reauthorization priorities for Title VIII Public Health Service Act (42 U.S.C. 296 et seq.). Retrieved from www.aacn.org/wd/practice/docs/publicpolicy/nursing_consensus_document .pdf - 2008-05-27

Orszag, P. R. (2009). Beyond Economics 101: Insights into healthcare reform from the Congressional Budget Office. *Healthcare Financial Management, 63*(1), 70–75.

Patients' Access to Responsible Care Alliance. (n.d.). Home page. Retrieved from http://www.accessparca.com/home.html

Peters, R. M. (2002). Nurse administrators' role in health policy: Teaching the elephant to dance. *Nursing Administration Quarterly, 26*(4), 1–8.

Phillips, S. J. (2015). 27th annual APRN legislative update: Advancements continue for APRN practice. *The Nurse Practitioner, 40*(1), 16–42.

Rains, J. W., & Carroll, K. L. (2000). The effect of health policy education on self-perceived political competence of graduate nursing students. *Journal of Nursing Education, 39*(1), 37–40.

Rice, R. (2002). Coalitions: A powerful political strategy. In D. J. Mason, J. K. Leavitt, & M. W. Chaffee (Eds.), *Policy and politics in nursing and healthcare* (pp. 121–140). St. Louis, MO: Saunders.

Robert Wood Johnson Foundation Health Policy Fellowships Program. (n.d.). *Alumni directory.* Retrieved from http://www.healthpolicyfellows.org/secure/alumni-search.php

Rowles, J. (2009). *Comments of the American Association of Nurse Anesthetists on financing healthcare reform to the Senate Finance Committee*. Park Ridge, IL: American Association of Nurse Anesthetists.

Rubotzky, A. M. (2000). Nursing participation in healthcare reform efforts 1993–1994: Advocating for the national community. *Advances in Nursing Science, 23*(2), 12–33.

Schroeder, S. A. (1993). The Clinton health care plan: Fundamental or incremental reform? *Annals of Internal Medicine, 119*(9), 945–947.

Senate Finance Committee. (2009). *Financing comprehensive health care reform: Proposed health system savings and revenue options*. Retrieved from http://www.finance.senate.gov/newsroom/ranking/release/?id=24d07772-b4b8-414d-811d-24cc1c75c2a8

Short, N. M. (2008). Influencing health policy: Strategies for nursing education to partner with nursing practice. *Journal of Professional Nursing, 24*(5), 264–269.

Silva, M. C. (2002). Ethical issues in health care, public policy, and politics. In D. J. Mason, J. K. Leavitt, & M. W. Chaffee (Eds.), *Policy and politics in nursing and healthcare* (pp. 177–184). St. Louis, MO: Saunders.

Spetz, J., Bates, T., Chu, L., Lin, J., Fishman, N. W., & Melichar, L. (2014). Creating a dashboard to track progress toward IOM recommendations for the future of nursing. *Policy, Politics, and Nursing Practice, 14*(3–4), 117–124.

Sudduth, A. L. (2008). Program evaluation. In J. A. Milstead (Ed.), *Health policy and politics: A nurse's guide* (pp. 171–196). Sudbury, MA: Jones and Bartlett.

Sullivan-Marx, E. M. (2008). Lessons learned from advanced practice nursing payment. *Policy, Politics, and Nursing Practice, 9*(2), 121–126.

Summary of Citizens United v. Federal Election Commission. (2010). Retrieved from https://www.cga.ct.gov/2010/rpt/2010-R-0124.htm

Taft, S. H., & Nanna, K. M. (2008). What are the sources of health policy that influence nursing practice? *Policy, Politics, and Nursing Practice, 9*(4), 274–287.

Tobin, M. (2001). State government regulation of nurse anesthesia practice. In S. Foster & M. Faut-Callahan (Eds.), *A professional study and resource guide for the CRNA* (pp. 111–131). Park Ridge, IL: AANA Publishing.

Trotter Betts, V. (1996). Nursing's agenda for healthcare reform: Policy politics and power through professional leadership. *Nursing Administration Quarterly, 20*(3), 1–8.

Twedell, D. M., & Webb, J. A. (2007). The value of the political action committee: Dollars and influence for nurse leaders. *Nursing Administration Quarterly, 31*(4), 279–283.

Wakefield, M. K. (2008). Government response: Legislation. In J. A. Milstead (Ed.), *Health policy and politics: A nurse's guide* (pp. 65–90). Sudbury, MA: Jones and Bartlett.

Glossary

Caucus: A group of members of Congress or a political party created to support a defined political ideology or interest; in Congress, often votes en bloc.

Continuing resolution: A type of appropriations legislation that financially supports the government until a formal appropriations bill can be passed by Congress and signed into law.

Drop: Submitting the committee report concerning proposed legislation to the appropriate desk in the Senate or the House of Representatives.

Final rule: A regulation that has been published in the Federal Register. Includes the date on which the regulation goes into effect.

Grassroots lobbying: Occurs when nonpaid individuals contact their legislators to influence policy. May be very effective when coming from a legislator's constituency.

Hearing: A public meeting of a legislative committee or regulatory body held for the purpose of taking testimony concerning proposed legislation or regulation.

Jurisdiction: The authority or power granted to a legislative or regulatory body to allocate resources and approve, execute, and enforce laws. Typically has defined areas of responsibility.

Legislative assistant (LA): An employee of a senator or representative who keeps the legislator informed, meets with constituents, drafts reports, and so forth.

Markup: A committee process that amends, debates, and rewrites proposed legislation.

Omnibus legislation: A single bill that is voted on once but contains diverse amendments to a variety of other laws. Notably used in spending bills.

Regulation: A principle, rule, or law designed to control or govern conduct.

Report out: The proposed legislation, along with the committee report, is sent out of committee to the floor of the House or Senate to be acted on.

Special interest group: A group of individuals who coordinate lobbying efforts around a common interest (e.g., nursing) and seek to influence policy makers.

Statute: A law that pertains to certain subject matters (e.g., tax code).

Chapter 6

Interprofessional Collaboration for Improving Patient and Population Health

Laurel Ash, Catherine Miller, and Mary E. Zaccagnini

Background

The *Consensus Model for APRN Regulation* (2008), prepared by the APRN Consensus Work Group and the National Council of State Boards of Nursing APRN Advisory Committee and endorsed by numerous nursing organizations, defined advanced practice registered nursing (APRN) as nurses practicing in one of four recognized roles: certified nurse practitioners, certified nurse midwives, clinical nurse specialists, and certified registered nurse anesthetists. The primary focus of the practice of an advanced practice registered nurse (APRN) includes provision of direct patient or population care. Conventionally, APRNs are prepared in accredited programs, sit for national certification, and meet regulatory requirements authorizing license to practice as an APRN. A number of nurses with advanced graduate preparation function in specialties that do not fall into these categories yet advance the health of an organization, population, or aggregate or provide indirect patient care. Such roles may include administration, informatics, education, and public health. Discussions are ongoing as to how these specialty practices fit into the traditional definition of APRN practice and subsequently the doctor of nursing practice (DNP) role. This chapter will use the term *APRN* to reflect all advanced roles of nursing practice.

Numerous research has well documented the impact that APRNs have on health outcomes, including the ability to deliver excellent quality, cost-effective care with high levels of patient satisfaction (Cunningham, 2004; Dailey, 2005; Horrocks, Anderson, & Salisbury, 2002; Ingersoll, McIntosh, & Williams, 2000; Lambing, Adams, Fox, & Devine, 2004;

Laurant et al., 2004; M. Miller, Snyder, & Lindeke, 2005; Mundinger et al., 2000; Oliver, Pennington, Revelle, & Rantz, 2014). The world is changing, and APRNs must position themselves to be at the table with other disciplines and professionals in order to emphasize the influence of nursing care on the health of an individual or population. The complexity of the current healthcare delivery system, trends in patient demographics, epidemiological changes of disease and chronic conditions, economic challenges, the need for improved patient safety, and the call for a redesign or reform of the healthcare delivery system will challenge all professionals to envision health care in new ways.

Healthcare reform is a prominent issue for health professionals, policy makers, and the public. During the 2008 presidential campaign, President Obama announced a comprehensive healthcare reform proposal (Kaiser Family Foundation [KFF], 2008). This proposal outlined key points regarding restructuring our present system. As a foundation, all individuals and communities must be guaranteed a set of essential preventive care services. Reform must include measures to improve health outcomes and safeguard patients from preventable medical error. President Obama's platform supports programs that use collaborative teams as a means to deliver comprehensive, cost-effective, and safe care to persons with chronic conditions (KFF, 2008). Access to safe, effective, and affordable health care is a concern shared by the American public and rated of significant importance in a national poll, released in January 2009, conducted by researchers from the KFF and the Harvard School of Public Health.

Health Care Reform, formally known as the Patient Protection and Affordable Care Act (PPACA) (Public Law 111-148), was signed into law March 23, 2010, by President Barack Obama. This comprehensive set of enactments aims to control healthcare expenditures, enhance access to care, and improve patient care delivery and quality of health care (KFF, 2011; PPACA, 2010). Nursing is highlighted throughout the Act as playing a key role in addressing multiple reforms. Shortages of primary care physicians, particularly in certain geographic and underserved areas, contribute to access problems. Because the Act intends to extend health coverage to many more millions of Americans, further burdens are placed on an already stressed system. This legislation recognizes advanced practice nurses, particularly nurse practitioners, as part of the solution to raise numbers of primary care providers and expands funding for nurse practitioner training and education. Additionally, a number of provisions specifically identify nurses as interprofessional team leaders and members. The Medical/HealthCare Home provision (KFF,

2011; PPACA Section 3502, 2010) explicitly identified interdisciplinary teams—to include nurses, nurse practitioners, physicians, pharmacists, social workers, and other allied health professionals—to provide coordinated, integrated, and evidence-based care to patients and families, particularly those with complex healthcare needs. The Public Health Services Act of PPACA was amended to support nurse-managed health centers (KFF, 2011; PPACA Section 5208, 2010). The grant appropriates funds and authorizes advanced practice nurses to coordinate and deliver comprehensive primary and wellness care to underserved, vulnerable populations. Nurses must be the major providers of services in a team led by an advanced practice nurse. Demonstration projects, such as Independence at Home (KFF, 2011; PPACA Section 3024, 2010), clearly designate nurse practitioners as leaders of and/or participants in healthcare teams aimed at improving health outcomes of and reducing costs to homebound Medicare beneficiaries. Additionally, clinical nurse specialists have been noted as leaders in measures that were proved to prevent hospital-acquired conditions in acute care settings. DNPs, at the highest level of clinical nursing practice, must fully participate as team leaders and members in innovative models of care delivery and document improved healthcare outcomes as a result of such collaboration and leadership.

The professions of nursing and medicine agree on the need to create organizational environments that promote interprofessional collaboration. The American Nurses Association (ANA) report *Nursing's Agenda for Health Care Reform* (2008) placed particular emphasis on the role of collaboration in chronic disease management and patient safety. The American College of Physicians (ACP, 2009) also acknowledged that the future of healthcare delivery requires interprofessional teams that are prepared to meet the diverse, multifaceted health issues of the population. Providers, policy leaders, and health systems will need to shift their mindset from traditional models of linear, disease-focused care to new delivery approaches. In a redesigned model, each discipline brings specialized skills and abilities, practices at the highest level of the individual provider's scope, assumes new roles, and participates in a collaborative manner with other professionals to provide high-quality, safe, cost-effective, patient-focused care. This call to action demands that APRNs perform at the highest level of clinical expertise, the DNP, and collaborate interprofessionally to improve patient and population health outcomes.

In 2008, the Institute of Medicine (IOM), in partnership with the Robert Wood Johnson Foundation (RWJF), convened an 18-member panel of physicians, nurses, educators, policy makers, economists, and public health experts to examine, debate, and problem solve critical health-care issues—in particular, the role that nurses play in transforming the healthcare system. In October 2010, the panel released its findings in an evidence-based report, "The Future of Nursing: Leading Change, Advancing Health" (IOM, 2011). This 500-plus-page document highlights nursing's reputation for safe, high-quality care and provides specific recommendations to further advance skills and expertise of nurses to lead change. The report proposed that nurses attain higher educational levels to address increasingly complex health issues; that outdated organizational and regulatory barriers be removed to allow nurses to practice to the full extent of their education and training; and that nurses be provided opportunities to assume leadership positions and be full collaborative partners with physicians and other healthcare professionals in redesigning health care in the United States (IOM, 2011).

To improve quality, maximize resources, and coordinate care, patients with complex health needs are best served by an interdisciplinary approach to care. To foster positive collaborative behaviors between professionals, reduce biases of other disciplines, and ultimately improve patient outcomes, nursing education needs to expand to include competencies in interprofessional teamwork and collaboration in clinical environments (IOM, 2011). All nurses will benefit from enhanced leadership, political suaveness, advocacy, and health policy development skills, all of which are components of DNP programs. Although the IOM is a highly regarded institution, not all health professions embrace the report. Mistrust between disciplines continues to persist. The American Medical Association issued a response to the *Future of Nursing* report that challenged nursing's role, iterated that a "physician-led team approach to care helps ensure high quality patient care and value for health care spending," and emphasized the differences in physician and nurse practitioner education, suggesting that nurses are less prepared to deliver primary care (American Medical Association, 2010). Full partnership is a work in progress; DNPs must embrace these challenges and practice to the highest level to design, collaborate, lead, and document results of innovative models of care and resultant improved healthcare outcomes.

Merriam-Webster's Collegiate Dictionary (2015) defined *collaborate* as "to work jointly with others or together especially in an intellectual endeavour." Leaders in the business world further described collaboration as a concept involving "strategic alliances" or "interpersonal networks" in an effort to accomplish a project (Ring, 2005). As healthcare professionals, we can learn from successful business and management practices and use the collaboration processes of communicating, cooperating, transferring knowledge, coordinating, problem solving, and negotiating to more effectively reach a healthcare goal or outcome. The ACP (2009) suggested that collaboration involves mutual acknowledgment; understanding; and respect for the complementary roles, skills, and abilities of the interprofessional team. Effective collaborative partnerships promote quality and cost-effective care through an intentional process that allows members to exchange pertinent knowledge and ideas and subsequently engage in a practice of shared decision making. The purpose of this chapter is to generate a better understanding of interprofessional collaboration, distinguish the elements that DNPs must possess to successfully collaborate with other professionals to improve the health status of persons or groups, and provide an overview of models of interprofessional collaboration in the real world.

Improving Health Outcomes

The IOM's 2001 report, *Crossing the Quality Chasm: A New Health System for the 21st Century*, identified four key issues contributing to poor quality of care and undesirable health outcomes: the complexity of the knowledge, skills, interventions, and treatments required to deliver care; the increase in chronic conditions; inefficient, disorganized delivery systems; and challenges to greater implementation of information technology. The report went on to outline 10 recommendations intended to improve health outcomes, one of which focuses on interprofessional collaboration. It emphasizes the need for providers and institutions to actively collaborate, exchange information, and make provisions for care coordination because the needs of any persons or population are beyond the expertise of any single health profession (IOM, 2001; Yeager, 2005). An earlier IOM report (1999), *To Err Is Human: Building a Safer Health System*, addressed issues related to patient safety and errors in health care. This report articulated interprofessional communication and collaboration as primary measures to improve quality and reduce errors. A newer IOM report focused on *Measuring the Impact of Interprofessional Education (IPE) on Collaborative Practice and Patient Outcomes* (2015).

Accrediting and regulatory bodies such as The Joint Commission (2015) recognize interprofessional collaboration as an essential component of the prevention of medical error. This organization's mission is to continuously improve the safety and quality of care through the measure and evaluation of outcomes data. It has targeted improved communication and collaboration among providers, staff, and patients as a means to better protect patients from harm. Improved patient safety outcomes can be additionally facilitated through collaborative efforts such as development of interdisciplinary clinical guidelines and interprofessional curricula that incorporate proven strategies of team management and collaboration processes. Doctorally prepared APRNs are well positioned to participate in and lead interprofessional collaborative teams in efforts to improve health outcomes of the individual patient or target population (American Association of Colleges of Nursing [AACN], 2006b).

Interprofessional Collaboration

The terms *interdisciplinary* and *interprofessional* are often interchanged in the literature about collaborative teams, but each has a slightly different connotation. Interprofessional collaboration describes the interactions among individual professionals who may represent a particular discipline or branch of knowledge but who additionally bring their unique educational backgrounds, experiences, values, roles, and identities to the process. Each professional may possess some shared or overlapping knowledge, skills, abilities, and roles with other professionals with whom he or she collaborates. Hence, the term *interprofessional* offers a broader definition than *interdisciplinary*, which is more specific to the knowledge ascribed to a particular discipline. DNPs are suited to serve as effective collaborative team leaders and participants not only because of the scientific knowledge, skills, and abilities related to their distinctive advanced nursing practice disciplines but also because of their comprehension of organizational and systems improvements, outcome evaluation processes, healthcare policy, and leadership. This new skill set will be critical for DNPs leading teams in the complex and ever-changing health arena. The AACN's *Essentials of Doctoral Education for Advanced Nursing Practice* (2006b) added that collaborative teams must remain "fluid depending upon the needs of the patient (population) . . . and [DNPs] must be prepared to play a central role in establishing interprofessional teams, participating in the work of the team and assuming leadership of the team when appropriate" (p. 14).

The concept of interprofessional collaborations to improve health outcomes is not new; it has been and continues to be the cornerstone of public health practice. Effective public health system collaborations are critical to protect populations from disease and injury and to promote health. Public health collaborations have involved not only vested professionals but also systems of communities, governmental agencies, nonprofit organizations, and private-sector groups to address a common goal or complex health outcome (Wilson & Bekemeir, 2004). DNPs can benefit from the experiences of public health colleagues and expand the definition of interprofessional panel collaboration. This is particularly relevant when considering potential stakeholders and in assembling the team. Successful implementation of a system or organizational improvement may require collaborations outside the typical healthcare team. The purpose or outcome of the project may dictate the need to include patient or family representation in accordance with their ability and willingness to participate, as well as professionals from information and technology, health policy, administration, governing boards, and library science.

Interprofessional Healthcare Teams

Many healthcare practitioners indicate that they practice within an interprofessional team. Often this involves each professional addressing a particular portion of patient or population care, working *independently* and in parallel or in sequence with one another, with the physician frequently assuming the role of team leader (RWJF, 2008). Drinka and Clark (2000) reinforced the need to function *interdependently* and engage in collaborative problem solving. All too often, competition exists between roles, with each discipline holding to the belief that it is the most qualified to manage the patient or problem, thus negatively influencing the functioning of the team. In effective interprofessional teams, members recognize and value dissimilar professional perspectives and overlapping roles, and they share decision making and leadership to best meet the needs of the patient or problem at hand (Drinka & Clark, 2000). To achieve optimal health outcomes, it is essential for DNPs and other health professionals to engage in true collaborative interprofessional practices. These types of collaborative practices will be most successful when (1) the complexity of the problem is high, (2) the team shares a common goal or vision for the outcome, (3) members have distinctive roles, (4) members recognize the value of each other's positions, and (5) each offers unique contributions toward the improved patient or population outcome (ACP, 2009; Drinka & Clark, 2000; RWJF, 2008). This model for interprofessional healthcare teams will require DNPs to have a thorough understanding of effective collaboration—in addition to a firm grounding in effective communication, team processes, and leadership—to bring forth innovative strategies to improve health and health care.

Benefits of Collaboration

The literature of the past two decades well documents the numerous benefits of collaborative practices, including reduced error, decreased length of stays, improved health, better pain management, improved quality of life, and higher patient satisfaction (Brita-Rossi et al., 1996; Chung & Nguyen, 2005; Cowan et al., 2006; D'Amour & Oandasan, 2005; Drinka & Clark, 2000; Grady & Wojner, 1996; IOM, 1999; The Joint Commission, 2008; Yeager, 2005). Nelson et al. (2002) and Sierchio (2003) noted the additional benefits to healthcare systems of cost savings and healthy work environments. High-performing collaborative teams promote job satisfaction (D'Amour & Oandasan, 2005; Hall, Weaver, Gravelle, & Thibault, 2007; Sierchio, 2003), support a positive workplace atmosphere, and provide a sense of accomplishment while valuing the unique work and contributions of team members. Additionally, Weller, Boyd, and Cumin (2014) noted that "interventions to improve teamwork in healthcare may be the next major advance in patient outcomes" (p. 149).

These issues are particularly relevant to nursing practice. Addressing concerns of nursing shortages, improving working environments, and promoting measures to increase job satisfaction all have been found to correlate with lower rates of nurse burnout (Vahey, Aiken, Sloane, Clarke, & Vargas, 2004) and in turn indirectly influence nurse retention and recruitment.

The concept of "value added" has been discussed as an indirect benefit of effective collaboration (Dunevitz, 1997; Kleinpell et al., 2002). The term *value added* indicates the growth or improvement experienced in a group, project, or organization over a period, which yields an indirect "value" gained by a patient or population. Such value-added contributions may be the improvement to patient care delivery over time due to the rich professional interactions and exchanges that occur within an interprofessional team meeting. This enhanced communication would be more beneficial than the communication required from professionals working independently of one another. Value-added benefits may additionally be evident from the process itself, such as the creative problem solving that occurs during a brainstorming session designed to address a community health problem.

Barriers to and Drivers of Effective Collaboration in Interprofessional Healthcare Teams

Barriers

In spite of the mandates or recommendations by the IOM, the RWJF, the ANA, and The Joint Commission, effective interprofessional collaboration has yet to be adopted in any widespread form in the United States to improve patient or population outcomes. Literature from both Canada and Britain also makes recommendations for interprofessional collaboration to improve care (Oandasan et al., 2004), along with current thinking as to why healthcare systems have not adopted interprofessional healthcare teams. Some of the barriers to interprofessional collaboration include (1) gender, power, socialization, education, status, and cultural differences between professions (Hall, 2005; Whitehead, 2007); (2) lack of a payment system and structures that reward interprofessional collaboration; (3) the misunderstanding of the scope and contribution of each profession; (4) turf protection (Patterson, Grenny, McMillan, & Switzler, 2002); and the existence of individual discipline-based teams (Weller et al., 2014). The DNP will need a comprehensive understanding of these barriers to provide fresh, creative thinking and leadership for the healthy development and sustainment of collaboration.

Nursing and medicine were and are often considered central players in healthcare teams; an examination of the issues related to these two professions is prudent. Nurse and physician role differences are easier to understand in light of the historical roles of gender. In the 19th century, nurses cared for patients in hospitals, while physicians cared for patients in their offices or patients' homes. According to Lynnaugh and Reverby's *Ordered to Care: The Dilemma of American Nursing 1850–1945* (1990), whereas physicians were "welcome visitors," hospitals were run by lay boards and often staffed by "live in" nurses (p. 26). That changed when medicine became more science oriented and doctors realized that hospitals were full of sick patients to whom they could apply their newly developed knowledge of science. Medicine soon controlled hospitals and defended this control with the argument that they owned "special knowledge" to diagnose and treat. Physicians were able to convince the public that nurses were not trustworthy enough to manage medications or capable of obtaining the "special knowledge" that physicians had (often because of the menstrual cycle). Nurses soon became handmaidens to physicians; they needed to be "self-less, knowledgeless and virtuous" (Gordon, 2005, p. 63).

Nursing education in the 20th century was designed to provide cheap labor for hospitals while educating its new workforce. Nurses came to view themselves as working for doctors, not patients. Nurses were valued for their virtue, not for their knowledge (Buresh & Gordon, 2006). Most nurse leaders either accepted this subjugated role or were unable to change it. As nursing lost power, medicine increased its social status by high-tech innovations in acute care (along with reimbursement for them). Healthcare delivery became fragmented based on physician specialty care for patients with acute care needs. Indeed, medicine dominated health care in the 20th century.

It can be argued that this physician-dominant, fragmented care has driven up healthcare costs, promoted polypharmacy, and encouraged "silo" practices. Wheatley (2005) compared organizations to the biological natural world. In the biological world, if a species becomes too dominant and loses its ability to work when the environment shifts, the entire system can collapse. According to *Healthy People 2020* (U.S. Department of Health and Human Services, 2010), the nation's healthcare system will be challenged to provide effective chronic disease prevention and treatment. The current system, which is based on episodic care, will not serve the needs of the population. To meet the needs of the early 21st century, DNPs will need to bring a full nursing perspective into the healthcare environment, along with the empowerment of other members of the team to improve the viability and strength of the healthcare system.

Physicians have also been closely aligned with the financial success of healthcare organizations (often hospitals) and therefore have often been designated leaders for any clinically based team. Even today, the ACP (2009) concluded that the "patient is best served by a multidisciplinary team where the clinical team is led by the physician" (p. 2). Although physicians may have the most training in diagnosis and treatment of disease, they may not always be the best choice to lead teams. Haas (1977) discussed the "cloak of competence" that is expected of physicians by society. Medical students are socialized to adopt this "cloak" or image of confidence and perceived competence to meet societal expectations and may bring this "decisiveness" to the interprofessional arena. This may lead the physician to believe that he or she must always make the final decision in the team, which may result in a professional power imbalance whereby physicians have more power than other members of the team.

The issue of "disruptive behavior" in the workplace has been studied in light of the connection between poor communication and adverse events (The Joint Commission, 2008). Rosenstein's (2002) qualitative study of physician–nurse relations found that almost all nurses in the study experienced some sort of "disruptive physician behavior," including verbal abuse. Rosenstein and O'Daniel (2008) repeated this work, expanded to include disruptive behavior by both nurses and physicians. This second report concluded that whereas "physician disruptive behavior is usually more direct and overt, nurse disruptive behaviors more frequently take the form of back-door undermining, clique formation, and other types of passive-aggressive behavior" (Rosenstein & O'Daniel, 2008, p. 467).

In its *Essentials of Doctoral Education for Advanced Nursing Practice*, the AACN (2006b) discussed the need for interprofessional healthcare teams to function as high-performance teams. High-performance teams are those that emphasize the skills, abilities, and unique perspective of each team member. If the nurses (or other team members) remain invisible, the overall effectiveness of the team will be impaired.

To work on interprofessional teams, nurses will need to articulate the role they play in improving patient care. The work that nurses perform is often not recognized by other healthcare professionals and reimbursement systems or found within the nomenclature of electronic health records. Many tasks that nurses perform are difficult to quantify, such as supporting a family through a crisis. A vital responsibility of the DNP (likely collaborating with other nursing PhD colleagues) is to articulate to the public, insurers, and policy makers the role that nurses play in promoting positive patient and family outcomes.

Another key factor in empowering nurses in interprofessional collaboration is the importance of role identification and clarity. In the United States, there is confusion about the education and titling of nurses. Although many states protect the title of "nurse," the public (including other healthcare professionals) continues to be confused about just who nurses are. Nurses in administration may not identify themselves as nurses, whereas some medical assistants may call themselves "nurses." Although the work that medical assistants do with patients is valuable, it is not nursing. The first step to getting our voices heard is to identify who we are and call ourselves "nurses" at all levels. It is important that as nurses work to gain visibility and voice, they remain open to listening to other voices on the team.

Drivers

Successful Team Development

What are the stages of development that transform groups of disparate professionals into high-performance teams? Tuckman and Jensen (1977) and many others believe that teams go through stages, including forming, storming, norming, performing, and adjourning. Amos, Hu, and Herrick (2005) recommended that nurses understand these developmental stages in order to promote the development of a successful team.

Forming is the stage when the team first comes together to serve a specific purpose. Team members come into the group as individuals and get to know each other while determining the mission of the team, along with their roles and responsibilities. The development of trust is key in this stage. Davoli and Fine (2004) suggested incorporating activities that are designed to show the human side of each team member, such as "icebreakers" or "member check-in" (p. 269).

In an interdisciplinary team, it is likely that there are members from diverse professions, each with its own culture and language. An important first task of an interdisciplinary team is to discuss and understand the scope of each profession represented (Hall, 2005). It is likely there will be both overlap and diversity of function and skills among the professions. It is also important to develop a sense of shared language by reducing the use of professional jargon. Although it may be unintentional, jargon can prevent knowledge sharing, hinder communication, and promote power imbalances. Standardized tools such as SBAR (situation, background, assessment, and recommendation), developed and used by Kaiser Permanente, can be used by interprofessional teams for discussion and problem solving regarding patient situations (Leonard, Graham, & Bonacum, 2004).

In the *storming* stage, team members have not fully developed trust, and conflict inevitably arises. Within interprofessional teams, members come from diverse disciplines and world views. It is highly likely that there will be a wide range of opinions and thoughts related to the issues and work of the team. It is important to face this conflict directly, however, to move on to the next stage. During the storming stage, it is vital that members learn to listen to one another with tolerance and patience (Lee, 2008). If the team does not go through this stage successfully, differences between individuals will not be brought into the team process and outcome. Conflict resolution will be discussed at length later in this chapter.

Norming is the stage in which team members begin to develop a team identity. It is still important for the team to elicit differences of opinion in order to prevent "groupthink." During this phase, team members develop a comfort level at which they can express their ideas freely and begin to gain respect for others on the team. Constructive criticism is acceptable, and members begin to resolve problems.

In the *performing* stage, team members work together to achieve team goals. Individual and professional turf needs will be set aside for the team to be effective in its mission. At this stage, the team members also learn to be flexible in tasks and roles in order to achieve the team's goals. There should now be a sense of commitment to the tasks and goals of the team.

Finally, the stage of *adjourning* concludes the formation of a team. The team evaluates its performance and progress by reviewing whether outcomes were met. Occasionally team members may lose focus on the actual task. It can, however, be a time of celebration of accomplishments.

The following factors assist teams to progress through the stages of team development:

- Shared purpose, goal, and buy-in of members
- Reciprocal trust in team members
- Recognition and value of the unique role or skills each brings

- Functioning at the highest level of *skill*, ability, or practice
- Clear understanding of roles and the responsibilities of team members to meet goals
- Work culture and environment that embrace the collaborative process
- Collective cognitive responsibility and shared decision making

Shared Purpose

For a team to be effective, there must be a shared purpose or vision (Kouzes & Pozner, 2007). The purpose of the interprofessional health-care team is based on improving some aspect of patient or population health outcomes. Competing needs of team members must be tabled in favor of the greater purpose. Turf wars and politicized thinking have no place in an effective interprofessional healthcare team. The leader must inspire this shared vision and elicit buy-in from each member. As Wheatley (2005) suggested, creativity is unleashed in people when they find "meaning" or purpose in "real" work. Meaningful teamwork can create synergistic solutions from members when the team has shared meaning or vision. Patterson et al. (2002) described how free-flowing dialogue helps "fill the pool" of shared meaning. By allowing dialogue to be safe, more people can add their meaning to the "shared pool," giving the group a higher IQ. Learning to make dialogue safe is a skill that drives trust.

Team Members and Reciprocal Trust

An effective team must include the development of reciprocal trust between members. According to Kouzes and Pozner (2007), members of a high-trust team must continue to work to maintain interpersonal relationships with one another. In addition to the group mission and goals, the work of the group must also include getting to know one another. The leader or facilitator who is willing to trust others in the group enough to show vulnerability and give up control often begins a culture of trust. The leader must have enough self-confidence to be the first to be transparent; because trust is contagious, others will likely follow. Team members and leaders need to listen intently and value the unique viewpoints of others in the group. If the group fails to develop trust or to listen to and value each other, it is likely that group members will resist and sabotage the group's efforts (Wheatley, 2005). Many authors describe this aspect of team leadership as leading with the heart: looking at how the heart can help shape dialogue and goals (Kouzes & Pozner, 2007; Patterson et al., 2002).

Because of growth in global businesses, along with economic and time constraints, many teams now meet in virtual formats. Virtual formats can unite team members from different cultural groups and social constructs. The question many have is: What components are necessary to build trust in virtual teams? Kouzes and Pozner (2007) proposed that a group will become a team only when they have met face to face four to five times. These authors suggested that "virtual trust, like virtual reality, is one step removed from the real thing" (Kouzes & Pozner, 2007, p. 241). Watkins (2013) believes that it is easier to build trust if the team meets physically early on. During this meeting, it would be imperative to build in social time in order for members to get to know each other. Watkins then suggested that there be occasional reconnection if possible. Other sources discussed the very real possibility of developing trust via virtual means (Grabowski & Roberts, 1999; Greenberg, Greenberg, & Antonucci, 2007; Kirkman, Rosen, Gibson, Tesluk, & McPherson, 2002). Mayer, Davis, and Schoorman (1995) proposed that trust consists of three dimensions: ability, benevolence, and integrity. There is some evidence that when teams meet face to face, they form trust based on benevolence, whereas virtual teams rely more on ability. For example, in teams that meet in person, benevolence or interpersonal trust is enhanced by informal personal meetings that occur at lunch or in the copy room. Virtual groups tend to develop trust based on performance and ability of team members.

Because of the lack of eye contact and body language in virtual interactions, communication patterns should be more deliberate. Greenberg et al. (2007) proposed that trust building in virtual teams intentionally includes activities that promote both cognitive and affective trust. Cognitive trust is implicated in the formation of "swift, but fragile trust" during the early development of the team (Greenberg et al., 2007, p. 325). For cognitive trust to develop, individual team members need to believe that group members have both ability (competence) and integrity. One action to promote a sense of competence in individual team members is to have the team leader introduce members, endorse their abilities, and note why they were chosen for the team. Another important asset for building the sense of integrity is for team members to keep deadlines and stay engaged in the process (no freeloading). Affective trust is essential during later stages of the team's development and is vital to the functioning of team members to complete the task. Development of affective trust is based on benevolence and relies on team members seeing the humanity in one another, with development of true caring and concern.

Holton (2001) recommended that virtual teams include time in "caring talk," which she defined as "personal conversations and storytelling" (p. 36). G. Boehlhower recommended that virtual teams begin their meeting time with "check in, story-telling, deep questioning and dialogue, and affirmation" (personal communication, April 10, 2009). He went on to state that he "sees the level of trust develop regularly" in online groups when the human side of individuals is shared. As discussed earlier in this chapter, this type of sharing may be started with icebreakers, check-ins, and checkouts.

DNPs will likely have experience with online relationship and team building during their education process and can continue to experiment with team building in face-to-face and virtual formats based on the current evidence. The use of video conferencing (which includes visual and nonverbal cues) enhances the richness of communication and thus decreases ambiguity and increases trust. It may be that the communication channel (face to face, video or audio conferencing, group chat, text, email, and so on) should be matched to the purpose of the communication (Clark, Clark, & Crossley, 2010).

Recognition and Value of Each Team Member

According to Burkhardt and Alvita (2008), "Each person is a moral agent and must be recognized as worthy of dignity and respect" (p. 219). Without respect, the work of the group cannot move forward; dialogue is halted. Respect among team members is vital because, as Patterson et al. (2002) noted, "Respect is like air. If it goes away, it is all people can think about" (p. 71). Each member's voice must be heard and respected regardless of whether he or she is the highest educated member. To do this, team members must recognize the moral agency of each member and his or her unique skills and abilities, often based on the individual's professional skill set.

Using structure in interprofessional team dialogue may be called for as a result of the entrenched perceived power and authority of individual members and the professions they represent. Such methods as the Indian talking stick and Johari window can be used proactively to be sure that all team members feel they have a voice, are understood, and are free to share their thoughts and feelings. The concept behind the talking stick is that only the person who is holding the stick may speak. When the person finishes speaking, the stick is passed to the next speaker. That next person may not argue or disagree with the former speaker but is to restate what has been said. This process allows for all team members to be and feel understood (Covey, 2004).

The Johari window is a tool developed in 1955 by Joseph Luft and Harry Ingham (Chapman, 2008). It is used to help build trust among group members by encouraging appropriate self-disclosure. The Johari window has four quadrants: the open area, the blind area, the hidden area, and the unknown area. The goal is to increase the open area so that team members can be more productive because communication is not hampered by "distractions, mistrust, confusion, conflict and misunderstanding" (Chapman, 2008, p. 4). One team member (the subject) is given a list of 55 adjectives and is told to pick 5 or 6 that describe himself or herself. A team member is given the same list and also picks out 5 or 6 words that describe the subject. The adjectives are then placed in the four quadrants:

1. Both team members know the open area.
2. Only the subject, not the other team member, knows the hidden area.
3. Only the team member, not the subject, knows the blind spot.
4. The unknown area includes adjectives picked by neither subject nor team member and may or may not be applicable to the subject. (Chapman, 2008)

The Johari tool can assist team members to learn about both themselves and each other. Appropriate and sensitive increases in the open area can be promoted by the use of team-building exercises and games, along with teams engaging in nonworktime activities.

Functioning at the Highest Level

American health care is expensive but not always effective. There is pressure for innovative models of care that are cost-effective and improve outcomes for patients. Many clinical systems have begun to use episodic treatment groups (ETGs) to measure patient outcomes and provider performance (Fortham, Dove, & Wooster, 2000). Introduced in 1993, "ETGs have become the industry standard for episodic patient classification" (OPTUM, 2015). Examples of ETGs are those for chronic diseases such as diabetes, asthma, depression, and hypertension. Guideline development by such groups as the Institute for Clinical Systems Integration (ICSI) can provide evidence-based pathways of care for the various ETGs.

In the past, physicians have felt the need to perform all the primary care tasks for patients. Given the current complexity and expense of health care, it is not possible for one group to do it all. This realization has led to the concept of having all healthcare providers work to the top of their licenses. This involves a shifting of tasks, often with each discipline giving up some tasks that can be done by another care provider more cost effectively. An example of working to the top of one's license is for advanced practice nurses to take more responsibility for routine chronic and acute care and health maintenance, while physicians perform the diagnosing and treatment of more complex unstable patients, and registered nurses (RNs) assume the role of care coordinator (including pre- and postvisit planning), coach, and educator. In this example, all disciplines may need to give up some tasks to be cost effective. An exemplar of a program that utilizes healthcare providers at the top of their licenses is the DIAMOND (Depression Improvement Across Minnesota, Offering a New Direction) project (ICSI, 2014). At the center of the DIAMOND project is a case manager (typically an RN) who has 150 to 200 patients with depression in an outpatient setting. The case manager works with a consulting psychiatrist to review patients on a weekly basis (typically 2 hours per week). This has proved to be a cost-effective model that provides better depression outcomes than standard care. The challenge is to provide a payment structure that rewards this type of innovative care.

Clear Understanding of Roles and Responsibilities

During the forming stage of the team (and beyond), it is vital that each team member understand his or her role and responsibilities. Role uncertainty can lead to conflict among team members and decrease team functioning (Baker, Baker, & Campbell, 2003). The leader should be certain that each team member has a clear understanding of his or her role by having the members restate their role to the team. This type of candid discussion can occur only if the team feels that open communication is safe. A clear understanding of each team member's role helps to prevent role overlap as well as tasks falling through the cracks (Lewis, 2007).

Work Culture That Embraces Collaboration

Some of the components of a work culture that embraces collaboration are: (1) providing psychological safety, (2) a flattened power differential (hierarchy), (3) administrative support and resultant resources allocated for collaboration (Kelly, 2008), and (4) physical space design that promotes collaboration, such as rooms for interdisciplinary interaction (Lindeke & Sieckert, 2005).

According to Gilbert (2006), organizations that support "upward voice" promote a culture of psychological safety. She went on to state that "upward voice is communication directed to someone higher in the organizational hierarchy with perceived power or authority to take action on the problem or suggestion" (p. 1). Some tangible evidence of this are leaders who walk around the organization and initiate conversation, suggestion boxes placed around the organization, and an open-door policy. Individuals must have the sense that they can readily ask questions, try out new ideas and innovations, and ask for support from others.

Another way to promote psychological safety within an organization centers on employee confidence that there will not be a penalty for admitting to mistakes. Safety culture research is shifting from focusing on only the role of individuals in errors to the role of systems. Healthcare leaders have had to explore other industry successes that promote safety, such as aviation, where the focus of safety improvement is on the systems in which individuals operate (Feldman, 2008). Authors such as Snijders, Kollen, Van Lingen, Fetter, and Molendijik (2009) have recommended a nonpunitive incident reporting system to improve safety standards. A nonpunitive incident reporting system helps ensure that issues are brought to the forefront so that improvements can be made. The Agency for Healthcare Research and Quality (2009) has developed evaluation tools for primary care offices, nursing homes, and hospitals with questions related to psychological safety and communication. However, in many institutions there remains the problem that individuals are discouraged from reporting adverse events (O'Reilly, 2012). It should be recognized that this fear could cause a decrease in safety. DNPs will be required to provide leadership and recommend resources to champion the culture of both psychological and systems safety within the organizations they serve.

Collective Cognitive Responsibility and Shared Decision Making

As fundamental as it is for each team member to have a clear understanding of individual roles and responsibilities, it is also essential for high-performance teams to have a culture of shared decision making or collective cognitive responsibility. Scardamalia (2002) described collective cognitive responsibility in terms of team members having responsibility not only for the outcome of the group but also for staying cognitively involved in the process as things unfold. She described the functioning of a surgical team, in which members not only perform their assigned tasks but also stay involved in the entire process. The responsibility for the outcome lies not just with the leader of the surgical team but with the entire team as a whole.

A key component of shared decision making is that it usually occurs at the point of service (Golanowski, Beaudry, Kurz, Laffey, & Hook, 2007; Porter-O'Grady, 1997). Porter-O'Grady stated that "the point of decision making in the clinical delivery system is the place where patients and providers meet" (p. 41), which has implications for including patients as collaborators on the interprofessional team.

Healthcare systems, as complex adaptive systems, require flexibility and continuous participation, learning, and sharing (Begun, Zimmerman, & Dooley, 2003). All the interprofessional healthcare team members must stay engaged in the process at the point of service for the outcome of care to be successful.

Strong Leadership

There is no dispute that redesigning health care will require strong leadership. As opposed to "management," which seeks to control and manage, leaders seek to create and inspire change (Kotter, 1990). Leadership theories generally fall under the classifications of behavioral, contingency, contemporary, and Wheatley's "new leadership" approaches (Kelly, 2008). Behavioral theories posit that leadership style or behavior is the most important factor in the outcome desired. Behavioral approaches include autocratic, democratic, and laissez-faire, based on where the power or decision making occurs and the type of worker or task involved. Contingency theories recognize that there is more to leadership than the leader's behavior. One type of contingency theory is situational leadership, developed by Blanchard (2008), in which follower maturity is evaluated and determines the amount of direction, support, or delegation from the leader to the follower. Contemporary theories include transformational leadership, which the IOM (2003) deemed vital to the achievement of the transformation of health care.

Transformational Leadership The IOM (2003) report recommended transformational leadership to make the necessary changes to improve patient safety. Transformational leadership, developed first by Burns (1978), is based on the concept of empowering all team members (including the leader) to work together to achieve a shared goal. This fits with Covey's (2004) definition of leadership: "Leadership is communicating to people their worth and potential so clearly that they come to see it in themselves" (p. 98).

The transformational leader need not be in a formal position of administration, but can lead from any position within the organization and operates through an ethical and moral perspective. Transformational leaders lead with a clear vision and use coaching, inspiring, and mentoring to transform themselves, followers, and organizations (Burns, 1978; Kelly, 2008).

Complexity Leadership or "New Leadership" Complexity leadership is the name given to the new paradigm of thinking about leadership that unites science and management to solve problems. Complexity has contributions from chaos theory and similarities to the thinking of such nurse theorists as Rogers, Newman, and Watson (Crowell, 2011). Margaret Wheatley (2005) described this "new way" of leadership, which is contrary to the Western style of linear, hierarchical organizations. She bases her view of organizations on biology, which is self-organizing and complex. Instead of seeing change as negative, Wheatley views change as life itself. She stated, "Nothing alive, including us, resists creative motions. However, all of life resists control. All of life reacts to any process that inhibits its freedom to create itself" (p. 28). She recommended that teams self-organize to build communities that are no longer ruled by "command and control" (p. 68). Instead of viewing organizations and workers as machines, Wheatley suggested that organizations model themselves after living systems, which are adaptive, creative, and depend on one another for growth and sustainability.

Leadership Versus Management Whereas management is the coordination of resources to meet organizational goals, leadership is built on relationships. Kouzes and Pozner (2007), in their seminal book *The Leadership Challenge*, examined leaders over 25 years and determined that leadership is a relationship in which leaders do five things:

1. *Model the way.* The leader must be aware of his or her own values and live a life that expresses those values.
2. *Inspire a shared vision.* The leader must be able to imagine the future and inspire others to share that vision.
3. *Challenge the process.* Leaders are engaged in the processes of the team and continually looking for innovations. They are willing to take risks and learn from experiences.
4. *Enable others to act.* Leaders help to build trust in relationships through collaboration and competence.
5. *Encourage the heart.* Leaders identify the contributions of each individual team member and encourage celebration when victories occur.

Anyone can be a leader; a formal title is not necessary.

Effective Communication

> *Remember not only to say the right thing in the right place, but far more difficult still, to leave unsaid the wrong thing at the tempting moment.*

—Benjamin Franklin

All the work of interprofessional collaborations involves communication. Success or failure of the team is dependent on the effectiveness of the communication processes. Communication is a complex process of transmitting a message between a sender and receiver. The sender must effectively deliver the content, and the receiver must in turn correctly interpret or decipher the message. Many sources of error can occur within this exchange, and skilled communicators must make a concerted effort to deliver clear, consistent messages to prevent misinterpretation and loss of meaning.

Communication is more than the exchange of verbal information; in fact, the majority of communication is nonverbal. The DNP must be accomplished not only in the art of verbal and written communication but also in the interpretation and effective use of nonverbal communiqués such as silence, gestures, facial expressions, body language, tone of voice, and space (Sullivan, 2004).

In addition to sending congruent verbal and nonverbal messages, it is vital for DNPs to employ strategies that enhance communication within the interprofessional team setting. Determining the timing and best medium for what, how, and when to deliver a message is a necessary skill (Sullivan, 2004). Appropriate timing of key messages increases the likelihood that the message will have the desired impact on the recipient. The message may be phrased well but rejected if the intended audience is not receptive. Consider the availability and state of mind of the recipient. Is there adequate time for the discussion? Is the recipient distracted, emotionally or physically? Are other issues more pressing now? Such factors may contribute to misinterpretation or lack of objectivity regarding the communication. Reflect as to whether an alternative time, venue, or medium may provide a more appropriate means by which to deliver the message. For instance, if the message is of a sensitive, confidential matter, face-to-face communication would be preferable to an email, voicemail correspondence, or team discussion (Sullivan, 2004). In group settings, it is imperative to allow participants enough time to provide objective information and express thoughts, viewpoints, and opinions about the situation in order for meaningful collaboration to occur.

Buresh and Gordon, in their book *From Silence to Voice: What Nurses Know and Must Communicate to the Public* (2006), suggested use of the "voice of agency" when communicating the role of nursing to others. Within the collaborative team, it is imperative that DNP members clearly communicate nursing's involvement in a patient care scenario or clinical project and, more important, articulate the level of clinical judgment and rationale required for such actions. It is important and necessary to embrace the opportunity to communicate to the team the role of the DNP in enhanced care delivery. This voice of agency is not boastful nor an attempt to be superior, but rather an accurate acknowledgment of the unique contributions, value added, and improved patient outcomes resulting from expert nursing care. Conversely, it may reflect the negative consequences or potential for error averted as a result of the expertise, skills, and knowledge of doctorally prepared nurses. Davoli and Fine (2004) offered a similar perspective and noted, "Collaboration gives providers an opportunity to be introspective and solidify their role through the contributions they make. A successful collaborative process will enhance one's professional identity" (p. 268). Draye, Acker, and Zimmer (2006), in their article on the practice doctorate in nursing, proposed that the educational preparation of DNPs include opportunity for the student to convene an interprofessional team. This experience allows the student to incorporate strategies to promote effective team functioning while communicating the unique contributions of nursing required for the improved health outcome.

Buresh and Gordon (2006) went on to discuss the role that self-presentation plays in communicating information regarding the competency and credibility of the DNP to team members, patients, or the public. Attire and manner of address influence the perceptions of others. What does dress communicate if Mary wears teddy bear scrubs rather than street clothes and a lab coat to a committee meeting? How might the DNP's role be valued if she is introduced as Mary from pediatrics versus Dr. Mary Jones, pediatric nurse practitioner? How are physician colleagues addressed in similar workplace encounters? Introductions using one's full name and credentials convey professionalism, respect, and credibility on par with other healthcare professional colleagues (Buresh & Gordon, 2006).

Ineffective communication is a major obstacle in interprofessional collaboration, is directly related to quality of patient care, and contributes to adverse health outcomes (Clarin, 2007; IOM, 1999). Some barriers that lead to communication breakdowns are specific to interactions between the sender and receiver, whereas others relate to the organizational system. Defensiveness on the part of either participant can hamper communications (Sullivan, 2004). These behaviors may result from lack of self-confidence, a fear of rejection, or perceived threat to self-image or status. Defensiveness impedes communication by displacing anger via verbal aggression or conflict avoidance. Awareness of this mechanism and developing an approach to manage it in the context of the collaborative team are necessary attributes of an effective DNP leader.

As healthcare teams become more global and virtual, the potential for language and cultural communication barriers increases. Misreading body language or misinterpretation of the spoken or written message often results from a lack of understanding regarding language (especially in translation) and cultural differences (Sullivan, 2004). What one group finds acceptable another may consider offensive, such as eye contact, physical touch, or the use of space. Room for misinterpretation exists in translation. Language used by Western cultures typically is direct and explicit, in which the background is not necessarily required to interpret the meaning of the message. This may differ from cultures that use indirect communication, in which the intent of the message often relies on the context in which it is used (Brett, Behfar, & Kern, 2006). DNPs and interprofessional colleagues have an obligation to increase their cultural competence and understanding of health issues and healthcare disparities to dispel any misconceptions, particularly if the team is composed of persons from diverse cultures or if the recipient of care is from another culture.

Jargon is another "language" that can pose a barrier to understanding (Davoli & Fine, 2004; Sullivan, 2004). Unfamiliar terms can lead to confusion and error and should be avoided to prevent unfavorable outcomes. Although professional jargon may serve as a type of verbal shorthand among some group members, it can also be a form of intimidation or exclusion and contribute to an imbalance of knowledge or power within the team (Davoli & Fine, 2004). Lindeke and Block (2001) stressed that collaborative teams communicate with a shared, inclusive (i.e., "we," "our") language to prevent this imbalance and promote participation of all members. Effective communication involves the use of a common, shared language that is understood by all members of the team.

Preconceived assumptions and biases prevent the listener from tuning in and focusing on the content (Sullivan, 2004). This hinders the communication process because the receiver has formulated a predetermined judgment or drawn a conclusion before all the information is shared or facts validated. Effective communicators need to suspend judgments until all viewpoints are shared.

Gender differences in style and approach to communication can also pose obstacles (Sullivan, 2004). Subtle differences exist in how men and women perceive the same message. In collaborative teams, women may strive for consensus, whereas men may place emphasis on hierarchy and "leading the team." Differences exist in the use of questions and interruptions in communications. An appreciation and understanding of these dissimilarities can prepare the DNP to function more effectively in teams of mixed gender.

Organizations and systems may pose additional obstacles to effective interprofessional communications. Outdated, limited, or unavailable technologies, such as video conferencing, messaging, or paging systems, or lack of electronic health record interoperability between systems can significantly impair the ability of members to communicate on a timely basis. This can be of vital importance to patient safety when attempting to communicate critical changes in patient status, medications, or lab values. The system further contributes to communication problems when the roles and responsibilities of team members are unclear. Participants may be hesitant or resistant to engage in exchanges or knowledge sharing. Clear designation of roles is of particular importance in virtual organizations and teams (i.e., electronically linked providers). In these collaborative environments, risks can be mitigated if members have a clear understanding of what is expected of each other and have a pre-established path of communication (Grabowski & Roberts, 1999) (see **Table 6-1**).

Table 6-1 Measures to Improve Communication

Maintain eye contact: Convey interest, attentiveness. (U.S./Canada)

Speak concisely: Avoid jargon.

Use questions wisely: Clarify or elicit further information.

Avoid qualifiers or tags (e.g., "sort of," "kind of," "I don't know if you would be interested"): These reduce the effectiveness of one's message.

Be aware of gestures, facial expressions, posture: Send positive nonverbal signals (e.g., smiling conveys warmth, leaning forward indicates receptivity, and open-palm gestures suggest accessibility).

Avoid defensiveness.

Avoid responding emotionally: Never raise your voice, yell, or cry.

Conflict Resolution

As both leaders and members of interprofessional teams, DNPs will need to develop and continue to refine skills related to conflict resolution. Conflicts are inevitable and are even vital for interprofessional team effectiveness. *Conflict* is defined in many ways but generally includes disagreement, interference, and negative emotion (Barki & Hartwick, 2001). If conflict is disruptive or dysfunctional, team efforts can decrease communication and thus team functioning. On the other hand, conflict that is constructive leads to superior results by including the "shared pool of meaning" of all team members. According to Patterson et al. (2002), the "larger the shared pool, the smarter the decisions" (p. 21).

As stated earlier, nurses over the last century have often used passive-aggressive methods to resolve conflict, such as avoidance, withholding, smoothing over, and compromising (Feldman, 2008). These methods do not promote dialogue, the most central means to attain the shared pool of meaning of the entire team. DNPs need to lead nurses and other professionals in techniques that promote dialogue and thus collaboration between professionals. The purposes of collaborative conflict management are to promote win-win versus win-lose solutions. The skills for conflict resolution and improving dialogue can be learned. According to Patterson et al. (2002) in their book *Crucial Conversations*, conflict resolution includes such methods as starting with the heart, making conversation safe, staying in dialogue when emotions are high, using persuasion, and promoting positive actions. Most of the skills related to collaborative conflict management are intertwined with effective communication skills and the development of emotional intelligence (EI).

Chinn (2008) offered suggestions that are foundational for the transformation of conflict into solidarity and diversity. These recommendations begin before there is any conflict in a group or team and include rotating leadership, practicing critical reflection, and adopting customs to value diversity. By rotating leadership, the team members all have a stake in the outcome of the team goals and processes. When a conflict arises, involved parties can step back while other members rise up to help lead the team. Critical reflection can be accomplished by incorporating a closing time at which all team members can share their thoughts and feelings about the team process. By practicing ways to value diversity, such as developing team processes during meetings that show appreciation and value for each individual, conflict can move from violence to peaceful recognition of the diversity of alternative views.

Emotional Intelligence

Emotional intelligence (EI) is yet another valuable attribute of successful interprofessional leadership. EI is the awareness of the role that emotion plays in personal relationships and the purposeful use of emotion to communicate, build rapport, and motivate self and others. These characteristics have been found to play a far greater role than cognitive abilities in the success or failure of a leader (Goleman, Boyzatsis, & McKee, 2002).

Goleman et al. (2002) outlined five realms of EI: self-awareness, self-regulation, motivation, empathy, and social skills. Self-awareness involves recognizing your own emotions and the effect your mood and confidence level have on persons. Maintaining your composure in high-emotion meetings or challenging clinical situations is an example of effectual self-regulation. Conflict is a natural process of interprofessional teamwork, which can lead to positive or negative group functioning, depending on leadership style. Emotionally intelligent leaders have the ability to adapt, withhold judgment, and exhibit self-control in emotionally charged situations. An optimistic attitude, passion, and commitment to pursuing the goals of the group and desire for excellence help provide the motivation factor of EI. Leaders who are sensitive and empathetic to the needs and perspectives of others encourage the group to carry on and perform to its best ability.

Drinka and Clark (2000) talked about the role of "reflective practice" in interprofessional team practice. This concept builds on the self-awareness and empathy qualities of EI: the understanding of how our professional cultures, preparations, and experiences shape how we function in teams, as well as the ability to appreciate the similar and dissimilar perspectives of other interprofessional team members.

A fifth element is that of social skill: the ability to build rapport, network, communicate, and facilitate change. As an effective leader, it is imperative to foster a system of open, timely communication—whether by face-to-face communication, phone, or electronic means—to meet the desired outcomes for the project, patient, or population successfully. Regularly practicing calming relaxation techniques and rehearsing responses before anticipated stressful encounters allow one to manage reactions in an emotionally intelligent manner. DNPs can develop these skills with regular practice, self-reflection, coaching, and feedback from colleagues and can use "EQ" (emotional intelligence quotient) as a tool to gauge their performance as leaders.

McCallin and Bamford (2007) suggested that EI is integral to effective interdisciplinary team functioning. Healthcare providers may be highly skilled in practicing emotionally intelligent interactions with their patients and families but may receive little preparation in promoting emotionally intelligent, healthy communication and functioning between professionals. K. L. Miller et al. (2008) specifically explored the role of EI in nursing practice as it relates to interprofessional team functioning. In this qualitative study, the ability of the nurse to effectively collaborate on interprofessional teams was influenced by his or her degree of EI. Nurses who engaged in *esprit de corps* (significant role embracing to the exclusion of other professionals) were considerably less able to function successfully on the team, less able to have other members appreciate nursing's contribution to patient care, and generally less engaged in team processes. These researchers support the need to address not only the cognitive aspects of interprofessional teamwork but also the emotional aspects of optimal team functioning. DNP leaders versed in EI work are well suited to recognize individual and personality differences among team members and can build on them, mentor colleagues, and use EI to influence the effectiveness of the team and improve patient outcomes and satisfaction among interprofessional team members.

Necessities for Collaboration

Change Agent: Lewin's Model

The objective of interprofessional collaboration is, of course, to generate a practice or systems enhancement to improve the health of an individual or population. Whether implementing an evidence-based practice effort or a quality improvement initiative, some sort of change is required. Even what many group members view as a desirable change will inevitably encounter some reluctance or resistance. The ability to facilitate change or serve as an agent of change is a key function required for successful collaboration. DNPs must be versed in one or more theories of change to effectively motivate and move the collaborative team to the optimal goal.

Lewin's force field analysis model (1951) is a classic framework for understanding the process of change within a group, system, or health initiative. Lewin's theory recognizes change as a constant factor of life ensuing from a dynamic balance of driving and opposing forces. The desired change results from the addition of driving forces or the diminishing of opposing forces and progresses over a series of three stages: unfreezing, moving, and refreezing. Unfreezing necessitates assessing the need and preparing members to move from the status quo to an improved level of practice, whereas the movement phase involves the addition of driving forces to motivate and empower members to adopt the improved perspective while simultaneously minimizing restraining forces that pose barriers to the desired change (Lewin, 1951; C. Miller, 2008). Driving forces must outweigh opposing forces to shift the equilibrium in the direction of the desired change. The improvements must then be secured, or allowed to refreeze, in order to maintain the desired change (Lewin, 1951; C. Miller, 2008).

Continuous Reflective Learning

The drivers of effective interprofessional teams discussed in this chapter will evolve in teams over time. Knowing the drivers is the first step in the development of both personal and team skills, but individual team members and the team as a whole will need continuous reflection. Each leader and follower should develop habits that build in time for personal reflection and growth. Many find that reading sacred texts or poetry, listening to music, practicing yoga, praying, meditating, exercising, connecting with spiritual leaders, or being in nature allows for deep reflective thinking and learning. Covey (1991) called this "sharpening the saw" (p. 38) and recommended that people proactively plan for daily time to renew themselves. The wholeness of each team member is vital for the best functioning of the entire team.

Teams within healthcare organizations in the 21st century will need to practice continuous reflective learning (developed by Senge, 1990) to adapt to the rapid changes taking place. Interprofessional teams can utilize the vast organizational behavior research on the significance of continuous reflective learning. Edmonson (1999) defined team learning as "the activities carried out by team members through which a team obtains and processes data that allow it to adapt and change" (p. 352). Spending some time on reflection regarding team functioning will be vital to learning. Structural practices that foster team learning include providing time during each meeting for reflection, leaving the worksite for retreats, conducting "critical incident" evaluations, discussing errors and failures, using patient satisfaction surveys and interviews, and celebrating successes.

The Patient and Family as Interprofessional Team Members

As health care reorganizes into interprofessional teams in which primary care is the hub of the system, central team members will be patients and their families. Patients and their families will need to be invited into and supported in the interprofessional collaboration process through actions that promote meaningful dialogue, patient empowerment, self-efficacy, and activation (Hibbard, Stockard, Mahoney, & Tusler, 2004). Some tools the DNP may want to recommend include patient or family focus groups, satisfaction surveys, personal health records, decisional guides such as the *Ottawa Personal Decision Guide* (O'Connor, 2006), and advance directives, along with ongoing patient education regarding the patients' and families' role in health care.

Models for Implementation: From Project to Practice

Value of Incorporating Collaborative Work into Educational Preparation Curricula

Although there is a growing body of evidence regarding the benefits of collaboration between disciplines in the delivery of optimal patient care, few healthcare professionals have received any formal training in this concept during their educational preparation. Students in health professional programs often are taught in both the classroom and clinical setting by faculty from the same professional background. They have little opportunity to learn about the work of other disciplines or participate in any shared learning experience. Brewer (2005) described this pattern of education as "silo" preparation, in which each discipline believes it is best qualified to care for the patient. Without a formal structure and support for learning and practicing a team approach to care delivery in the educational setting, negative attitudes, prejudices, and misunderstanding of roles can occur. This contributes to an inability to collaborate effectively and consult with other providers as practicing professionals and may lead to discipline overlap and competition rather than collaboration for delivery of care.

A Cochrane systematic review of interprofessional education interventions (Reeves et al., 2008) examined six studies—four randomized controlled and two controlled before-and-after designs in a variety of settings. Interprofessional education was defined as any type of educational experience or learning opportunity in which interactive learning occurred between two or more health-related disciplines. Although a number of positive outcomes were noted, further rigorous studies are needed to draw conclusive evidence supporting core elements of interprofessional education and the subsequent impact of interprofessional collaborative education on health outcomes.

In an effort to increase the ability of health professional teams to deliver optimal patient care, RWJF funded educational programs (Partnerships for Quality Education [PQE]) designed to improve interprofessional collaboration, chronic disease management, systems-based care, and quality (RWJF, 2008). These initiatives were developed to provide nurse practitioners, physicians, and other allied healthcare providers with educational experiences, skills, and attitudes to deliver better quality care than could be provided by any single discipline. One funded model was Collaborative Interprofessional Team Education (CITE); the objective of this program was to design collaborative clinical and educational interventions for health professional students from medicine, nursing, social work, and pharmacy (RWJF, 2008). The program did make some strides toward improvement in participants' understanding of and attitudes toward other professions.

Whitehead (2007) offered some insight into the challenges of engaging medical students in interprofessional educational programs. Real and perceived power, high degree of status, professional socialization, and decision-making responsibility can limit the ability of physicians to collaborate with other members of the healthcare team unless efforts to change the culture, flatten hierarchy, and share responsibility are promoted. A number of additional obstacles prevented full implementation of the CITE initiative, including differing academic schedules and a lack of faculty practicing in teams to effectively mentor and model for students (RWJF, 2008).

The primary objective of Achieving Competence Today (ACT), another PQE initiative, was to promote interprofessional collaboration and quality improvement in the curriculum of healthcare professionals within two academic health centers (Ladden, Bednash, Stevens, & Moore, 2006; RWJF, 2008). Four disciplines worked jointly to plan and implement a quality improvement project. As a result, core competencies necessary for successful interprofessional teams were identified, and researchers suggested measures for incorporating these competencies into the educational preparation of future students as a means to improve quality and safety in health care.

DNP programs can build on concepts of interprofessional education by allowing and encouraging programs to use faculty from a variety of disciplines to prepare DNP students. Interprofessional faculty can add a depth and richness to the DNP curriculum by bringing and sharing skills, knowledge, and the highest level of expertise in areas of clinical practice—whether it be business and management, pharmacy, public policy, psychology, medicine, or informatics (AACN, 2006a). Educational experience related to interprofessional collaboration as a means to improve quality or promote safety should be highly visible within the scholarly DNP project.

Role of the Scholarly Project: Real Interdisciplinary Collaboration

The Essentials of Doctoral Education for Advanced Nursing Practice (AACN, 2006b) refers to the final DNP scholarly project or capstone as a culminating immersion experience that affords the opportunity to integrate and synthesize all elements of doctoral education competencies within an interprofessional work environment. DNP-led scholarly projects provide a venue for students to assume leadership roles for effective interprofessional collaboration in order to improve health care, patient outcomes, and healthcare systems.

The DNP project "Optimal Use of Individualized Asthma Action Plans in an Electronic Health Record" (C. Miller, 2008) involved a number of opportunities for interprofessional collaboration. This process improvement project involved a systems change designed to improve pediatric asthma care delivery in a regional health system. An asthma action plan tool built into the electronic health record of a multispecialty regional health system served as a vehicle for the delivery of evidence-based practice. Distinct DNP-led interprofessional teams collaborated during various stages of program planning, implementation, and evaluation. Collaboration with nursing professionals and professionals in the fields of informatics, information technology, statisticians, and management was active throughout the project, particularly during tool development and in the implementation phase. Key to ensuring effective communication within this group was the use of a common language and developing a clear understanding of each other's roles and contributions. A second opportunity for interprofessional collaboration occurred during the implementation phase. Each member of the pediatric asthma team—the DNP, clinical nurse specialist, and physician—came to the project with his or her own agenda and perspective. Frequent revisiting of desired project outcomes, goals, and objectives was necessary early on to develop a cohesive, unified collaboration.

A third DNP-led collaboration took place at the pilot project site, a regional primary care clinic. This collaboration, which initially presented many challenges, involved physicians, nurses, administrative management, and administrative support. This site had recently been acquired by the parent organization. Previous quality improvement initiatives had been attempted and, because of a variety of factors, were not successfully implemented. A number of barriers to collaboration were anticipated at this site, including a sense of mistrust and resistance to change. Building trusting, nonthreatening relationships with staff and providers was a much-needed starting point. Issues of power were foreseeable between the physicians and the project manager. Initially, this group expressed hesitancy with the concept of anyone other than the physician being responsible for the optimal delivery of pediatric asthma care. It is important to acknowledge that providers might experience competing loyalties as they struggle to prioritize and balance the additional time needed to implement a project along with time required to see other patients or perform other duties. Avoiding these barriers requires mutual respect for each other's role, purpose, and workload. It is vital to continually clarify and communicate the shared vision of the collaborative project—in this case, improved asthma care for children. Building relationships, seeking team member input, and developing a shared vision play critical roles in negotiating hurdles for interprofessional collaboration and for effective project implementation and evaluation.

In the DNP project "Developing a Population-Focused Student Health Service" (Ash, 2005), interprofessional collaboration morphed from providers within the student health services (SHS) to a broad range of professionals. The ecologic approach (NASPA, 2004) was used in the final stages of the student DNP project, which broadened the stakeholders and thus the collaborating professionals. The ecologic perspective views the connections between health and learning within the campus setting (Sacher et al., 2005). The initial task force led by the DNP student included a project mentor who was an expert in group work as a result of his education and experience as a master of social work (MSW). His skills in the so-called softer side of team development molded the experience by bringing all the team members into the process. He was also continually willing to try new approaches and then evaluate the outcomes. He had direct access to the vice president of student affairs, who was also known to be innovative and skilled in human relationships because of his background in counseling. A current DNP student project, which is an offshoot of the former project, is preventing chronic disease through screening, nonpharmacologic and pharmacologic interventions, and healthcare coaching. This project will include nonhealthcare team members (coaches) to facilitate the attainment of healthcare goals.

Unlike many healthcare-related projects, there were no physicians on the interprofessional team. This may have changed the leadership and political issues that have plagued nurse–physician relationships in the past. The DNP student may have struggled to lead a team that included a physician. If, however, a physician was part of the team, increased efforts could have been made to develop reciprocal trust and to recognize and value each profession. Having a physician from outside the college may have afforded an opportunity for increased networking of the interprofessional team within the community in which the college is situated.

Some of the drivers of interprofessional team functioning, such as trust, recognition and value of team members, and a shared purpose, were already present on this team at some level. Team members knew each other and had passion for the team purpose: developing a culture that embraces health and well-being. The team members worked within a college that espouses "Benedictine values" (College of St. Scholastica, 2009), which include community, hospitality, and stewardship. This emphasis on Benedictine values provided a work culture that embraced collaboration, which is a driver of interprofessional teams.

One of the barriers that plagued the team was that there was no clear understanding of roles and responsibilities. The team met and formed ideas that the team leader and mentor needed to follow through on. This team structure has changed since the end of the DNP project and now comprises four separate working groups focused on student health, faculty and staff health, marketing, and academic integration, respectively. The project, now entitled Well U, has been in full swing for over four years.

The use of Wheatley's "new leadership" approach helps account for the success of this project. The college campus, in relationship to health, could be seen as chaotic; once the relationships were formed between team members, however, information and ideas flowed. The team came to understand that all connections were vital to the development of a collegewide culture that embraced health and well-being. A long-term approach to building cultural change continues in this project. **Table 6-2** shows interprofessional team members in the DNP project.

Table 6-2 Interprofessional Team Members

Initial Task Force	Final Multi-interprofessional Team
DNP student	DNP student
MSW mentor	MSW mentor
RN from SHS	RN from SHS
Student	Student
	Director of Institutional Research and Assessment
	VP for Enrollment Management
	Registrar
	Manager, Wellness Center
	International student advisor
	Department chair, Physical Therapy

Interprofessional collaboration is not limited to efforts in the United States. In two reports to the Minister of Health in Canada, the Health Provisions Regulatory Advisory Council (2008, 2009) reviewed the scope of practice of nurse practitioners and the need for interprofessional collaboration as a means to address primary care provider shortages and comprehensive, quality care. As a result, the Minister of Health supported initiatives for innovative practice models to improve access and quality of care for underserved Canadian residents. In the DNP-led project, "A Nurse Practitioner-Led Clinic in Thunder Bay" (Thibeault, 2011), a team of nurse practitioners, RNs, social worker, dietitian, pharmacist, administrator, and community representative designed and implemented a comprehensive primary care clinic that opened its doors to Thunder Bay residents in November 2010. The clinic's primary focus is comprehensive care across the life span, with a focus on health promotion, disease prevention, and chronic care delivery. The clinic has exceeded initial goals of increasing access for unattached patients and reducing costly emergency department visits.

Summary

Given their advanced preparation, DNPs are well positioned to participate and lead interprofessional teams. Recognizing obstacles and developing strategies to reduce such barriers are key functions of interprofessional team leadership. All members of the interprofessional team need to have preparation and opportunities to rehearse this new approach to patient care delivery. Incorporating shared interdisciplinary learning experiences into the educational preparation of healthcare professionals provides the foundation for forming partnerships rather than competition for patient care delivery. Further study is needed to demonstrate the most effective educational interventions to prepare healthcare providers for successful collaborative work.

Workforce and regulatory issues may present both challenges and opportunities for interprofessional collaborations. Shortages of physician primary care providers, particularly in rural settings, are likely to influence both the configuration and function of the interprofessional team (ACP, 2009; Minnesota Department of Health [MDH], 2009). DNP-prepared primary care providers can help to fill this gap but must be allowed to practice at the top of their education and scope; this will necessitate that physician colleagues reexamine and relinquish some of the responsibilities and tasks traditionally "owned" by medicine. Nursing and medicine will need to work together to devise a vision for this new collaborative practice model to most efficiently and effectively address the needs of the population and improve the quality of care provided.

The American Academy of Pediatrics' concept of a "medical home" suggests that all individuals, particularly those with complex or chronic health conditions, should receive a comprehensive, coordinated approach to health care and social services (MDH, 2009). The proposed Health Care Home initiatives expand the definition of primary care provider to include physicians, APRNs, and physician assistants (MDH, 2009). The primary care provider will lead and coordinate the efforts of the interprofessional team to best meet the needs of the patient. Nurse practice acts, regulations, and reimbursement issues must be reviewed and revised to support the ability of APRNs to assume this role and deliver comprehensive care. Continued research is needed to identify the full impact of workforce and regulatory issues on these collaborations as well as strategies to address these concerns. DNPs in both direct (certified nurse practitioner [CNP], clinical nursing specialist [CNS], certified registered nurse anesthetist [CRNA], certified nurse midwife [CNM]) and indirect provider roles (health policy makers, administrators, informatics specialists, public health experts) must continue to effectively work with other members of the healthcare team to deliver comprehensive, patient-centered care. Interprofessional collaborations are an important facet of a reformed healthcare delivery system and a vital step toward improving health outcomes and reducing medical error.

References

Agency for Healthcare Research and Quality. (2009). *Surveys on patient safety culture.* Retrieved from http://www.ahrq.gov/qual/patientsafetyculture/

American Association of Colleges of Nursing. (2006a). *DNP roadmap task force report, October 20, 2006.* Retrieved from http://www.aacn.nche.edu/dnp/roadmapreport.pdf

American Association of Colleges of Nursing. (2006b). *The essentials of doctoral education for advanced nursing practice.* Washington, DC: Author.

American College of Physicians. (2009). *Nurse practitioners in primary care* [Policy monograph]. Philadelphia, PA: Author.

American Medical Association. (2010, October 5). *AMA responds to IOM report on future of nursing.* Retrieved from http://www.ama-assn.org/ama/pub/news/news/nursing-future-workforce.page

American Nurses Association. (2008, February). *Nursing's agenda for health care reform.* Silver Spring, MD: Author. Retrieved from http://www.nursingworld.org/Content/HealthcareandPolicyIssues/Agenda/ANAsHealthSystemReformAgenda.pdf

Amos, M., Hu, J., & Herrick, C. (2005). The impact of team building on communication and job satisfaction of nursing staff. *Journal for Nurses in Staff Development, 21*(1), 10–16.

APRN Consensus Work Group & National Council of State Boards of Nursing APRN Advisory Committee. (2008, July). *Consensus model for APRN regulation: Licensure, accreditation, certification and education.* Retrieved from http://nursecredentialing .org/Certification/APRNCorner/APRN-ConsensusModelReport

Ash, L. (2005). *Developing a population-focused student health service* (Unpublished doctoral dissertation). Rush University, Chicago, IL.

Baker, S., Baker, K., & Campbell, M. (2003). *Complete idiot's guide to project management.* Indianapolis, IN: Alpha.

Barki, H., & Hartwick, J. (2001). Interpersonal conflict and its management in information system development. *MIS Quarterly, 25*(2), 195–228.

Begun, J., Zimmerman, B., & Dooley, K. (2003). Health care organizations as complex adaptive systems. In S. M. Mick & M. Wyttenbach (Eds.), *Advances in health care organization theory* (pp. 253–288). San Francisco, CA: Jossey-Bass. Retrieved from http://change-ability.ca/files/Complex_Adaptive.pdf

Blanchard, K. (2008). Situational leadership. *Leadership Excellence, 25*(5), 19.

Brett, J., Behfar, K., & Kern, M. (2006, November). Managing multicultural teams. *Harvard Business Review, 84*(11), 84–91. Retrieved from Business Source Premier database.

Brewer, C. (2005). The health care workforce. In A. Kovner & J. Knickman (Eds.), *Health care delivery in the United States* (pp. 320–326). New York, NY: Springer.

Brita-Rossi, P., Adduci, D., Kaufman, J., Lipson, S. J., Totte, C., & Wasserman, K. (1996). Improving the process of care: The cost-quality value of interdisciplinary collaboration. *Journal of Nursing Care Quality, 10*(2), 10–16.

Buresh, B., & Gordon, S. (2006). *From silence to voice: What nurses know and must communicate to the public.* Ithaca, NY: Cornell University Press.

Burkhardt, M., & Alvita, K. (2008). *Ethics and issues in contemporary nursing.* Clifton Park, NY: Thomson Delmar Learning.

Burns, J. (1978). *Leadership.* New York, NY: Harper & Row.

Chapman, A. (2008). *Johari window: Ingham and Luft's Johari window model diagrams and examples—for self-awareness, personal development, group development and understanding relationships.* Retrieved from http://www.businessballs .com/johariwindowmodel.htm

Chinn, P. (2008). *Peace and power.* Sudbury, MA: Jones and Bartlett.

Chung, H., & Nguyen, P. H. (2005). Changing unit culture: An interdisciplinary commitment to improve pain outcomes. *Journal for Healthcare Quality: Official Publication of the National Association for Healthcare Quality, 27*(2), 12–19.

Clarin, O. A. (2007). Strategies to overcome barriers to effective nurse practitioner and physician collaboration. *Journal for Nurse Practitioners, 3*(8), 538–548.

Clark, W., Clark, L., & Crossley, K. (2010). Developing multidimensional trust without touch in virtual teams. *Marketing Management Journal, 20*(1), 177–193.

collaborate. (2015). In *Merriam-Webster.com.* Retrieved from http://www.merriam-webster.com/dictionary/collaborate

College of St. Scholastica. (2009). *Guiding documents.* Retrieved from http://www .css.edu/About/Leadership/Guiding-Documents.html

Covey, S. (1991). *Principle-centered leadership.* New York, NY: Summit Books.

Covey, S. (2004). *The eighth habit: From effectiveness to greatness.* New York, NY: Free Press.

Cowan, M. J., Shapiro, M., Hays, R. D., Afifi, A., Vazirani, S., Ward, C. R., & Ettner, S. L. (2006). The effect of a multidisciplinary hospitalist/physician and advanced practice nurse collaboration on hospital costs. *Journal of Nursing Administration, 36*(2), 79–85.

Crowell, D. (2011). *Complexity leadership.* Philadelphia, PA: F. A. Davis.

Cunningham, R. (2004, March). Advanced practice nursing outcomes: A review of selected empirical literature. *Oncology Nursing Forum, 31*(2), 219–232. Retrieved from CINAHL Plus with Full Text database.

Dailey, M. (2005, April). Interdisciplinary collaboration: Essential for improved wound care outcomes and wound prevention in home care. *Home Health Care Management & Practice, 17*(3), 213–221. Retrieved from CINAHL Plus with Full Text database.

D'Amour, D., & Oandasan, I. (2005). Interprofessionality as the field of interprofessional practice and interprofessional education: An emerging concept. *Journal of Interprofessional Care, 19*, 8–20.

Davoli, G. W., & Fine, L. J. (2004). Stacking the deck for success in interprofessional collaboration. *Health Promotion Practice, 5*(3), 266–270.

Draye, M. A., Acker, M., & Zimmer, P. A. (2006). The practice doctorate in nursing: Approaches to transform nurse practitioner education and practice. *Nursing Outlook, 54*(3), 123–129.

Drinka, T., & Clark, P. (2000). *Health care teamwork: Interdisciplinary practice and teaching.* Westport, CT: Auburn House.

Dunevitz, B. (1997). Perspectives in ambulatory care. Collaboration—in a variety of ways—creates health care value. *Nursing Economic$, 15*(4), 218–219.

Edmonson, A. (1999). Psychological safety and learning behavior in work teams. *Administrative Science Quarterly, 44*(2), 350–383.

Feldman, H. (2008). *Nursing leadership: A concise encyclopedia.* New York, NY: Springer.

Fortham, M., Dove, H., & Wooster, L. (2000). Episodic treatment groups (ETGs): A patient classification system for measuring outcomes performance by episode of care. *Topics in Healthcare Information Management, 21*(2), 51–61. Retrieved from http://www.thedeltagroup.com/Corporate/Pubs/ETGs.pdf

Gilbert, S. J. (2006). Do I dare say something? *Harvard Business School Working Knowledge.* Retrieved from http://hbswk.hbs.edu/item/do-i-dare-say-something

Golanowski, M., Beaudry, D., Kurz, L., Laffey, W., & Hook, M. (2007). Interdisciplinary shared decision-making: Taking shared governance to the next level. *Nursing Administration Quarterly, 31*(4), 341–353.

Goleman, D., Boyzatsis, R., & McKee, A. (2002). *Primal leadership: Realizing the power of emotional intelligence.* Boston, MA: Harvard Business School Press.

Gordon, S. (2005). *Nursing against the odds.* Ithaca, NY: Cornell University Press.

Grabowski, M., & Roberts, K. (1999, November). Risk mitigation in virtual organizations. *Organization Science, 10*(6), 704–721. Retrieved from Business Source Premier database.

Grady, G. F., & Wojner, A. W. (1996). Collaborative practice teams: The infra-structure of outcomes management. *AACN Clinical Issues: Advanced Practice in Acute & Critical Care, 7*(1), 153–158.

Greenberg, P., Greenberg, R., & Antonucci, Y. (2007). Creating and sustaining trust in virtual teams. *Business Horizons, 50*(4), 325–333.

Haas, J. (1977). The professionalism of medical students: Developing a cloak of confidence. *Symbolic Interaction, 1*(1), 71–88.

Hall, P. (2005). Interprofessional teamwork: Professional cultures as barriers. *Journal of Interprofessional Care, 19*(Suppl. 1), 188–196.

Hall, P., Weaver, L., Gravelle, D., & Thibault, H. (2007). Developing collaborative person-centred practice: A pilot project on a palliative care unit. *Journal of Interprofessional Care, 21*(1), 69–81.

Health Professions Regulatory Advisory Council. (2008). *A report to the Minister of Health and Long Term Care on the review of the scope of practice for registered nurses in the extended class (nurse practitioners)*. Toronto, Ontario, Canada: Author.

Health Professions Regulatory Advisory Council. (2009). *Critical links: Transforming and supporting patient care: A report to the Minister of Health and Long Term Care on mechanisms to facilitate and support interprofessional collaboration and a new framework for the prescribing and use of drugs by non-physician regulated health professions*. Toronto, Ontario, Canada: Author.

Hibbard, J. H., Stockard, J., Mahoney, E. R., & Tusler, M. (2004). Development of the patient activation measure (PAM): Conceptualizing and measuring activation in patient and consumers. *Health Services Research, 39*(4), 1005–1026.

Holton, J. A. (2001). Building trust and collaboration in a virtual team. *Team Performance Management, 7*(3), 36–47.

Horrocks, S., Anderson, E., & Salisbury, C. (2002, April 6). Systematic review of whether nurse practitioners working in primary care can provide equivalent care to doctors. *British Medical Journal, 324*(7341), 819–823. Retrieved from CINAHL Plus with Full Text database.

Ingersoll, G. L., McIntosh, E., & Williams, M. (2000). Nurse sensitive outcomes of advanced practice. *Journal of Advanced Nursing, 32*(5), 1272–1281.

Institute for Clinical Systems Integration. (2014). *DIAMOND initiative: Depression improvement across Minnesota: Offering a new direction*. Retrieved from https://www.icsi.org/_asset/rs2qfi/DIAMONDWP0614.pdf

Institute of Medicine. (1999). *To err is human: Building a safer health system*. Washington, DC: National Academies Press.

Institute of Medicine. (2001). *Crossing the quality chasm: A new health system for the 21st century*. Washington, DC: National Academies Press.

Institute of Medicine. (2003). *Health professions education: A bridge to quality*. Washington, DC: National Academies Press.

Institute of Medicine. (2011). *The future of nursing: Leading change, advancing health*. Washington, DC: National Academies Press.

Institute of Medicine. (2015). *Measuring the impact of interprofessional education (IPE) on collaborative practice and patient outcomes*. Retrieved from http://iom.edu

The Joint Commission. (2008). Sentinel event alert, issue 40. Behaviors that undermine a culture of safety. Retrieved from http://www.jointcommission.org/SentinelEvents/SentinelEventAlert/sea_40.htm

The Joint Commission. (2015). *Accreditation program: Ambulatory health care national patient safety goals.* Retrieved from http://www.jointcommission.org/assets/1/6/2015_AHC_NPSG_ER.pdf

Kaiser Family Foundation. (2008). *President-elect Barack Obama's health care reform proposal.* Retrieved from http://www.kff.org/uninsured/upload/Obama_Health_Care_Reform_Proposal.pdf

Kaiser Family Foundation. (2011, April 15). *Summary of new health reform law.* Retrieved from http://www.kff.org/healthreform/upload/8061.pdf

Kaiser Family Foundation/Harvard School of Public Health Survey. (2009). *The public's health care agenda for the new president and congress* (Publication No. 7853). Retrieved from http://www.kff.org/kaiserpolls/upload/7853.pdf

Kelly, P. (2008). *Nursing leadership and management.* Clifton Park, NY: Delmar.

Kirkman, B., Rosen, L., Gibson, C. B., Tesluk, P., & McPherson, S. (2002). Five challenges to virtual team success: Lessons from Sabre, Inc. *Academy of Management Executive, 16*(3), 67–79.

Kleinpell, R. M., Faut-Callahan, M. M., Lauer, K., Kremer, M. J., Murphy, M., & Sperhac, A. (2002). Collaborative practice in advanced practice nursing in acute care. *Critical Care Nursing Clinics of North America, 14*(3), 307–313.

Kotter, J. (1990). What leaders really do. *Harvard Business Review, 68,* 104.

Kouzes, J., & Pozner, B. (2007). *The leadership challenge.* San Francisco, CA: Wiley.

Ladden, M., Bednash, G., Stevens, D., & Moore, G. (2006). Educating interprofessional learners for quality, safety and systems improvement. *Journal of Interprofessional Care, 20*(5), 497–509.

Lambing, A., Adams, D., Fox, D., & Divine, G. (2004, August). Nurse practitioners' and physicians' care activities and clinical outcomes with an inpatient geriatric population. *Journal of the American Academy of Nurse Practitioners, 16*(8), 343–352. Retrieved from CINAHL Plus with Full Text database.

Laurant, M., Reeves, D., Hermens, R., Braspenning, J., Grol, R., & Sibbald, B. (2004, December). Substitution of doctors by nurses in primary care. *Cochrane Database of Systematic Reviews.* Retrieved from CINAHL Plus with Full Text database.

Lee, S. (2008). *The five stages of team development.* Retrieved from http://ezinearticles.com/?The-Five-Stages-of-Team-Development&id=1254894

Leonard, M., Graham, S., & Bonacum, D. (2004). The human factor: The critical importance of effective teamwork and communication in providing safe care. *Quality and Safety in Health Care, 13*(Suppl. 1), 85–90.

Lewin, K. (1951). Frontiers in group dynamics. In D. Cartwright (Ed.), *Field theory in social science* (pp. 188–237). New York, NY: Harper.

Lewis, J. (2007). *Fundamentals of project management.* New York, NY: AMACOM.

Lindeke, L. L., & Block, D. E. (2001). Interdisciplinary collaboration in the 21st century. *Minnesota Medicine, 84*(6), 42–45.

Lindeke, L. L., & Sieckert, A. M. (2005). Nurse-physician workplace collaboration. *Online Journal of Issues in Nursing, 10*(1). Retrieved from http://www.nursingworld.org/MainMenuCategories/ANAMarketplace/ANAPeriodicals/OJIN/TableofContents/Volume102005/No1Jan05/tpc26_416011.aspx

Lynnaugh, J., & Reverby, S. (1990). *Ordered to care: The dilemma of American nursing 1850–1945.* New York, NY: Cambridge University Press.

Mayer, R. C., Davis, J. H., & Schoorman, F. D. (1995). An integrative model of organizational trust. *Academy of Management Review , 20*(3), 709–734.

McCallin, A., & Bamford, A. (2007). Interdisciplinary teamwork: Is the influence of emotional intelligence fully appreciated? *Journal of Nursing Management, 15*(4), 386–391.

Miller, C. (2008). *Optimal use of individualized asthma action plans in an electronic health record* (Unpublished doctoral dissertation). University of Minnesota, Minneapolis.

Miller, K. L., Reeves, S., Zwarenstein, M., Beales, J. D., Kenaszchuk, C., & Gotlib Conn, L. (2008). Nursing emotion work and interprofessional collaboration in general medicine wards: A qualitative study. *Journal of Advanced Nursing, 64*(4), 332–343.

Miller, M., Snyder, M., & Lindeke, L. (2005, September). Forces of change. Nurse practitioners: Current status and future challenges. *Clinical Excellence for Nurse Practitioners, 9*(3), 162–169. Retrieved from CINAHL Plus with Full Text database.

Minnesota Department of Health. (2009). *Health workforce shortage study report: Report to the Minnesota legislature 2009.* St. Paul, MN: Author.

Mundinger, M., Kane, R., Lenz, E., Totten, A., Tsai, W., Cleary, P., . . . Shelanski, M. L. (2000). Primary care outcomes in patients treated by nurse practitioners or physicians: A randomized trial. *Journal of the American Medical Association, 283*(1), 59–68. Retrieved from CINAHL Plus with Full Text database.

NASPA. (2004). *Leadership for a healthy campus: An ecological approach for student success.* Retrieved from http://www.longwood.edu/assets/health/leadership_for_a_healthy_campus.pdf

Nelson, E. C., Batalden, P. B., Huber, T. P., Mohr, J. J., Godfrey, M. M., Headrick, L. A., . . .Wasson, J. H. (2002). Microsystems in health care: Part 1. Learning from high-performing front-line clinical units. *The Joint Commission Journal on Quality Improvement, 28*(9), 472–493.

Oandasan, I., D'Amour, D., Zwarenstein, M., Barker, K., Purden, M., Beaulieu, M. D., . . . Tregunno, D. (2004). *Interprofessional education for collaborative patient-centred practice: An evolving framework* [Executive summary]. Retrieved from http://www.ferasi.umontreal.ca/eng/07_info/IECPCP_Final_Report.pdf

O'Connor, A. (2006). *Ottawa personal decision guide* [Pamphlet]. University of Ottawa, Ontario, Canada: Ottawa Health Research Institute.

Oliver, G. M., Pennington, L., Revelle, S., & Rantz, M. (2014). Impact of nurse practitioners on health outcomes of Medicare and Medicaid patients. *Nursing Outlook,* 1–8. http://www.nursingoutlook.org/article/S0029-6554(14)00150-X/fulltext

OPTUM. (2015). *Care points.* Retrieved from http://comparionanalytics.com

O'Reilly, K. (2012). *Fear of punitive response to hospital errors lingers.* Retrieved from http://www.amednews.com

Patient Protection and Affordable Care Act, Pub. L. No. 111–148, §2702, 124 Stat. 119, 318–319 (2010).

Patterson, K., Grenny, J., McMillan, R., & Switzler, A. (2002). *Crucial conversations: Tools for talking when stakes are high.* New York, NY: McGraw-Hill.

Porter-O'Grady, T. (1997). *Whole systems shared governance.* Gaithersburg, MD: Aspen.

Reeves, S., Zwarenstein, M., Goldman, J., Barr, H., Freeth, D., Hammick, M., & Koppel, I. (2008). Interprofessional education: Effects on professional practice and health care outcomes [Review]. *Cochrane Database of Systematic Reviews, 1,* CD002213. doi:10.1002/14651858.CD002213.pub2

Ring, P. (2005, January). Collaboration. In *Blackwell encyclopedic dictionary of organizational behavior.* Retrieved from Blackwell Encyclopedia of Management Library database.

Robert Wood Johnson Foundation. (2008, April). *Partnerships for quality education* (Robert Wood Johnson Grant Results Reports). Retrieved from http://www.rwjf.org/pr/product.jsp?id=17748

Rosenstein, A. (2002). The impact of nurse-physician relationships on nurse satisfaction and retention. *American Journal of Nursing, 102*(6), 26–34.

Rosenstein, A., & O'Daniel, M. (2008). A survey of the impacts of disruptive behaviors and communication defects on public safety. *The Joint Commission Journal on Quality and Patient Safety, 34*(8), 464–471.

Sacher, L., Moses, K., Fabiano, P., Haubenreiser, J., Grizzel, J., & Mart, S. (2005, March). *College health: Stretch your definitions of the core concepts, assumptions and practices.* American College Health Association. PowerPoint presentation at NASPA session, Student Affairs Administration in Higher Education, Washington, DC.

Scardamalia, M. (2002). Collective cognitive responsibility for the advancement of knowledge. In B. Smith (Ed.), *Liberal education in a knowledge society* (pp. 67–98). Chicago, IL: Open Court.

Senge, P. (1990). *The art and discipline of the learning organization.* New York, NY: Doubleday.

Sierchio, G. P. (2003). A multidisciplinary approach for improving outcomes. *Journal of Infusion Nursing, 26*(1), 34–43.

Snijders, C., Kollen, B., Van Lingen, R., Fetter, W., & Molendijik, H. (2009). Which aspects of safety culture predict incident reporting behavior in neonatal intensive care units? A multilevel analysis. *Critical Care Medicine, 37*(1), 61–67.

Sullivan, E. J. (2004). *Becoming influential: A guide for nurses.* Upper Saddle River, NJ: Pearson Prentice Hall.

Thibeault, L. (2011). *A nurse practitioner-led clinic in Thunder Bay* (Unpublished doctoral dissertation). College of St. Scholastica, Duluth, MN.

Tuckman, B. W., & Jensen, M. A. C. (1977). Stages of small-group development revisited. *Group & Organization Management, 2*(4), 419–427. doi:10.1177/105960117700200404

U.S. Department of Health and Human Services. (2010). *About Healthy People 2020.* Retrieved from http://www.healthypeople.gov/2020/about/default.aspx

Vahey, D. C., Aiken, L. H., Sloane, D. M., Clarke, S. P., & Vargas, D. (2004). Nurse burnout and patient satisfaction. *Medical Care, 42*(Suppl. 2), 1157–1166.

Watkins, M. (2013). Making virtual teams work: Ten basic principles. *Harvard Business Review.* Retrieved from http://hbr.org

Weller, J., Boyd, M., & Cumin, D. (2014). Teams, tribes and patient safety: Overcoming barriers to effective teamwork in healthcare. *Postgraduate Medical Journal, 90*(1061), 149–154.

Wheatley, M. (2005). *Finding our way: Leadership for an uncertain time.* San Francisco, CA: Berrett-Koehler.

Whitehead, C. (2007). The doctor dilemma in interprofessional education and care: How and why will physicians collaborate? *Medical Education, 41*(10), 1010–1016.

Wilson, J., & Bekemeir, B. (2004). Public health. In *Encyclopedia of leadership* (Vol. 3, pp. 1271–1274). Thousand Oaks, CA: Sage.

Yeager, S. (2005). Interdisciplinary collaboration: The heart and soul of healthcare. *Critical Care Nursing Clinics of North America, 17*(2), 143–148.

Chapter 7

Clinical Prevention and Population Health for Improving the Nation's Health

Diane Schadewald and Jeanne Pfeiffer

Introduction

The World Health Organization (WHO), in the preamble to its constitution, defines health as "a state of complete physical, mental and social well-being and not merely the absence of disease or infirmity" (2006, p. 1). The WHO constitution further advocates for the provision of measures that promote health and prevent disease in a population and notes that cooperation between the people of a nation and their governments in this endeavor is necessary for positive social and economic outcomes to occur within a nation as well as globally. To address health inequities and thereby promote health and prevent disease, WHO developed the Commission on Social Determinants of Health (CSDH) to identify social determinants of health, examine the impact of those determinants, and develop recommendations to address the determinants. Categories that WHO identified as social determinants of health include health behaviors, the physical and social environment, working conditions, healthcare coverage and infrastructure, and social protection. Recommendations developed by the CSDH to positively affect these social determinants include actions to address the following three principles:

1. Improve daily living conditions
2. Tackle the inequitable distribution of power, money, and resources
3. Measure and understand the problem and assess the impact of action (CSDH, 2008, p. 2)

The U.S. Department of Health and Human Services (USHHS) has proposed national goals for health each decade for the past several decades. *Healthy People 2020* represents the fourth time these national goals have been developed. Expansion of prevention interventions, to include focus on social and physical environments, use of health information technology in public health and in promotion of health literacy, and public health "all hazards" preparedness is recommended to reach *Healthy People 2020* goals. The overarching goals of *Healthy People 2020* are:

- Attain high-quality, longer lives free of preventable disease, disability, injury, and premature death.
- Achieve health equity, eliminate disparities, and improve the health of all groups.
- Create social and physical environments that promote good health for all.
- Promote healthy development and healthy behaviors across every stage of life (USHHS, 2010a, p. 1).

Healthy People 2020 also identified 26 *leading health indicators* (LHIs) in 12 topic areas that are considered to represent significant threats to public health. One of these topic areas is *clinical preventive service*. The indicators for this topic are the number of adults who received colorectal cancer screening, adults with hypertension whose blood pressure is under control, adults with diabetes whose A1c is greater than 9%, and children 19–35 months who have received recommended doses of vaccines. These LHIs will be monitored for goal attainment or, in the case of A1c levels, a decrease in the percentage of diabetic adults with elevation of their A1c to that level (USHHS, 2010a).

The two overarching goals of *Healthy People 2010* were were to improve quality of health and longevity and eliminate health disparities (USHHS, 2000). These goals were not met, as evidenced by their inclusion as the second goal in *Healthy People 2020* (USHHS, 2010a). In part to address this, *Healthy People 2020* includes several evidence-based interventions in each topic area to meet goals, along with the caveat that there are no one-size-fits-all interventions. These interventions are rooted in the evidence-based public health movement, which had its beginnings in the 1970s (USHHS, 2010b).

The U.S. Patient Protection and Affordable Care Act (a.k.a. the Affordable Care Act [ACA]) enacted in March 2010 called for the creation of a *national prevention strategy*. This represents a change in the focus of the U.S. healthcare system from one based on illness to one

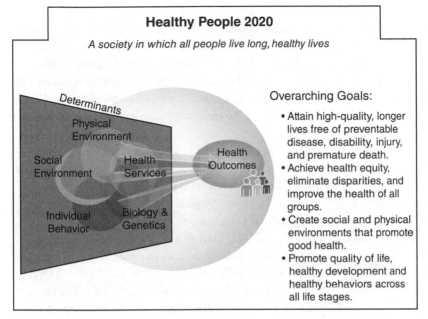

Healthy People 2020

A society in which all people live long, healthy lives

Determinants

Physical Environment

Social Environment

Health Services

Individual Behavior

Biology & Genetics

Health Outcomes

Overarching Goals:

- Attain high-quality, longer lives free of preventable disease, disability, injury, and premature death.
- Achieve health equity, eliminate disparities, and improve the health of all groups.
- Create social and physical environments that promote good health.
- Promote quality of life, healthy development and healthy behaviors across all life stages.

Figure 7-1 Social Determinants of Health and Overarching Goals
U.S. Department of Health and Human Services (2010). *Healthy People 2020*: Framework.
Retrieved from http://www.healthypeople.gov/sites/default/files/HP2020Framework.pdf page 3

based on prevention. Four strategic directions have been identified as foundational for prevention efforts: (1) healthy and safe community environments, (2) clinical and community preventive services, (3) empowered people, and (4) elimination of health disparities (Benjamin, 2011). This strategy reflects the goals of *Healthy People 2020* as well as the seventh essential of doctorate of nursing practice (DNP) education.

Social determinants of health that mirror those identified by WHO were included in the *Healthy People 2010* report and also used in *Healthy People 2020* (**Figure 7-1**). Actualizing the WHO principles identified by the CSDH that address social determinants of health will contribute to the eventual attainment of these goals. Nursing leadership is needed in developing, implementing, and evaluating clinical prevention and population health interventions that address these social determinants of health. Reaching these goals is the ultimate aim of the seventh essential of DNP education.

Background of the Development of the Seventh Essential

The American Association of Colleges of Nursing (AACN), in *The Essentials of Doctoral Education for Advanced Nursing Practice* (2006), uses the definitions of Allan et al. (2004) for both *clinical prevention* and *population health*. The term *clinical prevention* is understood to mean "health promotion and risk reduction/illness prevention for individuals and families" (AACN, 2006, p. 15). The term *population health* encompasses "aggregate, community, environmental/occupational, and cultural/socioeconomic dimensions of health" (AACN, p. 15). Aggregates consist of a set of individuals with similarities. Examples of aggregate similarities are similarities of age, diagnosis, or gender (AACN, 2006).

These definitions were developed by a task force made up of medical doctors, doctors of osteopathy, dentists, nurse practitioners, nurses, pharmacists, and physician assistants who met to identify curriculum recommendations in order to meet the goal of increasing health promotion content in educational programs for these various professions as outlined in *Healthy People 2010* (Allan et al., 2004; USHHS, 2000). Development of the framework task force was proposed in 2000 by the Association of Teachers of Preventive Medicine and the Association of Academic Health Centers (Allan, Stanley, Crabtree, Werner, & Swenson, 2005), and the task force first met in 2002 as the Healthy People Curriculum Task Force (HPCT) (Fincham, 2008). This task force developed interdisciplinary curriculum recommendations to address the need for education about clinical prevention and population health, which included four components: (1) evidence base for practice, (2) clinical preventive services–health promotion, (3) health systems and health policy, and (4) community aspects of practice. The document developed by the HPCT that describes these curricular recommendations is the *Clinical Prevention and Population Health Curriculum Framework*. It is recommended that all disciplines use the terminology of clinical prevention and population health (CPPH) when discussing this area of curriculum to improve interdisciplinary communication regarding subjects covered within the curriculum framework (Allan et al., 2004; Riegelman, Evans, & Garr, 2004). It has also been recognized that an interdisciplinary approach to education about clinical prevention and population health outside the traditional public health curriculum is necessary because prevention and population health interventions need to occur in all healthcare delivery settings if *Healthy People 2020* goals are to be realized (Zenzano et al., 2011). To accomplish this, an Education for Health framework has been included in *Healthy People 2020* for all health professionals. Evidence-based thinking and practice are integral to the Education for Health framework at the graduate level (Riegelman & Garr, 2011).

The Association of Teachers of Preventive Medicine has since changed its name to the Association for Prevention Teaching and Research

(APTR) and remains a leader in the field of health promotion and disease prevention education and research. The CPPH framework curriculum recommendations were updated by the HPCT in January 2008 and revised in January 2009, and the latest revision was completed in February 2015. The four components of the CPPH framework are now titled (1) foundations of population health, (2) clinical preventive services and health promotion, (3) clinical practice and population health, and (4) health systems and health policy (APTR, 2015). These four components are further divided into a total of 23 domains distributed among the components. (See **Table 7-1** for the complete framework.) The manner in which the CPPH framework recommendations are integrated into their curriculum is left to each discipline to decide.

Table 7-1 Clinical Prevention and Population Health Framework

Evidence-Based Practice

1. Problem Description—Descriptive Epidemiology
   - Burden of disease, e.g., morbidity and mortality
   - Course of disease, e.g., incidence, prevalence, and case fatality
   - Determinants of health and disease, e.g., genetic, behavioral, socioeconomic, environmental, health care (access and quality)
   - Distribution of disease, e.g., person, place, and time
   - Sources of data, e.g., vital statistics, active and passive public health surveillance

2. Etiology, Benefits, and Harms: Evaluating Health Research
   - Study designs, e.g., surveys, observational studies, randomized clinical trials
   - Estimation: magnitude of the association, e.g., relative risk/odds ratio, attributable risk percentage, number-needed-to-treat, and population impact measures
   - Inference, e.g., statistical significance test and confidence intervals
   - Confounding and interaction: concepts and basic methods for addressing
   - Quality and presentation of data, e.g., accuracy, precision, and use of graphics

3. Evidence-based Recommendations
   - Assessing the quality of the evidence, e.g., types and quality of studies and relevance to target population
   - Assessing the magnitude of the effect, e.g., incorporating benefits, harms, and values
   - Grading of the recommendations, e.g., combining quality of the evidence and magnitude of the effect

(continues)

Table 7-1 Clinical Prevention and Population Health Framework (*continued*)

4. Implementation and Evaluation

- Types of prevention, e.g., primary, secondary, tertiary
- At whom to direct intervention, e.g., individuals, high-risk groups, populations
- How to intervene, e.g., education, incentives for behavior change, laws and policies, engineering solutions
- Evaluation, e.g., quality improvement and patient safety, outcome assessment, reassessment of remaining problem(s)

Clinical Preventive Services and Health Promotion

1. Screening

- Assessment of health risks, e.g., biopsychosocial, environment
- Approaches to testing and screening, e.g., range of normal, sensitivity, specificity, predictive value, target population
- Criteria for successful screening, e.g., effectiveness, benefits and harms, barriers, cost, acceptance by patient
- Clinician–patient communication, e.g., patient participation in decision making, informed consent, risk communication, advocacy, health literacy
- Evidence-based recommendations
- Government requirements, e.g., newborn screening

2. Counseling for Behavioral Change

- Approaches to behavior change incorporating diverse patient perspectives, e.g., counseling skills training, motivational interviewing
- Clinician–patient communication, e.g., patient participation in decision making, informed consent, risk communication, advocacy, health literacy
- Criteria for successful counseling, e.g., effectiveness, benefits and harms, cost, acceptance by patient
- Evidence-based recommendations

3. Immunization

- Approaches to vaccination, e.g., live vs. dead vaccine, pre- vs. postexposure, boosters, techniques for administration, target population, population-based immunity
- Criteria for successful immunization, e.g., effectiveness, benefits and harms, cost, acceptance by patient
- Clinician–patient communication, e.g., patient participation in decision making, informed consent, risk communication, advocacy, health literacy
- Evidence-based recommendations
- Government requirements

4. Preventive Medication

- Approaches to chemoprevention, e.g., pre- vs. postexposure, time limited vs. long term

Table 7-1 Clinical Prevention and Population Health Framework (*continued*)

- Criteria for successful chemoprevention, e.g., effectiveness, benefits and harms, barriers, cost, acceptance by patient
- Clinician–patient communication, e.g., patient participation in decision making, informed consent, risk communication, advocacy, health literacy
- Evidence-based recommendations

5. Other Preventive Interventions

- Approaches to prevention, e.g., diet, exercise, smoking cessation
- Criteria for successful preventive interventions, e.g., effectiveness, benefits and harms, barriers, cost, acceptance by patient
- Clinician–patient communication, e.g., patient participation in decision making, informed consent, risk communication, advocacy, health literacy
- Evidence-based recommendations

Health Systems and Health Policy

1. Organization of Clinical and Public Health Systems

- Clinical health services, e.g., continuum of care: ambulatory, home, hospital, long-term care
- Public health responsibilities, e.g., public health functions (Institute of Medicine [IOM]); 10 essential services of public health
- Relationships between clinical practice and public health, e.g., individual and population needs
- Structure of public health systems

2. Health Services Financing

- Clinical services coverage and reimbursement, e.g., Medicare, Medicaid, employment based, the uninsured
- Methods for financing healthcare institutions, e.g., hospitals vs. long-term care facilities vs. community health centers
- Methods for financing public health services
- Other models, e.g., international comparisons
- Ethical frameworks for healthcare financing

3. Health Workforce

- Methods of regulation of health professionals and healthcare institutions, e.g., certification, licensure, institutional accreditation
- Discipline-specific history, philosophy, roles, and responsibilities
- Racial/ethnic workforce composition including underrepresented minorities
- Interdisciplinary health professional relationships
- Legal and ethical responsibilities of healthcare professionals, e.g., malpractice, HIPAA, confidentiality

Table 7-1 Clinical Prevention and Population Health Framework (*continued*)

- The role of public health professionals
- Interprofessional activities

4. Health Policy Process

- Process of health policy making, e.g., local, state, federal government
- Methods for participation in the policy process, e.g., advocacy, advisory processes, opportunities, and strategies to impact policy
- Impact of policies on health care and health outcomes including impacts on vulnerable populations and eliminating health disparities
- Consequences of being uninsured or underinsured
- Ethical frameworks for public health decision making

Population Health and Community Aspects of Practice

1. Communicating and Sharing Health Information with the Public

- Methods of assessing community needs/strengths and options for intervention, e.g., community-oriented primary care
- Media communications, e.g., strategies for using mass media, risk communication
- Evaluation of health information, e.g., websites, mass media, patient information (including literacy level and cultural appropriateness)

2. Environmental Health

- Sources, media, and routes of exposure to environmental contaminants, e.g., air, water, food
- Environmental health risk assessment and risk management, e.g., genetic, prenatal
- Environmental disease prevention focusing on susceptible populations

3. Occupational Health

- Employment-based risks and injuries
- Methods for prevention and control of occupational exposures and injuries
- Exposure and prevention in healthcare settings

4. Global Health Issues

- Roles of international organizations, e.g., the WHO, the Joint United Nations Programme on HIV and AIDS (UNAIDS), nongovernmental organizations, (NGOs), private foundations
- Disease and population patterns in other countries, e.g., burden of disease, population growth, health, and development
- Effects of globalization on health, e.g., emerging and reemerging diseases/conditions, food, and water supply
- Socioeconomic impacts on health in developed and developing countries

Table 7-1 Clinical Prevention and Population Health Framework (*continued*)

5. Cultural Dimensions of Practice
   - Cultural influences on clinicians' delivery of health services
   - Cultural influences on individuals and communities, e.g., health status, health services, health beliefs
   - Culturally appropriate and sensitive health care
6. Community Services
   - Methods of facilitating access to and partnerships for physical and mental healthcare services, including a broad network of community-based organizations
   - Evidence-based recommendations for community preventive services
   - Public health preparedness, e.g., terrorism, natural disasters, injury prevention
   - Strategies for building community capacity

Association for Prevention, Teaching and Research. (2009, January). Clinical prevention and health curriculum framework. Retrieved from http://www.atpm.org/resources/pdfs/Revised_CPPH_Framework_2009.pdf. Modified with permission.

Terminology Used for This Essential

The term *clinical prevention* is used in the title of the framework. The interdisciplinary nature of this task force probably influenced the terminology used. Actually, the original title planned for the framework was "Health Promotion–Disease Prevention" (Allan et al., 2005). The term *health promotion* includes all interventions focused on avoidance of health risks or illness as well as improvement of current and future health status. The term *clinical prevention* stems from the medical model of healthcare delivery. The term implies a power differential, with the dominant power belonging to the healthcare provider. This implied power delegation clashes with the nursing paradigm of patient-centered care, in which the nurse and the patient are equal partners in care activities. Eisler and Potter introduced a new framework for nursing and partnership-based health care that transforms these traditional partnerships "from hierarchies of domination and isolated professions into high-functioning interprofessional teams ready to be full partners with patients, families and one another" (Eisler & Potter, 2014, p. xxvii).

The term *clinical prevention* is not yet included as a subject heading in either the Cumulative Index to Nursing and Allied Health Literature (CINAHL) or Medline, whereas *health promotion* is included as a subject heading in both databases. CINAHL defines the subject heading of health promotion as "the process of fostering awareness, influencing attitudes, and identifying alternatives so that individuals can make informed choices and change their behavior to achieve an optimum level of physical and mental health and improve their physical and social environment." Medline defines the subject heading of health promotion as "encouraging consumer behaviors most likely to optimize health potentials (physical and psychosocial) through health information, preventive programs, and access to medical care." Nola Pender, a pioneer in health promotion theory, differentiates health promotion from disease prevention by equating health promotion with the desire to reach or maintain high-level wellness and by equating disease prevention with desire to avoid illness, discover it in early stages, or manage it well (Pender, Murdaugh, & Parsons, 2006). Thus, health promotion, by conventional understanding, tends to have an individual focus that could limit its application to populations, and disease prevention is not a subset of health promotion by definition.

Clinical preventive services are considered to include interventions such as immunizations, screenings, counseling for behavioral change, and chemoprevention (Fletcher & Fletcher, 2005). All these interventions are domains included under the component of clinical preventive services and health promotion within the CPPH curriculum framework. These domains are also consistent with the manner in which the U.S. Preventive Services Task Force (USPSTF) organizes its recommendations (Allan et al., 2004, 2005). *Clinical prevention* is also the terminology used in Institute of Medicine (IOM) reports (Allan et al., 2005). The term *clinical preventive services* has versatility in application, because these services can be focused on an individual or a population or both. Likewise, population health is inclusive of interventions focused on an individual or a population or both. Therefore, the term *clinical prevention* was purposefully chosen for these reasons (Allan et al., 2004, 2005; Riegelman et al., 2004).

Population health as it relates to nursing was defined by Radzyminski in 2007. She described population health as inclusive of the socioeconomic, cultural, and physical environments and their impact on health. Individual behaviors, beliefs, health policy, and media communications are all components factored into a nursing assessment that is based on a population health model. Concepts of both public health nursing and community health nursing are included within this definition of population health nursing. In performing an assessment, the nurse practicing within a population health perspective looks for factors that are antecedent to the development of a problem and develops health promotion interventions to address the problem at that level for the population at large as well as treating the problem on the individual level (Radzyminski, 2007).

Educational Focus for the Essential

Health promotion has been an essential component of nursing education since the days of Nightingale. Educational focus on prevention to improve health diminished with the rise of the use of technology in medicine and the accompanying increased emphasis on diagnosis and treatment of disease to improve health (Allan et al., 2005; Radzyminski, 2007). Nevertheless, nursing continued to include education on health promotion and disease prevention within its curriculum at all educational levels, with the depth of knowledge and expected degree of performance increasing for those with advanced degrees (Allan et al., 2005; AACN, 2006, 2008, 2011). What had been missing in many nursing educational programs was a population health perspective regarding health promotion (Radzyminski, 2007; Zahner & Block, 2006). The combination of the concept of clinical prevention and the concept of population health in this essential addresses this curricular deficiency. Clinical prevention and population health activities have become a primary part of the majority of nursing practice (Zenzano et al., 2011).

Essentials for advanced practice registered nurse (APRN) education were developed for DNP programs. The AACN (2006) lists the seventh essential of DNP education as the title of this chapter: "Clinical Prevention and Population Health for Improving the Nation's Health" (p. 15). According to the AACN, the graduate of a DNP educational program meets this essential by being able to do the following:

1. Analyze epidemiological, biostatistical, environmental, and other appropriate scientific data related to individual, aggregate, and population health.
2. Synthesize concepts, including psychosocial dimensions and cultural diversity, related to clinical prevention and population health in developing, implementing, and evaluating interventions to address health promotion/disease prevention efforts, improve health status, access patterns, and/or address gaps in care of individuals, aggregates, or populations.
3. Evaluate care delivery models and/or strategies using concepts related to community, environmental and occupational health, and cultural and socioeconomic dimensions of health. (AACN, 2006, p. 16)

Analysis of Data

Nursing's Use of Data Analysis Historically

Analysis of data is not new to the nursing profession. Florence Nightingale, as a founder of modern nursing, was in the vanguard concerning use of statistical models to improve health by improving sanitation. Her wedge diagram illustrating cause of death of soldiers in the Crimean War was a relatively new method for presentation of statistical information; her report is famous for changing the way British soldiers were housed, with the result being a decrease in illness and death among this population (Dossey, 2000). This may well have been the first documented clinical prevention intervention by a nurse. Nightingale continued to expand use of statistics to develop recommendations for a uniform method of collection of hospital and surgical data, analysis of which led to changes in hospital design and surgical practices (Dossey, 2000). Data analysis did not continue to be seen routinely as an important part of the education of nurses or in the practice of nursing despite calls for the need for nursing research to be recognized (Henderson, 1991). In addition, much of nursing research in the middle years of the past century focused on the process of nursing and the methods of nursing education rather than the outcomes of nursing practice (Cullum, Ciliska, Marks, & Haynes, 2008; Henderson, 1991). This paucity in nursing research changed around the 1980s, but analysis of raw data to improve health continued not to be emphasized in nursing education (Henderson, 1991); this type of education was reserved for the doctorally prepared nurse.

However, this did not stop nurses from being involved in research. Hospitals instituted infection prevention and control initiatives in the 1950s as the acceleration of new intensive care units was associated with an increase in hospital-acquired staphylococcal infections. Influential external agencies, namely the American Hospital Association and the Joint Commission (previously known as the Joint Commission on Accreditation of Hospitals and then the Joint Commission on Accreditation of Healthcare Organizations), exerted pressure on hospitals to institute formal infection prevention and control programs during the 1960s and early 1970s. Nurses employed in hospitals and exceptionally familiar with high-risk invasive procedures were recruited to lead this initiative in the United States (Friedman, 2014). To understand how these infections were occurring and to develop prevention control strategies, these nurses needed to gather and analyze data to identify risks associated with these infections.

The Centers for Disease Control and Prevention (CDC) initiated the National Nosocomial Infections System in 1970 to train professionals across the country about surveillance. The first evidence-based research instituted was the Study on the Efficacy of Nosocomial Infection Control (SENIC) Project, which compared baseline nosocomial (healthcare-associated infection [HAI]) rates in 1970 with rates in 1976. The CDC employed a stratified random sample of hospitals in the United States to collect their data. The CDC trained these evolving infection prevention experts in data collection and analysis using standardized definitions and criteria for identifying infections in the populations at risk for infections in U.S. hospitals (Haley, Quade, Freeman, & Bennett, 1980). In 1985, Haley and colleagues reported results of the SENIC study, noting that an effective infection prevention program must contain four key components operating simultaneously to reduce infections by at least 32% in the United States: (1) a knowledgeable infection prevention nurse per 250 hospital beds, (2) a standardized surveillance system designed to detect and quantify HAIs, (3) an effectual infection control physician to advise the program, and (4) a system to report surgical site infections to surgeons (Haley et al.,1985).

In 2008, the international Association for Professionals in Infection Control and Epidemiology (APIC) voted to adopt "infection preventionist" as the new name for these professionals nationwide. This title is representative of the primary work of the programs and is better understood by consumers who are increasingly fearful about their loved ones acquiring a HAI as an adverse effect of receiving health care. The contemporary infection preventionist is a public health professional employed by health systems across the country to prevent HAIs and to control infections in patients who are admitted from the community. They are generally nurses with several years of experience in patient care practices, though programs with more than one infection preventionist may employ physicians, medical technologists, and public health professionals (Friedman, 2014).

The IOM report *Nursing, Health, & the Environment* was published in 1995 (Pope, Snyder, & Mood, 1995). This report identified a strong role for nursing in the field of environmental health. The need for greater knowledge of data regarding the impact of the environment on health and the need for health promotion and disease prevention activities related to the data available regarding environmental risks led to the formation of the Alliance of Nurses for Healthy Environments (ANHE) in December 2008 (ANHE, 2008). The ANHE website not only links to information about the impact of the environment on health but also provides access to four main work groups of nurses interested in education, practice, research, and policy/advocacy in regard to the environment and health. The website also serves as a link to local environmental health nursing organizations and other communities of nurses who are interested in a variety of environmental health topics (ANHE, 2015). The ANHE provides an eTextbook on its website and in 2010 partnered with the American Nurses Association (ANA) to add an environmental health standard to the ANA's *Scope and Standards of Practice* as a desired competency for registered nurses at all educational levels (ANA, 2013; ANHE, 2015). Another nursing organization, the American Association of Occupational Health Nurses (AAOHN), identifies itself as the professional organization for occupational and environmental health nurses (AAOHN, n.d.). The AAOHN focuses on environmental health in the workplace, whereas the relatively newly formed ANHE has the much broader focus for nursing described in 1995 by the IOM report for its environmental health efforts (Pope et al., 1995).

APIC, founded in 1972, is the leading professional association for infection preventionists, with 15,000 members. APIC members benefit from education, evidence-based practice information, electronic networking, and publications. In the past, nurses seeking advanced degrees in this field enrolled in schools of public health for courses in the environmental sciences and epidemiology. Currently, the DNP-prepared nurse infection preventionist, educated in schools of nursing, is better positioned to utilize environmental sciences, epidemiology, and knowledge of change theory to improve prevention of infections in a wide variety of health settings (APIC, n.d.).

Data Analysis and the DNP

Courses on biostatistics and epidemiology are included as part of the DNP curriculum, therefore preparing the graduate to meet the first goal of this essential. An understanding of biostatistical and epidemiological methods prepares the DNP to analyze health statistics and environmental and other scientific data. That is, the DNP will be able to analyze census data, morbidity and mortality reports, data from the National Center for Health Statistics, and other sources of public health data in relationship to population health. The DNP has knowledge of how to perform rate adjustments, to determine number needed to treat (NNT), and to interpret confidence intervals. Knowledge of epidemiological principles of risk is also vital when considering prevention activities. An understanding of the difference between relative risk and attributable risk is necessary when working on the population health level to develop appropriate interventions and decrease any potential for causing harm by inappropriate prevention activities (Gévas, Starfield, & Heath, 2008). The DNP graduate is well prepared to do this. Data regarding the negative impact of environmental changes and toxins on health are becoming more prevalent, and analysis of these data may provide the basis for prevention interventions developed for use by the DNP in program project planning (Ashton & Green, 2008; Barrett, 2015; Liu & Lewis, 2014; Stanhope & Lancaster, 2012; Trasande, 2014). The DNP's ability to perform analysis of data is further enhanced by developing proficiency in the practice of evidence-based nursing. DiCenso, Guyatt, and Ciliska (2005) have provided a framework for utilization of evidence-based nursing in a text on implementation of evidence-based nursing in clinical practice. The development of any nursing intervention always begins with assessment. To practice evidence-based nursing, however, it is also necessary to develop a properly formulated question about the patient population, the intervention, a comparison, and outcome (PICO) to facilitate gathering the available evidence. Adding the element of time (PICOT) to the question formulation, if indicated by the condition or population of interest, has been suggested by others (Fineout-Overholt & Johnston, 2005; Flemming, 2008). Next, the evidence gathered in answer to these questions needs to be analyzed to determine whether it is appropriate to use for the particular individual or population of interest. This is where additional background from coursework in statistics and epidemiology is so vital for the DNP graduate. By developing skill in these areas, all DNP graduates will be prepared to analyze data at individual, aggregate, and population health levels in order to use such data appropriately when developing interventions.

Psychosocial Dimensions and Cultural Diversity in Clinical Prevention and Population Health

Health Promotion and Disease Prevention

The USPSTF published its first recommendations about preventive services in 1989. An update to these recommendations was made in 1996; since then, guidelines have been updated annually, with a guide released in 2014 containing clinical preventive services recommendations (Agency for Healthcare Research and Quality [AHRQ], n.d.). The pocket guide is available by download from the AHRQ. The most up-to-date recommendations are available online at www.uspreventiveservicestaskforce.org/Page/Name/tools-and-resources-for-better-preventive-care.

In addition, USPSTF recommendations include clinical prevention guidelines regarding chemoprevention, such as use of aspirin for cardio protective benefit for those at risk for heart attack. Other professional specialty organizations, such as the American Cancer Society, the American College of Obstetrics and Gynecology, the American Academy of Pediatrics (AAP), and the Academy of Family Physicians, also have guidelines regarding clinical prevention.

The ACA of 2010 emphasized prevention as a means to improve health. The task force created to identify essential preventive services utilized preventive measures identified as Grade A or B recommendations by the guidelines of the USPSTF, Bright Futures recommendations of the AAP, and immunization recommendations of the APIC as the baseline for these essential services. In 2011, guidelines for essential preventive services for women identified by this task force were released (IOM, 2011a). The guidelines for preventive services for women have continued to be recognized as essential services, with some faith-based exemptions related to the contraceptive coverage guidelines by U.S. Supreme Court ruling (*Burwell v. Hobby Lobby Stores, Inc.*, 2014). However, the USPSTF, APA, and APIC recommendations have retained their role as guidelines for preventive healthcare provision.

Clinical prevention services focus on the primary, secondary, and/or tertiary level of prevention. Primary prevention activities focus on prevention of illness and can be conducted in many settings, including schools, businesses, and county fairs, and sponsored by public health agencies, such as providing a class on hand-washing for kindergartners, or setting up an immunization clinic. Primary prevention in a hospital setting would involve implementation of environmental and individual processes, including maintaining a sterile field, safe reprocessing of instruments, proper timing of prophylactic antibiotics, and standardized wound care protocols aimed at preventing surgical site infections (Garcia, Schaffer, & Schoon, 2014). Secondary prevention activities are directed at early detection of illness and traditionally can be done in an ambulatory or acute care setting. Secondary prevention activities center on implementation of USPSTF screening recommendations. Tertiary prevention activities are those intended to prevent worsening of a condition that is already present (Aschengrau & Seage, 2008; Fletcher & Fletcher, 2005; Garcia et al., 2014). Tertiary prevention activities, such as diabetes education classes, cardiac rehabilitation programs, and lactation consultation, take place at the individual or group level based on patient need. Both secondary and tertiary prevention activities have been integrated into the community settings, such as screenings at health fairs, in schools, in the work setting, and in home care services focused on prevention of complications. Tertiary prevention activities help stabilize the patient's condition and prevent rehospitalization from chronic illness. Lactation consultation services, another tertiary prevention strategy, promote the continuation of breastfeeding when the mother has symptoms such as cracked nipples or breast engorgement from this healthy behavior (Garcia et al., 2014; Nies & McEwen, 2014).

Use of Psychosocial Dimensions

Understanding how psychosocial dimensions affect health promotion practice has been in the forefront since Nola Pender began developing her nursing theory of health promotion (Pender, 1975). The first version of her health promotion model (HPM) was published in 1982 (Pender et al., 2006) and revised in 1996. The HPM is described as a theory that "integrates constructs from expectancy-value theory and social cognitive theory" (Pender, Murdaugh, & Parsons, 2011, p. 44). The theory incorporates personal biologic, psychological, and sociocultural considerations within factors that need to be taken into account for success in planning health promotion activities (**Figure 7-2**). Her middle-range nursing theory has been used as an introduction to the health promotion theory needed for planning and providing care in the clinical setting. The APRN uses this theory to assess a patient's readiness to engage in health-promoting behaviors and to plan where to intervene in the model to affect health behaviors.

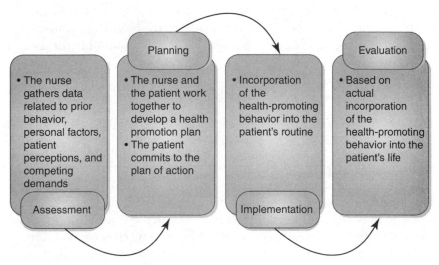

Figure 7-2 Nola Pender's Health Promotion Model

Another assessment model for use in planning health promotion activities by APRNs working in public health, community health, and population health is the PRECEDE-PROCEED model, which was developed by Green and Kreuter for use in planning public health activities. The dimension of health promotion was added to this model in 1999 (Green & Kreuter, 1999).

Knowledge about change theory is included in APRN educational programs because readiness to change is an important concept to understand when developing plans of care for health promotion that include behavioral change. In assessing readiness to change, one of the theories the APRN may use is the transtheoretical model of change (TTM). This theory was developed by DiClemente and Prochaska and is based on identification of stages of readiness to change (Prochaska, Norcross, & DiClemente, 1994). The stages are precontemplation, contemplation, preparation, action, maintenance, and relapse. Assessment regarding the stage of the target population is used to help direct intervention.

In addition to the previously discussed theories, the APRN may have used various other middle-range nursing theories in planning health promotion activities, such as the health belief model, modeling and role-modeling, self-efficacy theory, and the theory of planned behavior (Frisch, George, Giovoni, Jennings-Sanders, & McCahon, 2003; Peterson & Bredow, 2012).

APRNs and Cultural Competence

Nursing theorist Madeleine Leininger (1981) was the first to introduce nursing to the concept of the need for transcultural understanding in the provision of patient care and is considered the founder of transcultural nursing. Her sunrise model (**Figure 7-3**) depicts how her theory can be used for assessment to develop culturally congruent interventions (Leininger & McFarland, 2006).

Purnell developed a model for use in assessing culture in order to advance culturally acceptable healthcare interventions. The Purnell model for cultural competence (**Figure 7-4**) is made up of 12 domains that need to be assessed: overview/heritage, communications, family roles and organization, workforce issues, biocultural ecology, high-risk health behaviors, nutrition, pregnancy, death rituals, spirituality, healthcare practices, and healthcare practitioners (Purnell, 2002, 2009). Purnell and Paulanka (2005) developed a handbook for healthcare providers that contains information about each of these domains for various religious and ethnic groups. An updated third edition of this handbook has been released (Purnell, 2014).

The question could be asked as to whether cultural considerations are really vital to planning appropriate health promotion interventions.

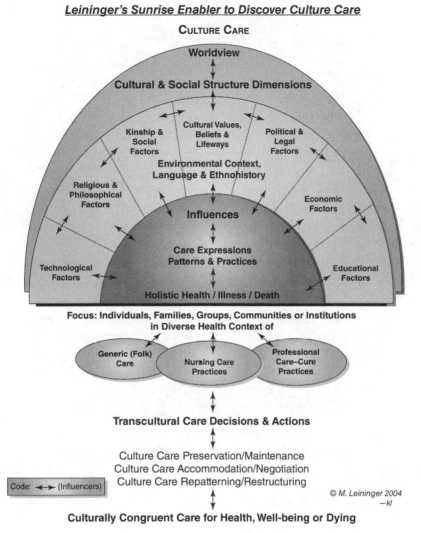

Figure 7-3 Madeleine Leininger's Sunrise Model

Leininger, M. M. and McFarland, M. (2006). Culture care diversity and universality: A worldwide nursing theory (2nd ed., p. 25). Sudbury, MA: Jones & Bartlett.

Anne Fadiman, author of *The Spirit Catches You and You Fall Down*, the famous account of an adverse healthcare outcome that occurred when aspects of Hmong culture were not considered during care provision, addressed this question in a lecture at the University of Minnesota (personal communication, March 2, 2009). She recommended that cultural competence be considered an assessment tool, like an otoscope, that healthcare providers need to develop the ability to use. This recommendation was made secondary to concern that the concept of being

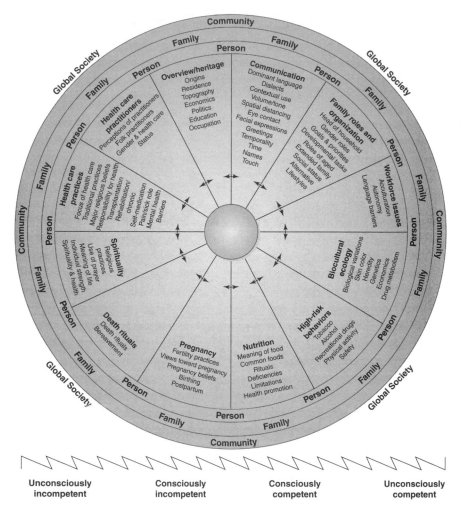

Figure 7-4 The Purnell Model for Cultural Competence
Purnell, L. (2002). The Purnell model for cultural competence. *Journal of Transcultural Nursing,* *13*(3), 194. Reproduced with permission.

culturally competent may be devalued as the "politically correct" manner of behavior or a fad rather than recognized as an important assessment tool that healthcare providers need to use routinely to develop expertise in its use and provide proper care.

Role of the DNP in Health Promotion and Disease Prevention

Individual-based interventions for health promotion and disease prevention performed by the DNP continue to be guided by the USPSTF recommendations. The DNP also may find *The Guide to Community Preventive*

Services, an online resource (www.thecommunityguide.org), useful in planning health promotion and disease prevention activity for population health-based interventions (Briss, Brownson, Fielding, & Zaza, 2004). Knowledge of materials in national and state health planning documents has also been recommended as essential for planning of population health-related activity (Zahner & Block, 2006). In addition, the DNP can assess the population of interest to identify which objective topic areas of *Healthy People 2020* might contain the most appropriate and timely health promotion and disease prevention interventions in order to improve the health of the given population (see **Table 7-2**). Clearly the topic area of

Table 7-2 Healthy People 2020 Objective Topic Areas

Access to Health Services

Adolescent Health

Arthritis, Osteoporosis, and Chronic Back Conditions

Blood Disorders and Blood Safety

Cancer

Chronic Kidney Disease

Dementias, including Alzheimer's Disease

Diabetes

Disability and Health

Early and Middle Childhood

Educational and Community-Based Programs

Environmental Health

Family Planning

Food Safety

Genomics

Global Health

Health Communication and Health Information Technology

Healthcare-Associated Infections

Health-Related Quality of Life and Well-Being*

Hearing and Other Sensory or Communication Disorders

Heart Disease and Stroke

HIV

Immunization and Infectious Diseases

Injury and Violence Prevention

Lesbian, Gay, Bisexual, and Transgender Health*

(continues)

Table 7-2 Healthy People 2020 Objective Topic Areas (*continued*)

Maternal, Infant, and Child Health

Medical Product Safety

Mental Health and Mental Disorders

Nutrition and Weight Status

Occupational Safety and Health

Older Adults

Oral Health

Physical Activity

Preparedness

Public Health Infrastructure

Respiratory Diseases

Sexually Transmitted Diseases

Sleep Health

Social Determinants of Health*

Substance Abuse

Tobacco Use

Vision

*Objectives under development

U.S. Department of Health and Human Services (2010). Healthy People 2020 Summary of Objectives. Retrieved from http://www.healthypeople.gov/2020/topicsobjectives2020/default

immunization and infectious disease has many goals and interventions that would be widely appropriate (see **Table 7-3**). When using these guides and documents, the DNP will also be aware of the need to synthesize psychosocial and cultural dimensions of the target population into the planning of any clinical prevention and population health interventions and can provide leadership in this area of project planning. For example, preventing diseases covered by vaccine is a U.S. public health goal. Measles was on the list to eradicate over a decade ago, but the U.S. measles outbreak January 2015 demonstrated that the population is no longer meeting the vaccine goals of *Healthy People 2020*; 154 cases of measles were reported from 17 states between January 1 and February 20, 2015. These cases were exposed to an index case in Disneyland (CDC, 2015). Consumer social networking groups concerned about the health effects of vaccinations have contributed to the downward vaccination trends. Another global event that impacted the population occurred in 2014, when the Ebola virus disease epidemic erupted in Western Africa. The Ebola virus has caused 23,539 cases and has been associated with a 40% mortality rate

Table 7-3 Healthy People 2020 Objectives for Immunization and Infectious Diseases

Immunization and Infectious Diseases

IID–1: Reduce, eliminate, or maintain elimination of cases of vaccine-preventable diseases.

IID–2: Reduce early onset group B streptococcal disease.

IID–3: Reduce meningococcal disease.

IID–4: Reduce invasive pneumococcal infections.

IID–5: Reduce the number of courses of antibiotics for ear infections for young children.

IID–6: Reduce the number of courses of antibiotics prescribed for the sole diagnosis of the common cold.

IID–7: Achieve and maintain effective vaccination coverage levels for universally recommended vaccines among young children.

IID–8: Increase the proportion of children aged 19 to 35 months who receive the recommended doses of DTaP, polio, MMR, Hib, hepatitis B, varicella and PCV vaccines.

IID–9: Proportion of children in the United States who receive zero doses of recommended vaccines by 19 to 35 months.

IID–10: Maintain vaccination coverage levels for children in kindergarten.

IID–11: Increase routine vaccination coverage levels for adolescents.

IID–12: Increase the proportion of children and adults who are vaccinated annually against seasonal influenza.

IID–13: Increase the percentage of adults who are vaccinated against pneumococcal disease.

IID–14: Increase the percentage of adults who are vaccinated against zoster (shingles).

IID–15: Increase hepatitis B vaccine coverage among high-risk populations.

IID–16: (Developmental) Increase the scientific knowledge on vaccine safety and adverse events.

IID–17: Increase the proportion of providers who have had vaccination coverage levels among children in their practice population measured within the past year.

IID–18: Increase the proportion of children under age 6 years of age whose immunization records are in fully operational, population-based immunization information systems.

IID–19: Increase the number of States collecting kindergarten vaccination coverage data according to CDC minimum standards.

IID–20: Increase the number of States that have 80 percent of adolescents with two or more age-appropriate immunizations recorded in immunization information systems (adolescents aged 11 to 18 years).

IID–21: Increase the number of States that use electronic data from rabies animal surveillance to inform public health prevention programs.

IID–22: Increase the number of public health laboratories monitoring influenza-virus resistance to antiviral agents.

(continues)

Table 7-3 Healthy People 2020 Objectives for Immunization and Infectious Diseases (*continued*)

IID–23: Reduce hepatitis A.

IID–24: Reduce chronic hepatitis B virus infections in infants and young children (perinatal infections).

IID–25: Reduce hepatitis B.

IID–26: Reduce new hepatitis C infections.

IID–27: Increase the proportion of persons aware they have a hepatitis C infection.

IID–28: (Developmental) Increase the proportion of persons who have been tested for hepatitis B virus within minority communities experiencing health disparities.

IID–29: Reduce tuberculosis (TB).

IID–30: Increase treatment completion rate of all tuberculosis patients who are eligible to complete therapy.

IID–31: Increase the treatment completion rate of contacts to sputum smear positive cases who are diagnosed with latent tuberculosis infection (LTBI) and started LTBI treatment.

IID–32: Reduce the average time for a laboratory to confirm and report tuberculosis cases.

U.S. Department of Health and Human Services (2010). Healthy People 2020 Summary of Objectives. Retrieved from http://www.healthypeople.gov/2020/topics-objectives/topic/immunization-and-infectious-diseases/objectives

(CDC, 2015). Previous outbreaks in African countries were quite small and regionally isolated as compared with this epidemic and were not picked up by the media. Because several continents were impacted by the 2014 public health emergency, there is global pressure to create a vaccine to protect the population in Africa and to mitigate its effects worldwide.

DNP-Level Synthesis of Psychosocial Dimensions and Cultural Diversity

The DNP-prepared APRN will be able to synthesize the various theoretical concepts and models described previously in this chapter when planning any health promotion intervention. Coursework in the DNP curriculum enables the DNP to synthesize the body of knowledge regarding the impact of psychosocial and cultural factors on health promotion and disease prevention in a way not previously promoted. Knowledge of the impact of health policy on access to healthcare and the intersection of these factors with cultural diversity and psychosocial dimensions allows the DNP to perform an in-depth analysis regarding how to develop and implement health promotion and disease prevention interventions appropriately for individuals and groups in the target population. In developing interventions, the DNP will also integrate concepts of change theory and leadership theory determined by analysis to be appropriate for the target population. The DNP develops familiarity with concepts of program planning and evaluation. Use of these concepts is vital to plan programs and properly evaluate outcomes of program interventions. All these abilities are actualized in DNP scholarly projects.

Another strength the DNP brings to the development of clinical prevention interventions is an increased depth of knowledge regarding how to implement programs. As discussed previously in this chapter, whether clinical prevention would be best delivered at the individual or the population level or simultaneously at both levels is a question that the DNP is able to assess. In performing a needs assessment while planning a project, the DNP is prepared to identify stakeholders and examine threats and barriers to planned project intervention. Such information will help determine the appropriate level for intervention. The DNP is also aware that planning for evaluation of the process of implementation of an intervention is also vital in understanding what went wrong if a program is not successful (Issel, 2014).

Health promotion and disease prevention interventions can be focused on an individual level, an aggregate level, or a population level and at the primary, secondary, or tertiary level. Psychosocial and cultural diversity factors will be considered by the DNP when planning what level or levels on which to provide intervention for a particular health need. Pender's HPM and Green and Kreutzer's PRECEDE-PROCEED model (**Figure 7-5**)

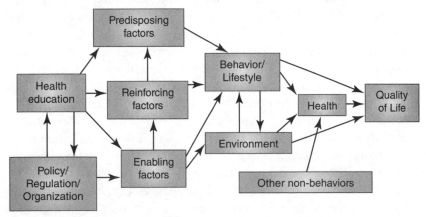

Figure 7-5 The PRECEDE-PROCEED Model as Used for Development of Health Promotion Planning

Wilson and Kolander (2011). Modified from L. W. Green and M. W. Kreuter, Health promotion planning: an educational and environmental approach, 2e. Mayfield Publishing Company, 1991, ISBN 978-0874847796, p. 1. Reprinted by permission of McGraw-Hill Education.

are examples of models that can be used as a theoretical basis for individual, aggregate, or population assessment regarding clinical prevention and population health project interventions planned and implemented by the DNP. Data on cultural diversity factors that already exist in the literature (for example, Monsen, 2009; Purnell, 2014) may be used in developing interventions. However, the DNP will also gather data on cultural diversity factors that are unique to the population of interest while performing a needs assessment as one of the initial steps in project planning.

The following are examples of some questions that may be considered in a needs assessment: Will the need respond to an educational intervention? If so, is the intervention best delivered on an individual level during a routine health maintenance visit, on an aggregate level, such as by providing a diabetes class in the clinic or the community, or on a population level by print media or broadcast media for the particular need and the population of interest? Is the population of interest of varied cultures? If so, are different approaches to intervention delivery needed to reach all population group members? Are there socioeconomic factors that would necessitate modifications in intervention plans?

In planning health promotion interventions, the DNP will also synthesize theoretical concepts related to the readiness of the target audience to change. The DNP has become familiar with many change theories in his or her previous coursework and will learn more about how to use these theories appropriately. For example, Lewin's change theory is one such theory that may be applicable for use by the DNP when planning health promotion activities. Three processes that occur during any change are included in Lewin's theory: unfreezing, moving, and refreezing (Geraci, 2004; Lewin, 1951, 1975). When performing a needs assessment, the DNP may assess driving and restraining factors to change and will need to overcome restraining forces first in order to unfreeze the situation and implement change. Many of the questions presented earlier integrate Lewin's concepts. In assessing readiness to change, the DNP may also use the TTM theory discussed previously in this chapter (Geraci, 2004).

Another change theory the DNP may use in health promotion project planning takes into consideration factors that might influence the rate of change to expect in response to an intervention and provides information on how to best promote the intervention. Everett Rogers's (2002, 2003) diffusion of innovation theory addresses how the process of change is influenced by the rate of acceptance of change. He categorized population groups responding to change as consisting of innovators, early adopters, early majority, late majority, and laggards. This theory was used in development of the Stop Aids program in San Francisco in the 1980s (Rogers, 2003), thereby demonstrating proven utility for health promotion intervention in a population. It has been recommended that the focus of initial promotion in a community be on the innovators in an attempt to use this population to accelerate the change within the community of interest (Haider & Kreps, 2004).

Focus of DNPs' Health Promotion and Disease Prevention Interventions

Improvement in Health Status

Evaluation of the impact of socioeconomic factors and cultural beliefs on health status is necessary to formulate an intervention that will be successful for the target population. The DNP will synthesize concepts from the theories discussed previously while formulating these interventions. For example, if, while using Pender's HPM, it is discovered that the population of interest is not able to attend a class because of lack of transportation, then provision of transportation may be the first step needed to improve health status for this population. The DNP will also assess for antecedent factors that contribute to the lack of transportation for this population and develop interventions to address the problem at that level. Likewise, if, while performing a cultural assessment using Leininger's sunrise model, it is discovered that a cultural belief exists that factors in life are predetermined and nothing can be done to change one's fate, then the first step in intervening to improve health status for this population will need to focus on how to work within this belief. Leadership in addressing social determinants of health that are adversely affecting improvement in health status in the areas of health promotion and disease prevention is another way in which the DNP will improve health status.

Access Patterns

One factor recognized as a contributor to limitation of access to care is limitation in the supply of providers (USHHS, 2013). In recent years, there has been a steady decrease in the number of primary care providers (Colwill, Cultice, & Kruse, 2008; DesRoches, Buerhaus, Dittus, & Donelan, 2015; Walker, 2006); fewer and fewer medical students are choosing family practice, internal medicine, and pediatrics as a specialty because of the decreased potential for income in this type of practice. One solution the medical community has proposed is for primary providers to charge patients an extra fee in order to make primary care practice more lucrative and therefore attract an increased number of medical school graduates to the field (Walker, 2006). Unfortunately, this proposed solution will do nothing to meet the needs of the underserved and uninsured and lacks focus on the needs of the patient.

DNPs can improve access by direct care provision of preventive services on the individual level in the primary care setting. Mundinger et al. (2000), in a randomized trial performed in the 1990s, provided evidence that care delivered by nurse practitioners was equivalent to care provided by physicians. Pohl, Barkauskas, Benkert, Breer, and Bostrom (2007) further validated and promoted the efficacy of nurse practitioners as primary care providers with findings that academic nurse-managed centers (ANMCs) produced a quality of care that was seen by patients as superior to care provided by physicians. This superiority was related to care being perceived by patients as secondary to the following care characteristics: "health (not just medical) care, comprehensive care and follow-through with problems and concerns, prevention, teaching, and listening" (Pohl et al., 2007, p. 273). That patients included provision of information on prevention in a list of characteristics that defined the superior care received in ANMCs highlights the importance that patients place on preventive services.

ANMCs that serve underprivileged populations have been around since the 1970s, but they rarely have been able to function without an outside funding source and usually have operated in the red, making it difficult to expand such services (Barkauskas et al., 2004; Hansen-Turton, Bailey, Torres, & Ritter, 2010). Improvement in access to care for the underprivileged continues to be necessary. The American College of Physicians' (ACP) 2009 policy statement on care provision by nurse practitioners advocated for inclusion of nurse-managed demonstration projects for the "medical home" model for primary care services (called "health care homes" in Minnesota), yet maintained that physician management of such primary care services would most likely prove to be the better model (ACP, 2009). The ACA has a provision for development of care delivery through accountable care organizations (ACOs) in which the organization's reimbursement for patient care services is linked to quality metrics and reductions in the total cost of care for an assigned panel of patients. When enacted, the law did not exclude APRNs from being designated as a patient's primary care provider. However, when the final rule for ACOs was written, the APRN was not recognized as a provider eligible to be the primary care provider for a panel of patients new to a clinic. An APRN may be the designated primary provider in ACOs only for those patients who were already under the care of the APRN (ANA, 2011a). This rule essentially eliminates new nurse-managed ACOs from opening. If nurse-managed ACO demonstration projects had been allowed and proved successful, as historical information suggests would be the case, they could have improved access to care for the underserved populations that are often the focus of nurse-managed clinics.

Nursing has a long history of patient-centered care delivery, and the DNP is poised to fill the gap in primary care. However, improving access to preventive service care by expansion of ANMCs will not be fully realized unless current restrictions on independent practice and restrictions on reimbursement for APRNs are dealt with legislatively (Barkauskas et al., 2004; Hansen-Turton, Ritter, Rothman, & Valdez, 2006; Hansen-Turton et al., 2010). One of the key messages of *The Future of Nursing* report released in 2011 was the recommendation that nurses, including APRNs, should be able to practice to the full extent of their education and training (IOM, 2011b). The report went on to recommend that regulatory barriers existing in some states that are restricting access to care provided by APRNs be removed. Barriers to practice have been removed in a number of states recently, such as Nevada in 2013 and Minnesota in 2014, but still remain in others. Nurse-managed health centers (NMHCs) have been acknowledged as a possible vehicle to improve access for underserved populations by the Senate Committee of Appropriations in 2005 (Newland, 2006).

Familiarity with how health policy is developed and how best to influence policy will be crucial for the DNP in removing barriers to practice. Inclusion of health policy in the curriculum framework for clinical prevention and population health is part of HPCT recommendations but is not included as part of the AACN goals for this DNP essential. Instead, the AACN made health policy advocacy a separate essential. Nevertheless, these two essentials intersect, and a change in health policy to improve access to NMHCs is one way in which the DNP can improve access to health care.

Gaps in Care

A gap in care for the underinsured and uninsured has been partially met by retail-based clinics. These clinics have become financially successful, and their numbers have grown (Hansen-Turton, Ryan, Miller, Counts, & Nash, 2007; Nelson, 2007). These clinics not only provide easy access to care, given that they function as a walk-in form of service, but also have become useful to provide care to the uninsured for at least a limited number of minor acute illnesses, therefore providing a form of tertiary prevention by decreasing risk for complications from untreated illness. These clinics also administer primary prevention services by providing immunizations for a reasonably affordable fee. Retail clinics have been staffed mainly with nurse practitioners and will be well served by the leadership expertise of the DNP.

Evaluate Care Delivery Models

Evaluation is the last step of the nursing process of assessment, diagnosis, planning, implementation, and evaluation of intervention outcomes. It is done to determine if a care delivery model is working as intended. That is, are the interventions effective in meeting desired outcomes? If they are not effective, would a modification of the planned intervention be warranted, or does an entirely new model of care delivery need to be developed?

Public health interventions are also primary, secondary, or tertiary in focus and usually address all three of the main functional concepts: (1) assessment, (2) policy development, and (3) assurance. These interventions can be delivered at the individual, community, or systems level (Keller, Strohschein, Lia-Hoagberg, & Schaffer, 1998). Models have been developed to illustrate how community and public health nurses plan and develop interventions (see **Figure 7-6** for diagrams of two such models). The community health nurse /public health nurse is an activist, is resourceful, prioritizes prevention, considers the client as an equal partner, is population focused, works collaboratively, and bases interventions on the concept of the greatest good (Allender, Rector, & Warner, 2014).

Occupational and environmental health nursing, as mentioned earlier in the chapter, have been linked in the past. However, the health promotion and disease prevention objectives for both *Healthy People 2010* and *Healthy People 2020* included, among many other objectives, specific separate objectives for occupational health nursing and environmental health nursing (**Table 7-4**). The National Institute of Environmental Health Sciences, the Agency for Toxic Substances and Disease Registry (ATSDR), and the National Institute for Nursing Research met in August 2002 to consider measures to increase involvement of nurses in environmental health (O'Fallon, 2003). Environmental health nursing seems poised to become a specialty of its own, but no nursing certifying organization currently offers certification in this area as a specialty. However, graduate-level education in environmental health nursing is offered at several universities.

Nevertheless, nurses have done environmental risk assessments for many years. Knowledge of the exposure risks of toxic chemical substances and other environmental factors was generally not stressed in nursing education until the end of the last century even though the writings of nursing pioneers such as Florence Nightingale and Lillian Wald include multiple references to the importance of the environment to health (Stanhope & Lancaster, 2012). For a number of years, assessment for environmental risk for exposure of children to lead has been done in pediatrics, but it is now recommended that nursing assessments for environmental

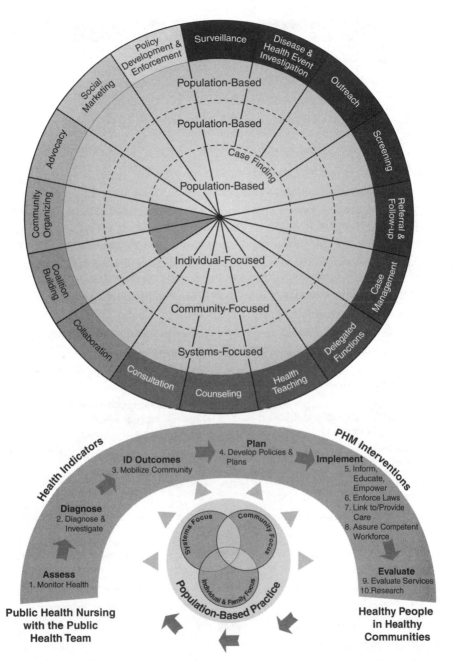

Figure 7-6 (a) Minnesota's Public Health Intervention Wheel (b) Los Angeles
County's Public Health Nursing Practice Model
(a) Cornerstones of Public Health Nursing, revised 2007, p. 7. Minnesota Department of Health,
Division of Community Health Services, Public Health Nursing Section.
(b) Public Health Nursing Practice Model. Los Angeles County Department of Health. Copyright
2007 by Los Angeles County DPH Public Health Nursing.

Table 7-4 Healthy People 2020 Objectives for Occupational and Environmental Health

Occupational Health

OSH–1: Reduce deaths from work-related injuries.

OSH–2: Reduce nonfatal work-related injuries.

OSH–3: Reduce the rate of injury and illness cases involving days away from work due to overexertion or repetitive motion.

OSH–4: Reduce pneumoconiosis deaths.

OSH–5: Reduce deaths from work-related homicides.

OSH–6: Reduce work-related assaults.

OSH–7: Reduce the proportion of persons who have elevated blood lead concentrations from work exposures.

OSH–8: Reduce occupational skin diseases or disorders among full-time workers.

OSH–9: (Developmental) Increase the proportion of employees who have access to workplace programs that prevent or reduce employee stress.

OSH–10: Reduce new cases of work-related, noise-induced hearing loss.

Environmental Health

EH-1: Reduce the number of days the Air Quality Index (AQI) exceeds 100.

EH-2: Increase use of alternative modes of transportation for work.

EH-3: Reduce air toxic emissions to decrease the risk of adverse health effects caused by airborne toxics.

EH-4: Increase the proportion of persons served by community water systems who receive a supply of drinking water that meets the regulations of the Safe Drinking Water Act.

EH-5: Reduce waterborne disease outbreaks arising from water intended for drinking among persons served by community water systems.

EH-6: Reduce per capita domestic water withdrawals with respect to use and conservation.

EH-7: Increase the proportion of days that beaches are open and safe for swimming.

EH-8: Reduce blood lead levels in children.

EH-9: Minimize the risks to human health and the environment posed by hazardous sites.

EH-10: Reduce pesticide exposures that result in visits to a healthcare facility.

EH-11: Reduce the amount of toxic pollutants released into the environment.

EH-12: Increase recycling of municipal solid waste.

EH-13: Reduce indoor allergen levels.

EH-14: Increase the percentage of homes with an operating radon mitigation system for persons living in homes at risk for radon exposure.

EH-15: Increase the percentage of new single family homes (SFH) constructed with radon-reducing features, especially in high-radon-potential areas.

(continues)

Table 7-4 Healthy People 2020 Objectives for Occupational and Environmental Health (*continued*)

EH-16: Increase the proportion of the Nation's elementary, middle, and high schools that have official school policies and engage in practices that promote a healthy and safe physical school environment.

EH-17: (Developmental) Increase the proportion of persons living in pre-1978 housing that has been tested for the presence of lead-based paint or related hazards.

EH-18: Reduce the number of U.S. homes that are found to have lead-based paint or related hazards.

EH-20: Reduce exposure to selected environmental chemicals in the population, as measured by blood and urine concentrations of the substances or their metabolites.

EH-21: Improve quality, utility, awareness, and use of existing information systems for environmental health.

EH-22: Increase the number of States, Territories, Tribes, and the District of Columbia that monitor diseases or conditions that can be caused by exposure to environmental hazards.

EH-23: Reduce the number of new schools sited within 500 feet of an interstate or Federal or State highway.

EH-24: Reduce the global burden of disease due to poor water quality, sanitation, and insufficient hygiene.

U.S. Department of Health and Human Services (2010). *Healthy People 2020* Summary of Objectives. Retrieved from http://www.healthypeople.gov/2020/topics-objectives/topic/occupational-safety-and-health/objectives & http://www.healthypeople.gov/2020/topics-objectives/topic/environmental-health/objectives

exposures be broadened beyond lead and beyond pediatrics. The mnemonic I PREPARE is used for an assessment tool recommended by the ATSDR for nurses to perform an appropriate environmental assessment (**Figure 7-7**) (CDC, n.d.; Stanhope & Lancaster, 2012). Beyond risk assessment, other roles suggested for the environmental health nurse are community involvement/public participation, individual and population risk assessment, risk communication, epidemiological investigations, and policy development (Stanhope & Lancaster, 2012).

The Role of the DNP Regarding Evaluation of Care Delivery Models

The DNP will identify strategies that lead to good outcomes within care delivery models. An unsatisfactory outcome may be the impetus for such an evaluation. In-depth preparation in program planning and evaluation

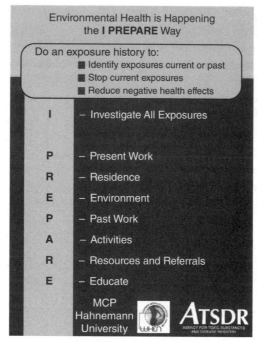

Figure 7-7 Environmental Assessment Tool: I PREPARE
Centers for Disease Control and Protextion. (n.d.). I PREPARE. Retrieved from http://www.atsdr
.cdc.gov/asbestos/site-kit/docs/IPrepareCard.pdf

methods makes the DNP able to evaluate a care delivery model. While performing this evaluation, the DNP may use concepts from the field of quality improvement in addition to psychosocial and cultural concepts. Concepts from community, environmental, and occupational health, such as the primacy of prevention, surveillance for exposures, and need for the greatest good, may also be used in evaluation of care delivery models and strategies.

One theory that can be used for outcomes assessment is the theory of quality assessment developed by Avedis Donabedian (1966, 1980). Donabedian provided an easy-to-use framework for evaluation of care delivery outcomes that consists of three concepts: structure, process, and outcome. According to Donabedian, when evaluating an outcome, the structure of an organization must be examined. The structure includes available finances, staff, and resources. The process also needs to be examined to formulate an intervention to affect outcome. In his theory, process includes such factors as utilization of care and timeliness of care (Donabedian, 1980). This simple but elegant theory can provide a framework for evaluation of the organizational aspects of care delivery models.

The DNP might also use the PRECEDE-PROCEED model. Green and Kreuter's PRECEDE-PROCEED model was developed for program planning and evaluation in the community health arena. The PRECEDE portion of this model assesses behavioral, social, and environmental factors that influence health. The PROCEED portion of this model is where evaluation of the implemented program occurs. The model guides evaluation of the process of implementation of interventions, the impact of interventions, and the outcomes from interventions. It is an excellent model for the DNP to use in evaluation of care delivery models or strategies and has been used for evaluation of many health promotion programs (Green & Mercer, 2006).

Familiarity with evidence-based practice and the economics of health care also helps prepare the DNP to evaluate care delivery models or strategies. Knowledge regarding the strength of evidence at each level is necessary to evaluate the suitability of the level of evidence for a given care delivery model. The DNP is prepared to identify the appropriateness of the evidence for the population of interest or the appropriateness of any evidence-based intervention chosen to improve an existing care delivery model. Consideration of the economic dimensions of cost-effectiveness, cost utility and cost-benefit ratios, cost minimization, and cost consequences of the continued use of or proposed change to a current delivery model is also a necessary component for thorough evaluation.

In their DNP scholarly projects, students at the University of Minnesota evaluated care delivery models, identified needed change, and developed interventions to change these models. Examples of interventions developed that have improved care delivery or strategies include access to care for truckers, continuity of care for those using retail clinics, patient flow patterns in an emergency department, timeliness in reporting abnormal test results to patients, and immunization rates in healthcare providers. These projects have incorporated concepts of community health as well as cultural and socioeconomic factors. The project that focused on implementing a new delivery strategy to improve immunization rates for healthcare providers addressed an important concept of occupational health.

Conclusions

Future Roles for DNPs in Clinical Prevention and Population Health

The acronym DNP, doctor of nursing practice, means that the practice of nursing, regardless of setting, has been brought to the doctoral level of expertise. There are vast opportunities for leadership and service for each individual DNP. The DNP graduate should be well prepared to lead in the development, implementation, and evaluation of interventions to meet the goals of *Healthy People 2020*. The advisory committee for *Healthy People 2020* developed a model to illustrate how these goals can be addressed (**Figure 7-8**). For each example, the population level of intervention is also identified.

Individual Level

The DNP as the expert provider in the area of health promotion and disease prevention is a role proposed by Burman et al. (2009). These authors maintain that "disease prevention has always been the soul of nursing, while health promotion has been its heart" (p. 14), and that the nursing educational curriculum for the DNP should focus on the fields of health promotion and disease prevention rather than just borrowing much of its curriculum from the medical field. In the view of Burman et al., this borrowing of the curriculum model from medicine has contributed to the view of the APRN as a "substitute for a physician," with titles such as *physician extender* or *midlevel provider*. Titles such as these may contribute to an impression of an accompanying need for dependent practice rather

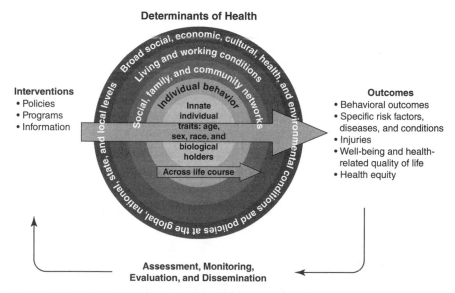

Figure 7-8 Action Model to Achieve *Healthy People 2020's* Overarching Goals
U.S. Department of Health and Human Services, Secretary's Advisory Committee on Health Promotion and Disease Prevention Objectives for 2010. (2008). Phase I Report: Recommendations for the framework and format of Healthy People 2020 (p.8). Retrieved from https://www .healthypeople.gov/sites/default/files/PhaseI_0.pdf

than visualization of an independent unique profession with ability to practice in its own right. This proposed change in the focus of education for the DNP graduate to one of health promotion and disease prevention would produce providers of care who are fundamentally different from medical providers, lead to improved patient satisfaction (see Pohl et al., 2007), and provide patients with a highly desirable type of care that is currently missing. Of course, Burman et al. acknowledged that each profession will continue to have some intersection regarding care provided, but each will also have its unique focus that is reflected in its educational preparation. Prevention of disease and promotion of health are key to decreasing healthcare costs, improving quality of life, and increasing longevity. Having a provider whose focus of care and educational preparation is devoted to prevention of disease and health promotion could enhance the potential for these outcomes to be realized. This role would promote healthy development and healthy behaviors across the life span.

This proposed change in curriculum focus works in parallel with this essential but may not be welcomed by all APRNs or medical providers because both may perceive the recommendation as limiting their respective roles in some manner. APRNs may see the proposed change as taking away from their ability to provide independent primary care services, and primary care medical providers may be reluctant to be limited in providing health promotion services.

Aggregate Level

The Human Genome Project, completed in 2003, holds promise to provide new opportunities for clinical prevention. The project, in addition to identifying all the genes that make up the human genome, also makes possible identification of gene defects that may indicate disease or disease risk. Unfortunately, merely testing for the presence of a gene defect is not sufficient in many cases to develop disease preventive interventions because the presence or absence of a defect is not diagnostic of the presence or absence of future risk for disease or diagnostic of current disease condition (Janssens et al., 2008; Monsen, 2009; Tranin, 2006).

Because of this ambiguity and the potential for psychosocial and cultural stressors for the patient considering genetic testing, in her 2006 Oncology Nursing Society Clinical Lectureship, Tranin advised that counseling regarding genetic testing is best done by nurses. Her reasoning was that nurses take a holistic view of a patient, have a wealth of experience in communicating with patients and their families, and know how to access the resources a patient might need to deal with test results. Provision of genetic counseling is within the scope of practice of the APRN certified in oncology nursing who has also obtained specialty training in genetics and genomics (ANA, 2011b). This is a role in which the educational preparation of the DNP in analysis of data, synthesis of psychosocial and cultural diversity concepts, and evaluation of care strategies can be well utilized. This role for the DNP would also help meet a *Healthy People 2020* goal, given that the goal of genetic testing and counseling is to eliminate preventable disease, disability, injury, and premature death. *Healthy People 2020* includes two specific goals under the topic area of genomics: increasing genetic counseling of women who have a family history of breast or ovarian cancer, and increasing genetic testing for Lynch syndrome in those persons newly diagnosed with colorectal cancer (USHHS, 2010a).

Population Level

With the importance of the environment to health recently coming to the forefront in nursing practice, the field of environmental health nursing holds much opportunity for the DNP to provide leadership in planning and evaluation of care delivery models or strategies that will decrease adverse health outcomes at the population level related to environmental risks. Possibly the greatest area of opportunity and need in environmental health nursing at the population level is in the area of climate change. Environmental risks related to climate change threaten everyone in the population, and population health–focused interventions will need to be developed to address these risks. Climate change health risks that have been identified by the Environmental Protection Agency (EPA) include extreme heat waves, other extreme weather events, increases in climate-sensitive diseases, air pollution, adverse effects on agricultural production, social disruption, adverse economic impacts, and displacement of populations (EPA, 2012). Barbara Sattler, in a presentation on global warming, identified the following factors that will contribute to increased health risks: increased sea levels, increased storms, problems with food security secondary to agricultural changes, fires related to increased episodes of drought, heat waves, problems with access to potable water, refugees created by climate change, and resulting increases in morbidity and mortality rates (Sattler, 2008a). She has also articulated her concern about the health impact of using chemicals in the environment (Sattler, 2008b) and more recently lobbied for nurses to join the Alliance for Nurses for Healthy Environments to advocate on behalf of their patients for chemical policies to be "based primarily on the protection of human health with rigorous pre-market testing, access to research results, and full disclosure of ingredients" (Sattler, 2010, para. 6). The role of the National Institutes of Health in supporting research on the health effects of climate change has also been explored, with a recommendation to increase support (Jessup et al., 2013). The DNP, with nursing's holistic focus, grounding in community and public health concepts, consideration for psychosocial and cultural dimensions, and strong background in health promotion when planning interventions, is best suited for the task of addressing these risks to populations that threaten to arise from climate change. If they were alive today, this may be the area of nursing on which Nightingale and Wald would be focusing.

DNP Outcome Potentials Related to Improving the Nation's Health

Broad dissemination of knowledge regarding effective health promotion and disease prevention measures is needed to reach the goal of improving the nation's health. The APTR provides all healthcare providers interested in prevention education, including the DNP, with the potential to communicate easily within an interdisciplinary healthcare community about clinical prevention and population health interventions and programs with its Web-based resource, the Prevention Education Resource Center (PERC). The PERC website (www.teachprevention.org) is a place where registered members can submit prevention-related educational material, access materials submitted by others, and evaluate the quality of these materials (Fincham, 2008). This site serves as a portal for speedy and broad dissemination of information to the prevention education and research community as well as peer evaluation of submitted prevention-based activities. The DNP graduate could submit any prevention-related scholarly project to this site to be used as a resource for others who may be dealing with similar problems. The potential for others to more quickly benefit from broader use of successful health promotion interventions through the PERC website provides a positive impetus toward reaching the goal of improving the nation's health.

Proof as to whether DNP graduates will exceed the abilities of master's-prepared APRNs in practice has yet to be determined, and opinion as to whether improvement in practice ability will result from the additional coursework provided to the DNP graduate is mixed (Dreher, 2009; Ford, 2009; Kaplan & Brown, 2009). But consideration of the expanded potential the DNP brings for improvements in outcomes related to clinical prevention and population health interventions as discussed in this chapter leads to the conclusion that the DNP will help propel the nursing profession to new horizons while promoting improvement in the nation's health.

Clinical prevention interventions developed, implemented, and evaluated by the DNP and directed at the levels of individual, aggregate, and population health hold much promise to improve health status at all these levels and may reach beyond improvements in health status. The WHO's (n.d.) agenda includes six points focused on improvement of population health: "promoting development; fostering health security; strengthening health systems; harnessing research, information, and evidence; enhancing partnerships; and improving performance." Within the description of the goal of "promoting development" is the need for access to health-promoting interventions to ensure the health of populations. This WHO goal is parallel to a portion of one of the AACN educational goals of this essential. The DNP is prepared to develop health promotion interventions focused on improving access patterns for health care. The WHO also closely ties good health to the socioeconomic development of nations; that is, good health is needed for a worker to be productive. If large portions of the population of a nation are in poor health, it will be difficult for that nation to improve its socioeconomic status because of the lack of a capable workforce. This is a concept well known to occupational health nurses. Ill health leads to absenteeism and increased risk for workplace injury. By meeting the goals of this essential, the DNP may hold promise to improve not only the nation's health but also its socioeconomic status. Truly, the potential for contribution by the DNP to improvement in the health of individuals, families, communities, and beyond is enormous for this nation as a whole.

References

Agency for Healthcare Research and Quality. (n.d.). *U.S. Preventive Services Task Force: About the USPSTF*. Retrieved from http://www.ahrq.gov/clinic/uspstfab.htm

Allan, J., Barwick, T. A., Cashman, S., Cawley, J. F., Day, C., Douglass, C., . . . Wood, D. (2004). Clinical prevention and population health: Curriculum framework for health professions. *American Journal of Preventive Medicine, 27*(5), 471–476.

Allan, J. D., Stanley, J., Crabtree, M. K., Werner, K. E., & Swenson, M. (2005). Clinical prevention and population health curriculum framework: The nursing perspective. *Journal of Professional Nursing, 21*(5), 259–267.

Allender, J. A., Rector, C., & Warner, K. D. (2014). *Community health nursing: Promoting and protecting the public's health* (8th ed.). Philadelphia, PA: Lippincott Williams & Wilkins.

Alliance of Nurses for Healthy Environments. (2008). *About ANHE.* Retrieved from http://envirn.org/pg/groups/4104/alliance-of-nurses-for-healthy-environments/

Alliance of Nurses for Healthy Environments. (2015). Retrieved from http://envirn.org/

American Association of Colleges of Nursing. (2006). *The essentials of doctoral education for advanced nursing practice.* Retrieved from http://www.aacn.nche.edu/DNP/pdf/Essentials.pdf

American Association of Colleges of Nursing. (2008). *The essentials of baccalaureate education for professional nursing practice.* Retrieved from http://www.aacn.nche.edu/education/pdf/BaccEssentials08.pdf

American Association of Colleges of Nursing. (2011). *The essentials of master's education in nursing.* Retrieved from http://www.aacn.nche.edu/education-resources/MastersEssentials11.pdf

American Association of Occupational Health Nurses. (n.d.). *About AAOHN.* Retrieved from http://www.aaohn.org/aaohn-aboutus-files.html

American College of Physicians. (2009). *Nurse practitioners in primary care* [Policy monograph]. Philadelphia, PA: Author.

American Nurses Association. (2011a). *Final ACO rules adopt ANA's recommendations on nursing leadership, patient-centered care: ANA contends improvements can be made on care coordination provisions.* Retrieved from http://www.nursingworld.org/MainMenuCategories/Policy-Advocacy/Positions-and-Resolutions/Issue-Briefs/ACOs/ACO-Rules-Adopt-ANAs-Recommendations.pdf

American Nurses Association. (2011b). *Essential genetic and genomic competencies for nurses with graduate degrees.* Retrieved from http://www.nursingworld.org/MainMenuCategories/EthicsStandards/Genetics-1/Essential-Genetic-and-Genomic-Competencies-for-Nurses-With-Graduate-Degrees.pdf

American Nurses Association. (2013). *Scope and standards of practice: Public health nursing* (2nd ed.). Silver Spring, MD: Author.

Aschengrau, A., & Seage, G. R. (2008). Screening in public health practice. In A. Aschengrau & G. R. Seage III, *Essentials of epidemiology in public health* (2nd ed., pp. 411–438). Sudbury, MA: Jones and Bartlett.

Ashton, K., & Green, E. S. (2008). *The toxic consumer: Living healthy in a hazardous world.* New York, NY: Sterling.

Association for Prevention Teaching and Research. (2009, January). *Clinical prevention and population health curriculum framework.* Retrieved from http://c.ymcdn.com/sites/www.aptrweb.org/resource/resmgr/HPCTF_Docs/Revised_CPPH_Framework_2009.pdf

Association for Prevention Teaching and Research. (2015, February). *Clinical prevention and population health curriculum framework.* Retrieved from http://c.ymcdn.com/sites/www.aptrweb.org/resource/resmgr/HPCTF_Docs/Revised_CPPH_Framework_2.201.pdf

Association for Professionals in Infection Control and Epidemiology, Inc. (n.d.). *About APIC.* Retrieved from http://apic.org/About-APIC/About-APIC-Overview

Barkauskas, V. H., Pohl, J., Breer, L., Tanner, C., Bostrom, A. C., Benkert, R., & Vonderheid, S. (2004). Academic nurse-managed centers: Approaches to evaluation. *Outcomes Management, 8*(1), 57–66.

Barrett, J. R. (2015). Seeds of toxicity? *Environmental Health Perspectives, 123*(3), A42.

Benjamin, R. M. (2011). Surgeon general's perspective: The national prevention strategy: Shifting the nation's health-care system. *Public Health Reports, 126*, 774–776.

Briss, P. A., Brownson, R. C., Fielding, J. E., & Zaza, S. (2004). Developing and using the Guide to Community Preventive Services: Lessons learned about evidence-based public health. *Annual Review of Public Health, 24*, 281–302.

Burman, M. E., Hart, A. M., Conley, V., Brown, J., Sherard, P., & Clarke, P. N. (2009). Reconceptualizing the core of nurse practitioner education and practice. *Journal of the American Academy of Nurse Practitioners, 21*, 11–17.

Burwell v. Hobby Lobby Stores, Inc. 13-354, U.S. 573 (2014).

Centers for Disease Control and Prevention. (n.d.). *I PREPARE*. Retrieved from http://www.atsdr.cdc.gov/asbestos/site-kit/docs/IPrepareCard.pdf

Centers for Disease Control and Prevention. (2015). *2014 Ebola outbreak in West Africa—Case counts*. Retrieved from http://www.cdc.gov/vhf/ebola/outbreaks/2014-west-africa/case-counts.html

Colwill, J. W., Cultice, J. M., & Kruse, R. L. (2008). Will generalist physician supply meet demands of an increasing and aging population? *Health Affairs, 27*(3), w232–w241.

Commission on Social Determinants of Health. (2008). *Closing the gap in a generation: Health equity through action on the social determinants of health*. Final report of the Commission on Social Determinants of Health. Geneva, Switzerland: World Health Organization. Retrieved from http://whqlibdoc.who.int/publications/2008/9789241563703_eng.pdf

Cullum, N., Ciliska, D., Marks, S., & Haynes, B. (2008). An introduction to evidence-based nursing. In N. Cullum, D. Ciliska, R. B. Haynes, & S. Marks (Eds.), *Evidence-based nursing: An introduction* (pp. 1–8). Hong Kong: Blackwell.

DesRoches, C. M., Buerhaus, P., Dittus, R. S., & Donelan, K. (2015). Primary care workforce shortages and career recommendations from practicing clinicians. *Academic Medicine, 90*(2), 1–7.

DiCenso, A., Guyatt, G., & Ciliska, D. (2005). *Evidenced-based nursing: A guide to clinical practice*. St. Louis, MO: Elsevier Mosby.

Donabedian, A. (1966). Evaluating the quality of medical care. *Milbank Quarterly, 44*(3), 166–203.

Donabedian, A. (1980). *Explorations in quality assessment and monitoring: The definition of quality and approaches to its assessment* (Vol. 1). Ann Arbor, MI: Health Administration Press.

Dossey, B. M. (2000). *Florence Nightingale: Mystic, visionary, healer*. Springhouse, PA: Springhouse Corporation.

Dreher, H. M. (2009). Education for advanced practice. In L. A. Joel (Ed.), *Advanced practice nursing: Essentials for role development* (2nd ed., pp. 58–71). Philadelphia, PA: F. A. Davis.

Eisler, R., & Potter, T. (2014). *Transforming interprofessional partnerships: A new framework for nursing and partnership-based health care*. Indianapolis, IN: Sigma Theta Tau International.

Environmental Protection Agency. (2012). *Climate change: Health and environmental effects*. Retrieved from http://www.epa.gov/climatechange/effects/health.html

Fincham, J. E. (2008). Clinical prevention and population health enabled through the prevention education resource center. *Journal of Public Health Management Practice, 14*(4), 396–399.

Fineout-Overholt, E., & Johnston, L. (2005). Teaching EBP: Asking searchable, answerable clinical questions. *Worldviews on Evidence Based Nursing, 2,* 157–160.

Flemming, K. (2008). Asking answerable questions. In N. Cullum, D. Ciliska, R. B. Haynes, & S. Marks (Eds.), *Evidence-based nursing: An introduction* (pp. 18–23). Hong Kong: Blackwell.

Fletcher, R. W., & Fletcher, S. W. (2005). Prevention. In *Clinical epidemiology: The essentials* (4th ed., pp. 147–167). Baltimore, MD: Lippincott Williams & Wilkins.

Ford, J. (2009). The doctorate of nursing practice: Coming into focus. *Advance for Nurse Practitioners, 17*(1), 31–38.

Friedman, C. (2014). Infection prevention and control programs. In P. Grota (Ed.), *APIC text of infection control and epidemiology* (4th ed., pp. 1–9). Washington, DC: APIC.

Frisch, N. C., George, V., Giovoni, A. L., Jennings-Sanders, A., & McCahon, C. P. (2003). Teaching nurses to focus on the health needs for populations: A master's degree program in population health nursing. *Nurse Educator, 28*(5), 212–216.

Garcia, C. M., Schaffer, M. A., & Schoon, P. M. (2014). *Population-based public health clinical manual: The Henry Street model for nurses* (2nd ed.). Indianapolis, IN: Sigma Theta Tau International.

Geraci, E. P. (2004). Planned change. In S. J. Peterson & T. S. Bredow (Eds.), *Middle range theories: Application to nursing research* (pp. 323–340). Philadelphia, PA: Lippincott Williams & Wilkins.

Gévas, J., Starfield, B., & Heath, I. (2008). Is clinical prevention better than cure? *Lancet, 372,* 1997–1999.

Green, L. W., & Kreuter, M. W. (1999). *Health promotion planning: An educational and ecological approach* (3rd ed.). Mountain View, CA: Mayfield.

Green, L. W., & Mercer, S. L. (2006). PRECEDE-PROCEED model. In L. Breslow & G. Cengage (Eds.), *Encyclopedia of public health.* Retrieved from http://www.enotes.com/precede-proceed-model

Haider, M., & Kreps, G. L. (2004). Forty years of diffusion on innovations: Utility and value in public health. *Journal of Health Communication, 9,* 3–11.

Haley, R. W., Culver, D. H., White, J. W., Morgan, W. M., Emori, T. G., Munn, V. P., & Hooten, T. W. (1985). The efficacy of infection surveillance and control programs in preventing nosocomial infections in U.S. hospitals. *American Journal of Epidemiology, 121*(2), 182–205.

Haley, R. W., Quade, D., Freeman, H. E., & Bennett, J. V. (1980). Study on efficacy of nosocomial infection control (SENIC Project): Summary of study design. *American Journal of Epidemiology, 111*(5), 472–485.

Hansen-Turton, T., Bailey, D. N., Torres, N., & Ritter, A. (2010). Nurse-managed health centers. *American Journal of Nursing, 110*(9), 23–26.

Hansen-Turton, T., Ritter, A., Rothman, N., & Valdez, B. (2006). Insurer policies create barriers to health care access and consumer choice. *Nursing Economic$, 24*(4), 204–211.

Hansen-Turton, T., Ryan, S., Miller, K., Counts, M., & Nash, D. B. (2007). Convenient care clinics: The future of accessible health care. *Disease Management, 10*(2), 61–73.

Henderson, V. A. (1991). *The nature of nursing: Reflections after 25 years.* New York, NY: National League for Nursing.

Institute of Medicine. (2011a). *Clinical preventive services for women: Closing the gaps.* Washington, DC: National Academies Press.

Institute of Medicine. (2011b). *The future of nursing: Leading change, advancing health.* Washington, DC: National Academies Press.

Issel, L. M. (2014). *Health program planning and evaluation: A practical, systematic approach for community health* (3rd ed.). Sudbury, MA: Jones and Bartlett.

Janssens, A. C., Gwinn, M., Bradley, L. A., Oostra, B. A., van Duijn, C. M., & Khoury, M. J. (2008). A critical appraisal of the scientific basis of commercial genomic profiles used to assess health risks and personalize health intervention. *American Journal of Human Genetics, 82,* 593–599.

Jessup, C. M., Balbus, J. M., Christian, C., Haque, E., Howe, S. E., Newton, S. A., . . . Rosenthal, J. P. (2013). Climate change, human health, and biomedical research: Analysis of the National Institutes of Health research portfolio. *Environmental Health Perspectives, 121*(4), 399–404.

Kaplan, L., & Brown, M. (2009). Proud to be a pioneer: Perspectives of a first cohort of DNP students. *American Journal for Nurse Practitioners, 13*(3), 10–20.

Keller, L. O., Strohschein, S., Lia-Hoagberg, B., & Schaffer, M. (1998). Population-based public health nursing interventions: A model from practice. *Public Health Nursing, 15*(3), 207–215.

Leininger, M. (1981). Transcultural nursing: Its progress and its future. *Nursing and Health Care, 2*(7), 365–371.

Leininger, M., & McFarland, M. R. (2006).*Culture care diversity and universality: A worldwide nursing theory* (2nd ed.) Sudbury, MA: Jones and Bartlett.

Lewin, K. (1951). *Field theory in social science.* London: Harper & Row.

Lewin, K. (1975). *Field theory in social science.* Westport, CT: Greenwood Press.

Liu, J., & Lewis, G. (2014). Environmental toxicity and poor cognitive outcomes in children and adults. *Journal of Environmental Health, 76*(6), 130–138.

Monsen, R. B. (2009). *Genetics and ethics in health care: New questions in the age of genomic health.* Silver Spring, MD: American Nurses Association.

Mundinger, M. O., Kane, R. L., Lenz, E. R., Totten, A. M., Tsai, W., Cleary, P. D., . . . Shelanski, M. L. (2000). Primary care outcomes in patients treated by nurse practitioners or physicians: A randomized trial. *Journal of the American Medical Association, 283*(1), 59–68.

Nelson, R. (2007). Retail health clinics on the rise. *American Journal of Nursing, 107*(7), 25–26.

Newland, J. (2006). Nurse managed health centers: Strengthening the healthcare safety net. *The Nurse Practitioner, 31*(2), 5.

Nies, M. A., & McEwen, M. (2014). Health: A community view. In M. McEwen & M. A. Nies, *Community/public health nursing: Promoting the health of populations* (6th ed., pp. 1–18). St. Louis, MO: Saunders Elsevier.

O'Fallon, L. (2003). NIEHS extramural update: Nursing and environmental health roundtable. *Environmental Health Perspectives, 111*(2). Retrieved from http://www.niehs.nih.gov/about/boards/naehsc/february_2003.pdf#xml

Pender, N. J. (1975). A conceptual model for preventive health behavior. *Nursing Outlook, 23*, 385–390.

Pender, N. J., Murdaugh, C. L., & Parsons, M. A. (2006). Introduction. In *Health promotion in nursing practice* (5th ed., pp. 1–12). Upper Saddle River, NJ: Pearson Prentice Hall.

Pender, N. J., Murdaugh, C. L., & Parsons, M. A. (2011). Individual models to promote health behavior. In *Health promotion in nursing practice* (6th ed., pp. 35–66). Upper Saddle River, NJ: Pearson Education.

Peterson, S. J., & Bredow, T. S. (Eds.). (2012). *Middle range theories: Application to nursing research* (3rd ed.). Philadelphia, PA: Lippincott Williams & Wilkins.

Pohl, J. M., Barkauskas, V. H., Benkert, R., Breer, L., & Bostrom, A. (2007). Impact of academic nurse-managed centers on communities served. *Journal of the American Academy of Nurse Practitioners, 19*, 268–275.

Pope, A. M., Snyder, M. A., & Mood, L. H. (1995). *Nursing, health, & the environment*. Washington, DC: National Academy Press.

Prochaska, J. O., Norcross, J. C., & DiClemente, C. C. (1994). *Changing for good: The revolutionary program that explains the six stages of change and teaches you how to free yourself from bad habits*. New York, NY: William Morrow.

Purnell, L. (2002). The Purnell model for cultural competence. *Journal of Transcultural Nursing, 13*(3), 193–196.

Purnell, L. (2009). *Guide to culturally competent health care* (2nd ed.). Philadelphia, PA: F. A. Davis.

Purnell, L. (2014). *Guide to culturally competent health care* (3rd ed.). Philadelphia, PA: F. A. Davis.

Purnell, L., & Paulanka, B. J. (2005). *Guide to culturally competent health care*. Philadelphia, PA: F. A. Davis.

Radzyminski, S. (2007). The concept of population health within the nursing profession. *Journal of Professional Nursing, 23*(1), 37–46.

Riegelman, R. K., Evans, C. H., & Garr, D. R. (2004). Why a clinical prevention and population health curriculum framework? *American Journal of Preventive Medicine, 27*(5), 477.

Riegelman, R. K., & Garr, D. R. (2011). Healthy People 2020 and education for health: What are the objectives? *American Journal of Preventive Medicine, 40*(2), 203–206.

Rogers, E. M. (2002). The nature of technology transfer. *Science Communication, 23*, 323–341.

Rogers, E. M. (2003). *Diffusion of innovations* (5th ed.). New York, NY: Free Press.

Sattler, B. (2008a). *Global warming and public health*. Presented at the 136th APHA annual meeting and exposition, San Diego, CA.

Sattler, B. (2008b). Bodies and the legacy of "Better Living Through Chemistry." *Pennsylvania Nurse, 63*(3), 22.

Sattler, B. (2010). *Why nurses need chemical policy reform.* Retrieved from http://www.psr.org/environment-and-health/environmental-health-policy-institute/responses/why-nurses-need-chemical-policy-reform.html

Stanhope, M., & Lancaster, J. (2012). *Public health nursing: Population-centered health care in the community* (8th ed.). St. Louis, MO: Mosby Elsevier.

Tranin, A. S. (2006). The bridge from genomic discoveries to disease prevention. *Oncology Nursing Forum, 33*(5), 891–900.

Trasande, L. (2014). Further limiting Bisphenol A in food uses could provide health and economic benefits. *Health Affairs, 33*(2), 316–323.

U.S. Department of Health and Human Services. (2000). *Healthy People 2010: Understanding and improving health* (2nd ed.). Washington, DC: U.S. Government Printing Office.

U.S. Department of Health and Human Services. (2010a). *Healthy People 2020 framework.* Retrieved from http://www.healthypeople.gov/2020/about/default.aspx

U.S. Department of Health and Human Services. (2010b). *Evidence-based clinical and public health: Generating and applying evidence.* Retrieved from http://www.healthypeople.gov/sites/default/files/EvidenceBasedClinicalPH2010.pdf

U.S. Department of Health and Human Services, Health Resources and Services Administration. (2013). *Projecting the supply and demand for primary care practitioners through 2020.* National Center for Health Workforce Analysis. Rockville, MD: U.S. Department of Health and Human Services.

Walker, H. K. (2006). Primary care is dying in the United States: *Mutatis mutandis. Medical Education, 40,* 9–11.

World Health Organization. (n.d.). *The WHO agenda.* Retrieved from http://www.who.int/about/agenda/en/index.html

World Health Organization. (2006). *Constitution of the World Health Organization, basic documents* (45th ed., Suppl.). Retrieved from http://www.who.int/governance/eb/who_constitution_en.pdf

Zahner, S. J., & Block, D. E. (2006). The road to population health: Using *Healthy People 2010* in nursing education. *Journal of Nursing Education, 45*(3), 105–108.

Zenzano, T., Allan, J. D., Bigley, M. B., Bushardt, R. L., Garr, D. R., Johnson, K., . . . Stanley, J. M. (2011). The roles of healthcare professionals in implementing clinical prevention and population health. *American Journal of Preventive Medicine, 40*(2), 261–267.

Part II

Doctor of Nursing Practice Roles

Chapter 8

Traditional Advanced Practice Roles for the DNP

I have an almost complete disregard of precedent, and a faith in the possibility of something better. It irritates me to be told how things have always been done. I defy the tyranny of precedent. I go for anything new that might improve the past.

—Clara Barton

Clinical Nurse Specialist

Mary E. Zaccagnini

It is apparent that these are tumultuous times in health care. Currently the United States is experiencing a flood of problems associated with health care and healthcare delivery systems. According to a U.S. Census Bureau report (2009), the numbers of Americans without insurance rose to 46.3 million in 2008, and healthcare premiums have grown faster than inflation. The United States allocates more of its economy to health care than any other developed country (Kaiser Family Foundation, 2009). The Centers for Medicare and Medicaid Services (CMS) reported that national healthcare expenditures are expected to reach 20.3% of the gross domestic product by 2018 (CMS, 2012). According to the Institute of Medicine (IOM) report *Crossing the Quality Chasm* (2001, p. 1), "The American healthcare delivery system is in need of fundamental change." The report additionally states that "in its current form, habits, and environment, American health care is incapable of providing the public with the quality health care it expects and deserves."

The doctor of nursing practice (DNP) degree is currently evolving into the terminal degree for advanced practice nursing and as such is lauded as the preparation nurses need to face the new complexities of patient care, healthcare delivery, and additional local and national healthcare concerns. According to the American Association of Colleges of Nursing (AACN, 2008), although the new degree will not alter the scope of practice of advanced practice nurses (APNs), transitioning to the DNP will better prepare them for the "growing complexity of health care." Because the clinical nurse specialist (CNS) is educated as a systems thinker and a practitioner who is primarily answerable for challenges and changes at the population, disease, or organizational level, the CNS is at the forefront of complex emerging issues in health care and at the cusp of shaping reform.

The CNS is a registered nurse functioning in an advanced role. The American Nurses Association (ANA) outlines the scope of practice for all nurses and the expectations of the professional roles within which all nurses must practice. A practicing CNS must first obtain a graduate degree and certification as a CNS within a chosen field. A clinical nurses specialist then enters a role that is multifaceted. The CNS is a clinical specialist, consultant, educator, and has expertise in project development, and quality management. He/she is an autonomous advanced practicitioner who assesseses diagnosis and manages patients, and whose clients can be an individual, institution, or community. The CNS is often responsible for the clinical education of nurses in multiple areas. Research and theory is the foundation of CNS practice. Research into CNS practice describes multiple interventions that are linked to a reduction of costs and lengths of stay in hospital settings. It is also notable that this care is safe and is reported as increasing patient satisfaction.

The National Association of Clinical Nurse Specialists (NACNS) articulates CNS practice competencies, educational guidelines, and credentialing requirements. This organization describes the essence of CNS practice as clinical nursing expertise in diagnosis and treatment to prevent, remediate, or alleviate illness and promote health, with a defined specialty (NACNS, 2004). A type of health problem, a disease or medical subspecialty, a type of care or problem, a specific setting or unit, a disease, or a population can define the specialty. Currently, over 72,000 APNs are prepared and credentialed to practice as CNSs (ANA, 2009; NACNS, 2012). Additionally, approximately "70% of CNSs work with adult patients from the age of 19–85 years of age," and "approximately 70% of CNSs work in some type of inpatient hospital setting" (NACNS, 2012).

History

Florence Nightingale has often been identified as the founder of modern nursing practice. She identified concepts that are the basis of contemporary CNS practices, including the identification of the differences of nursing and medicine; the understanding that an incorrect diagnosis would lead to an unwanted consequence; the recognition of nursing responsibilities, including disease prevention; the philosophy that nursing should be based in scientific evidence; a conviction that nursing competencies would ensure quality care; and the recognition that nurses could and should impact health care (NACNS, 2004).

Specialized nursing practice began with a psychiatric nursing program in 1880 at McLean Hospital in Massachusetts (Critchley, 1985). There was more formal attentiveness to this role in the 1940s, when it was ascertained that many soldiers returning from World War II were burdened with mental illness (Hamric, 2009). This was most likely posttraumatic stress syndrome, which had not yet been defined. This diagnosed illness was originally treated with electroshock therapy, which required the assistance of nurses with specialized training.

Dr. Hildegard Peplau is considered the "founding mother" of CNS practice (NACNS, 2009a). She was a psychiatric nurse and professor who described the CNS as an APN having expertise in the nursing care of complex patients. She established the first master's program at Rutgers University in 1954. This program in psychiatric nursing was considered the first CNS program and made more evident the link between academia and specialization.

In the 1960s, CNS practice took its modern form. In 1965, Dr. Peplau "contended that development of areas of specialization is preceded by three social forces: (1) an increase in specialty-related information; (2) new technological advances; and (3) a response to public need and interest" (Hamric, 2009, p. 15). These could be correlated to current issues in health care and the call for the further evolution of advanced practice specialized nurses.

The need for and growth of psychiatric CNS programs was instrumental in defining and developing the CNS role. Psychiatric CNSs continued to proliferate during the 1970s, and the specialties of critical care and oncology emerged (Keeling, 2009). It was not until the mid-1970s that the ANA officially recognized the CNS role and title. Initially, ANA defined the CNS as an expert practitioner and a change agent; at the same time, it included a master's degree as a requirement for CNS practice.

CNS expansion continued in the 1980s as researchers studied outcomes related to CNS practice. CNS practice began to include the practice of nursing staff development and organizational aspects of nursing care. In the 1990s, CNS roles were challenged because of changes in the healthcare landscape regarding financial reimbursement in organizations and the increased need for primary care practitioners. A major step in the specialty occurred in 1995, when the NACNS was established. In the same period, Medicare reimbursement was expanded to include direct payment to CNSs.

Historically, CNS practice was described by subroles of skills and activities. These included expert practitioner, educator, researcher, change agent, administrator, and consultant. In recent years, CNS practice has been described conceptually by integration of these subroles across the three spheres of influence: the patient/client sphere, the nurses/nursing sphere, and the system/organizational sphere. Direct care (the patient/client sphere) is the inner core of CNS practice.

Educational Preparation

CNS practice has expanded exponentially into more than 40 specialties. The master's degree has always been an entry-level requirement for CNS practice. Only since the 1990s have the foundational specialty competencies been defined. Educational preparation may vary; however, it is desirable that the foundational graduate education prepare the CNS as a proficient APN regardless of venue. It is then the intent that specialization education follow the core graduate tutelage. The curriculum dedicated to the expert portion should include a minimum of 500 hours of supervised clinical experience, not including prescriptive preparation hours, and a CNS in the same or similar specialization should provide the supervision. The clinical hours ensure that the practitioner meets the criteria for certification.

Certification

The purposes of certification are to validate knowledge and competency for CNS entry into practice and to meet emerging regulatory trends (NACNS, 2007). Required certification is defined by individual states and may require one or both of the following: CNS certification and specialty certification. The predominant trend is to require certification as a validation of attainment of initial advanced practice competencies and of recognition and authority to practice (NACNS, 2005). This may also be a factor in the application process for credentialing and prescriptive authority.

Currently, the American Nurses Credentialing Center (ANCC, 2012a) offers certification exams in adult health, gerontology, adult psychiatric and mental health, child and adolescent psychiatric and mental health, advanced diabetes management, home health, pediatric, and public/community health. The Adult Health CNS and the Gerontological CNS exams were retired in 2014. A new certification exam, Adult-Gerontology CNS certification, was launched in 2013–2014 to replace the two that were eliminated (ANCC, 2012b). Currently, all CNSs and nurse practitioners (NPs) must provide evidence that 25 out of the required 75 continuing education hours are in pharmacotherapeutics.

In addition to the ANCC certification process, many professional organizations offer examinations in specialty areas. However, not all specialties offer a process or examination. Many, if not all, states now require certification to practice in a specialty area as an APN, although generally, the current ANCC exams suffice, and the CNS educational preparation includes elements of a specialty practice. It should be noted that many states also require not only certification and a license as a registered nurse but also a second license as an advanced practice registered nurse (APRN).

Core Competencies

The core competencies for the CNS practice were developed by the NACNS and are applicable to all specialty areas. These competencies provide the foundation for practice and are written to reflect the three spheres of influence, with the patient/client sphere envisioned as the largest area of practice. It is expected that the competencies are then actualized within the specialty practice, across populations and settings. These competencies include educational requirements and outcomes. The core competencies were developed from evidence-based best practices, evidence from literature, and expert opinion. They were validated by a national study in 2005 and by Baldwin, Clark, Fulton, and Mayo (2009), who further validated and defined the entry-level core competencies' use in practice, their importance, and the potential gaps between competency and practice. The competencies were placed under the scrutiny of more than 30 national organizations, which were invited to provide critique and review (Baldwin, Lyon, Clark, Fulton, & Dayhoff, 2007), and they were presented to the organizations' membership for response. The competencies include a behavioral statement, the sphere(s) of influence, and nurse characteristics for the following competencies: direct care, consultation, systems leadership, collaboration, coaching, research, ethical decision making, moral agency, and advocacy.

On June 12, 2009, the NACNS board of directors approved a set of CNS core competencies for the DNP degree. As with the original core competencies, they encompassed the three spheres of influence, although the subject matter is much broader and far reaching. In the client sphere, the competencies speak to advanced clinical judgment and include pharmacologic interventions and prescribing. The nursing sphere dictates leadership and healthcare team processes that may affect both fiscal and clinical outcomes. Finally, the organizational/system sphere of influence includes areas such as organizational and systems theory, and care that is evidence based, cost effective, and ethical. Again, in the evolution of the competencies, public scrutiny and feedback were solicited. The competencies are meant to be used in conjunction with the core competencies and the AACN essentials of doctoral education for advanced nursing practice (NACNS, 2009b). According to the NACNS (2009b), the competencies are intended to "reflect CNS practice across all specialties, populations and settings." Although the competencies were not intended to be an endorsement of the DNP degree, they acknowledged that this degree is more than likely the terminal degree in the future of advanced practice nursing. Recently, the NACNS released a position statement endorsing the DNP degree as an entry into practice by 2030 (NACNS, 2015). This is consistent with other national statements and recommendations. The national association stated that "DNP preparation for practice in the CNS role will better position the CNS to meet the demands of an evolving healthcare system" (NACNS, 2015).

In March 2010, the AACN, in collaboration with the NACNS, published the adult-gerontology CNS competencies. These competencies are meant to build on both the APRN and the CNS core competencies and include a comparative behavioral statement to the core competencies, as well as the sphere of influence reflected within each statement. They are delineated using the model of the CNS core competencies and are intended to present the differing stages of acute and wellness care across a spectrum, from adult to older adult.

The Role and Scope of Practice

According to Hamric, Spross, and Hanson (2009), the role of the CNS has been dynamic and has moved from a listing and definition of roles (expert practitioner, educator, researcher, change agent, administer, and consultant) to the impact and influence that CNSs have on their clients and environment. This delineation of influences was intended to diminish role ambiguity and "to distinguish CNSs from other APNs" (NACNS, 1998).

CNS role genesis is specialization, and the client sphere is at its core. Direct clinical practice is at the heart of care, as with all APNs, although the CNS will most likely be found in the inpatient setting. Direct care not only is the mainstay of practice but also directs and influences all spheres and outcomes. The CNS, in this sphere, will most likely oversee care for his or her population or area of practice and directly manage those clients whose needs are multifaceted, complicated, challenging, or unique. Direct care refers to CNS activities and responsibilities that occur within the patient–nurse interface (Sparacino & Cartwright, 2009). The goal of CNS patient care is to decrease or prevent symptoms and suffering and improve the functioning of the individual patient or population. Outcomes related to this role could include direct reduction in costs for the institution as well as improved quality of care. Studies have reinforced the realization that CNS involvement in patient care has consistently improved outcomes. The amount of direct care practice, however, varies from institution to institution and CNS to CNS. The direct care practice role may be overemphasized or underemphasized depending on the institution's needs and the availability of other expert resources.

In the nurse/nursing sphere of influence, the CNS affects practice through the integration of evidence-based interventions into nursing care. This includes the leadership and expert coaching the CNS provides for nursing, and the education furnished regarding the current science of practice and technology. CNSs also develop and provide nursing education to improve practice and assist the institution in meeting goals of safety and quality. In addition, it is generally incumbent on the CNS to assist with the key indicators of magnet status accreditation.

In the organizational/system sphere, CNSs are skilled at "assessing organizational processes, including interdepartmental relationships/ functioning, professional climate, multi-disciplinary collaboration, external relationships and regulations, and health policy to identify facilitators and barriers to effective patient care" (McKinley, 2007, p. 53). In this context, CNSs work within the culture and mission of the institution and are in alignment with the organizational goals. CNSs lead multidisciplinary teams in developing new and inventive programs that improve care and are fiscally responsible. Given the complexity of health care and the need for expert clinical practice change agents, the practice doctorate enhances the CNS's effectiveness in the nurse/nursing practice and organization/system spheres.

The Future of CNS Practice

Regulatory Challenges

As with all APNs, the CNS is confronted with legislative and regulatory challenges that can restrict practice and withhold care. CNSs do not currently hold prescriptive authority in all states even though they are recognized as APNs. This is beginning to change, and it is hoped that the issue will be resolved so that CNSs can practice within their scope as APNs. It is important that all CNS curricula contain the content necessary for prescriptive practice so that CNSs will be prepared even if their state does not currently allow this provision of care.

Currently, APN groups, which include CNSs, are debating with regulatory agencies in many areas regarding the supervision verbiage contained in the standards of practice of many state boards of nursing. There is consensus that all APNs, including CNSs, should have autonomy in practice and not be required to have physician supervision or formalized collaborative practice agreements. This is supported by the IOM's *Future of Nursing* report, which states that "nurses should practice to the full extent of their education and training" (IOM, 2010).

Titling issues specific to the CNS also exist. There is significant inconsistency among various state boards of nursing regarding the recognition of the title of clinical nurse specialist. This includes the criteria necessary for attainment and use of the title. For example, in the state of Minnesota, a nurse may not use the title clinical nurse specialist unless he or she has graduated from a CNS program within a college or university and obtained a board of nursing-accepted national accreditation as a CNS. The NACNS (2004) has stated, and advocates, that the CNS title should be protected in the statute of all boards of nursing.

The Future Role of the CNS and the DNP Degree

> *Patients, health care professionals, and policy makers are becoming all too painfully aware of the shortcomings of our current care delivery systems and the importance of finding better approaches to meeting the health care needs of all Americans.*
>
> —William C. Richardson

According to the NACNS, CNSs can meet the need to "increase the effectiveness of transitioning care from hospital to home and prevent readmissions; improve the quality and safety of care and reduce health care costs; educate, train and increase the nursing workforce needed for an improved health system; increase access to community-based care; increase the availability of effective care for those with chronic illness; and improve access to wellness and preventative care" (NACNS, 2009a). This assertion reflects many of the changes needed to help reform the current healthcare system. For example, according to a 2007 Milken Institute report, "people with chronic health conditions cost the United States more than $1 trillion a year. This figure could jump to nearly $6 trillion by 2050 unless the provision of preventive health services substantially improves" (Bedroussian & DeVol, 2007). At the heart of APN practice is preventive care, and APN-led chronic care clinics developed to better manage chronic illness and prevent hospital readmissions are a current and imminent trend. The CNS is skilled in symptom management and has commonly acquired program management skills within the foundation of education and practice. This affords the CNS the proficiency necessary to ensure positive outcomes related to the chronic care process or clinic. As a DNP graduate, the CNS possesses additional expertise in areas such as policy and economics, which undoubtedly improves the prospect for the success of such ventures.

Studies have shown that those elders who received care from gerontological CNSs had fewer readmissions and fewer rehospitalization days (NACNS, 2009a). A study demonstrated a decrease in costs and complications when CNSs used evidence-based guidelines to reduce pain and to reduce the incidence of pulmonary complications in the intensive care unit setting (NACNS, 2009a). Several studies laud the success of the CNS as a practitioner who currently addresses healthcare needs and who will be an indispensable leader in healthcare reform in the future.

According to Hathaway, Jacob, Stegbauer, Thompson, and Graff (2006), "Graduates of DNP programs are already practicing upmarket and making important contributions. Their coursework and practical experiences acquired through doctoral study help prepare them for this phase of practice. For example, the study of policy and economics enables DNP graduates to knowledgeably and effectively represent the interests of nursing before regulatory agencies and legislative bodies. Epidemiology and advanced evidence-based practice courses help position DNP graduates for leadership in the burgeoning quality improvement movement" (p. 494). The CNS is currently knowledgeable in many of these matters, and the additional DNP degree will reinforce and strengthen those skills.

The CNS will continue to have extensive involvement in many healthcare settings. "The CNS is uniquely prepared to be the transprofessional collaborator, change agent, evidence-based practice integrator, and patient/client outcomes driver who will ensure safety and quality outcomes for patients now and into the future" (Goudreau et al., 2007, p. 319).

Nurse Practitioner

Gwendolyn Short

Transforming health care delivery recognizes the critical need for clinicians to design, evaluate, and continuously improve the context within which care is delivered. . . . Nurses prepared at the doctoral level with a blend of clinical, organizational, economic and leadership skills are most likely to be able to critique nursing and other clinical scientific findings and design programs of care delivery that are locally acceptable, economically feasible, and which significantly impact health care outcomes. (AACN, 2004, p. 3)

These words in the AACN's 2004 position paper on the practice doctorate in nursing describe the need and rationale for, and the timeliness of, the creation and development of the DNP degree. Included in the AACN position paper is the recommendation that by 2015, the DNP become the terminal degree for nursing practice.

From its inception, demand for the DNP has been strong. The first DNP program began at the University of Kentucky in the fall of 2001 with a cohort of 13 students. Several other schools had similar programs or were in the process of developing them, including the University of Tennessee and Columbia University (AACN, 2004). Interest quickly proliferated around the country, and within 8 years, 91 schools of nursing were accepting students into their newly developed DNP programs, and another 50 schools were planning such a program (AACN, 2009). By October 2014, over 250 schools were admitting students into their DNP programs, with accelerating movement toward offering the BSN to DNP option only, and discontinuation of the master's-level APRN program (Auerbach et al., 2014).

The AACN commissioned RAND Health to conduct a study to investigate and evaluate the progress toward implementation of the DNP as the terminal degree for nursing practice (Auerbach et al., 2014). As of April 2014, nearly half of nursing schools offering any graduate level nursing education offered a DNP program. Student demand for the master's-to-DNP degree continues to be robust, while that for the BSN-to-DNP is more variable (Auerbach et al., 2014).

Institute of Medicine Recommendations

Economics, technology, and politics have all affected and challenged the evolution of nursing education and practice. Important factors surrounding the development of the DNP are those that affect society at large: the rising costs of health care, the increasing complexity of disease care and healthcare delivery, the decline in the number of medical doctors entering primary care, and the integration of technology into patient care. The IOM's groundbreaking 1999 report, *To Err Is Human: Building a Safer Health System*, argued for the need to improve patient safety as well as the overall quality of healthcare organizations and systems (IOM, 1999). Subsequent work by the IOM (2001, 2003a, 2003b) provided additional direction on how to make these improvements and addressed the roles of specific groups of healthcare workers, including nurses. The IOM (2003a) proposed development of core competencies for all health professionals in the 21st century. These competencies will allow the health professional to provide patient-centered care, work in interdisciplinary teams, employ evidence-based practice, apply quality improvement, and utilize informatics.

The IOM competencies provide a supportive framework and share some common themes with the eight essentials of doctoral education for advanced nursing practice as developed and proposed by the AACN (2006). Both emphasize the goal of providing evidence-based, patient-centered health care to populations within systems of care that support collaboration between the different health disciplines.

More recently, the IOM, in its article *The Future of Nursing: Leading Change, Advancing Health* (2010), issued a set of recommendations to key governmental bodies (Congress, state legislatures, CMS, the Office of Personnel Management, the Federal Trade Commission, and the Antitrust Division of the Department of Justice) outlining strategies that would improve the effectiveness of the nursing workforce in this country (IOM, 2010). Included in these recommendations are those that advocate for nurses to be able to practice to the full extent of their education, participate as full partners with physicians and other healthcare professionals in providing patient care, and, specifically for APNs, recommendation for state legislatures to remove barriers to their scope of practice. Slow but steady progress is being made by NPs around the country as legislative changes grant full practice authority to APRNs. As of January 1, 2015, 18 states and Washington, D.C., had full practice and prescriptive authority, with six of these states requiring a postlicensure certification period of supervision or collaboration (Phillips, 2015).

Birth of a Movement

The first NPs began their education in 1965 at the University of Colorado as part of a demonstration project to determine whether nurses, working in an expanded role, could provide well-child care in community-based settings (Komnenich, 2005). Development of this program was the result of a collaborative effort by Loretta Ford, pioneer of the NP movement, and pediatrician Henry K. Silver (**Figure 8-1**) in direct response to an existing physician shortage and to the recognition among nursing leaders of a need to prepare graduate nurses for clinical specialization (Komnenich, 2005). The role of the graduate NP was fully grounded in nursing, with a focus on well-child care, health promotion, and disease prevention, preparing the NP to "assess autonomously, innovate, and work collaboratively with families and physicians" (p. 29) to provide health care. These graduates were certified in the area of pediatrics and assumed the title of pediatric NP.

Nurses soon began to request educational preparation in the care of populations other than pediatrics, spawning the development of NPs who focused on other groups, including adults, the family, older adults, and women. NPs currently constitute by far the largest group of APNs—192,000 (American Association of Nurse Practitioners [AANP], 2015b).

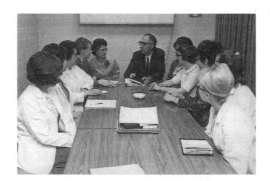

Figure 8-1 Early NP students meeting to discuss cases in the clinic and in the field. Photo taken in 1967. Seated left to right are: Audrey Dalen Clinton, Heather Walters Hull, Maddie Nichols, Susan Stearly (the first PNP graduate), Dr. Loretta Ford, Dr. Henry Silver, Mary Alexander Murphy, Jane Corwin Reeves, Rose Marie Egli, Nancy Brown, Mary Alice Rode.
Courtesy of University of Colorado College of Nursing, Anschutz Medical Campus.

An estimated 14,000 new NPs completed their studies in the 2011–2012 school year, with 87% of those completing their studies within a primary care focus (AANP, 2015b).

Educational Requirements and Specialty Areas

Early NP graduates received certificates as proof of their successful program completion, awarded jointly by the ANA and the American Academy of Pediatrics. Schools of nursing soon began to offer master's degree programs, and by the early 1970s, these programs began to out-number those granting certificates (Bullough, 1995). By 1990, 90% of NP programs were either master's degree programs or post–master's degree programs (Pulcini & Wagner, 2001).

A significant driving force for the development of the DNP is the amount of education required to earn a master's in an NP program, which has increased over the years to 45–50 semester credits. The average number of credit hours required to earn a master's degree in almost any other specialty is 30 semester credits (Chase & Pruitt, 2006). Even at the level of 45–50 credits, many leaders in NP education have voiced their concern that increased complexity in the healthcare environment continues to drive the need for additional content in the educational curricula for NPs.

Areas of focus within the master's program determine the type of specialty area the graduate will enter, the most common being family, adult, pediatrics, gerontology, psychiatry, women's health, and acute care. The newly graduated student then takes a certification exam within the specialty area, administered by an accredited certification body, and on passing this exam can become eligible for state licensure.

Core Competencies

The National Organization of Nurse Practitioner Faculties (NONPF) has developed and published a set of nine core competencies that reflect skills that doctorally prepared NPs are expected to learn and master by the completion of their DNP program of studies (NONPF, 2011). These core competencies build on and refine earlier versions of educational competencies for the master's-prepared NP and the DNP NP, and they are informed by and consistent with recommendations of the IOM's report, *The Future of Nursing* (IOM, 2010). As clinical practitioners in an increasingly complex healthcare environment, graduates of a DNP program will be expected to obtain expertise and increased knowledge in the following nine core areas: scientific foundation of advanced practice nursing; leadership; quality of clinical practice; practice inquiry; technology and information literacy; policy; healthcare delivery systems; ethics; and independent practice.

Certification, Licensure, and Credentialing

Certification, licensure, and credentialing constitute the often-complicated regulatory process that governs nursing, with the goal of maintaining standards of practice to protect the public and patients.

Certification is the process used by national professional nursing organizations to recognize advanced practice (ANA, 2010). Certification requires graduation from an accredited program and successful completion of a certification examination recognized nationally by the advanced practice specialty's professional organization (ANA, 2010). A total of 47 of the 50 states and Washington, D.C., require some type of certification for APN practice (Phillips, 2015). Certification of the NP can occur following graduation from either the master's program or the DNP program. As schools adopt the DNP and drop their master's-level curricula, completion of the DNP will be required prior to certification. Some schools, however, are choosing to continue a master's-level program of study while adding the DNP; for students in these programs, certification would continue to occur following completion of the master's course of study.

Licensure is the process whereby a state agency grants authority to an individual to practice as an NP. For NPs, licensing is granted following completion of an accredited educational program and passing of a national exam. The NP is first licensed as a registered nurse and in many states must then obtain an additional license to practice as an NP (ANA, 2010; Hanson, 2009).

Credentialing is an additional step, required by a state regulatory agency or local institution, to ensure that an individual can provide all the documentation necessary to practice in a professional capacity, with a given title. The credentialing process for NPs not only assures the public that the individual meets professional practice standards (Hanson, 2009) but also is required before the NP can be reimbursed for services rendered. Certification and licensure are just two components of the credentialing process.

Accreditation

There is no uniform model of regulation of NPs across states, and currently each state independently determines the NP's scope of practice, recognized roles, criteria for entry into advanced practice, and certification examinations accepted for entry-level competence assessment. This lack of standardization has restricted the mobility of NPs and has created a barrier to health care for patients (APRN Joint Dialogue Group, 2008). However, this is gradually changing. In an attempt to help standardize the regulatory process, representatives from a number of nursing organizations organized a working group to develop a plan for the licensure, accreditation, certification, and education of APNs. The outcome of this process—the Consensus Model for APRN Regulation, or the APRN Regulatory Model—addresses the licensure, accreditation, certification, and education (often referred to as LACE) of the four categories of APRNs: nurse anesthetists, nurse-midwives, CNSs, and NPs. Recommendations are included to clarify and improve the regulatory processes for each group, with an anticipated target date of 2015 for full implementation of the model (APRN Joint Dialogue Group, 2008). As of January 2015, much progress has been made toward implementation of the Consensus Model, but full implementation remains. According to Lisa Summers, senior policy fellow with the ANA, the Consensus Model was designed to guide implementation of the four components of LACE so that they all work together to provide support for APRN practice (L. Summers, personal communication, January 15, 2015). The model continues to be reassessed and revised according to the changes that have occurred.

The National Council of State Boards of Nursing (NCSBN) Model Nursing Practice Act and Model Nursing Administrative Rules (NCSBN, 2009) describe and clarify the relationship between licensure, accreditation, certification, and education of the NP (Article XVIII, Chapter 18) and are consistent with the Consensus Model. A further endorsement of the model is made by the IOM in *The Future of Nursing: Leading Change, Advancing Health* (2010); one of its recommendations is to limit federal funding for nursing education programs to only those programs in states that have adopted the NCSBN Model Nursing Practice Act and Model Nursing Administrative Rules.

Scope of Practice

Scope of practice describes the limits and boundaries of those practice activities within which nurses in the various advanced practice nursing specialties may legally practice (Hanson, 2009). Each advanced practice nursing specialty has its own scope of practice, based on its professional purpose and educational foundation. Furthermore, scope of practice differs from state to state and is based on state law described in the nurse practice acts and rules and regulations for APNs (Hanson, 2009; Phillips, 2015).

NPs have traditionally focused on health and wellness in a community-based primary care setting, their practice characterized by autonomy in clinical decision making, systematic collection of data through history taking, appropriate diagnosing and treatment, illness and injury prevention, patient advocacy, health counseling, and patient education (ANA, 2010; Komnenich, 2005). According to the AANP (2015c), NPs are "licensed independent practitioners who practice in ambulatory, acute, and long term care as primary and/or specialty care providers. They provide nursing and medical services to individuals, families, and groups."

The scope of practice for NPs has changed over time in response to the demands of the healthcare system and the natural evolution of the nursing profession. Scope of practice for NPs—and all APNs—is an area of NP practice debated in many state legislatures. Through legislation, NPs strive to ensure an environment in which they can practice to the limit of their skills, whereas others (frequently physicians) attempt to limit and place restraints on their practice activities (Safriet, 2002).

As cost containment strategies become an even greater focus nationally, with special emphasis on limiting the rising burden of healthcare costs, influential healthcare experts have proposed inventive ways of reeling in costs that may impact legislative restrictions on healthcare providers. One example of this is editor Susan Denzler's discussion in a September 2011 *Health Affairs* editorial of a telehealth program in the Northwest that showed significant Medicare savings for a group of chronically ill patients. She asked the question about the political viability of a federal law that allows major provider systems to override state medical licensure laws to implement intervention regionally or nationally (Denzler, 2011). Such a proposal would have lasting impact not just on medical licensure but also on that for the NP.

The DNP is not intended to increase the NP's level of clinical expertise, but rather to increase the NP's organizational, economic, and leadership skills (Chism, 2009). Although the master's degree has proved to be adequate preparation for a practitioner to function in an advanced nursing capacity, the healthcare environment is increasing in its complexity, requiring additional skills on the part of healthcare workers to improve the delivery of healthcare services. The DNP offers additional preparation to enable nurses to improve these services, especially in the areas of organizational leadership, project development and implementation, and quality improvement, all within the context of providing population-based health care. The DNP-prepared NP should be poised to assume a substantial role in an era of healthcare reform.

Role of the DNP Nurse Practitioner

The NP has much to add to the national discussion of healthcare delivery and reform and may very well become a key component of solutions to the challenges of improving and sustaining an effective and efficient health delivery system. The NP who has obtained a DNP, with its additional focus on providing health care within complex systems, will have an even greater impact on the improvement of patient care delivery and patient outcomes. Indeed, the first three essentials of doctoral education for advanced nursing practice specifically deal with systems improvement based on scientific evidence:

1. Scientific underpinnings for practice
2. Organizational and systems leadership for quality improvement and systems thinking
3. Clinical scholarship and analytical methods for evidence-based practice (AACN, 2006)

The DNP is a degree, not a role (AACN, 2004). The role of the APN with the DNP degree will continue to reflect the specialty practice of the APN as nurse anesthetist, nurse-midwife, CNS, or NP. The DNP-prepared NP will continue to provide health care through assessment, diagnosis, and treatment of the complex responses of individuals, families, or communities to actual or potential health problems, prevention of illness and injury, maintenance of wellness, and provision of comfort (ANA, 2010).

NPs have ample opportunity to provide care to newly insured patients under the Affordable Care Act. The bill language is mostly provider neutral, recognizes NPs as primary care providers and leaders in medical home care, and includes nondiscrimination language that covers NPs (AANP, 2015a). With fewer physicians entering primary care and increasing numbers of NPs graduating from master's and doctoral programs, NPs are well positioned to provide care to the increasing number of Americans accessing health care. With additional education at the doctoral level, the NP will be better prepared to navigate, and to help his or her patients navigate, the increased complexity of the healthcare environment. DNP curricula focus on organizational leadership, project development and implementation, quality improvement, and the use of evidence-based health care through use of existing research. Addition of these skills to the NP's existing skill set of providing patient-centered care, patient advocacy, and service coordination will ensure an even more competent NP and improved patient outcomes.

Certified Registered Nurse Anesthetist

Garrett J. Peterson

History

The first professional group to provide anesthesia services to surgical patients in the United States were nurses (**Figure 8-2**). In the late 1800s, nurse anesthesia became the first recognized clinical nursing specialty (Bankert, 1989). Surgeons were frustrated over the morbidity and mortality rates of their surgical patients and felt that it was associated with the administration of anesthesia (Bankert, 1989).

The initial methods of anesthesia delivery to surgical patients were dangerous because they involved either a handkerchief soaked in chloroform or an ether-soaked sponge held over the patient's nose and mouth (Bankert, 1989). These techniques allowed for minimal air inhalation by the patient, leading to death by suffocation. Surgeons therefore viewed nurses as practitioners with the ability to provide undivided attention to patients during administration of anesthesia. This resulted in nurses emerging as pioneers in anesthesia administration, providing anesthesia for all surgical specialties.

First-Known Anesthetic Documentation by Nurses

Virginia S. Thatcher researched the history of nurse anesthetists and discovered that significant contributions to the profession of nurse

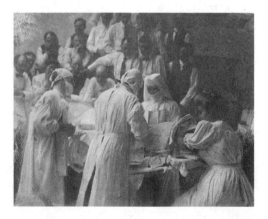

Figure 8-2 Nurse Anesthetist Alice McGaw Administers Anesthesia During Surgery at St. Mary's Hospital, Rochester, Minnesota, Circa 1910
American Association of Nurse Anesthetists Archives. Reproduced with permission.

anesthesia were made by the religious nursing sisters. The code of canon law required
detailed documentation of each individual
nun, which revealed that these nursing nuns
were involved in anesthesia administration
(Bankert, 1989). In 1877, a Catholic nun
named Sister Mary Bernard (**Figure 8-3**)
provided anesthesia administration at
St. Vincent's Hospital in Erie, Pennsylvania.
Her anesthetic documentation became the
first-known documentation of a nurse administering an anesthetic (Bankert, 1989).

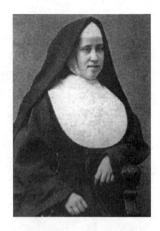

Figure 8-3 Sister Mary
Bernard
American Association of Nurse
Anesthetists Archives. Repro-
duced with permission.

In a textbook written by Isabel Adams
Hampton Robb in 1893, *Nursing: Its Principles
and Practice; For Hospital and Private Use*, an entire chapter was titled "The Administration
of Anesthetics." Robb explained that "a nurse
is often called upon in private practice to
administer an anaesthetic" (Robb, 1893, p. 331). The Third Order of the
Hospital Sisters of St. Francis established St. John's Hospital in Spring-
field, Illinois, which provided a place where the sisters were instructed in
the administration of anesthesia by surgeons. Additional hospitals were
built for employees of the Missouri Pacific Railroad, which were also
managed by the Sisters of St. Francis, allowing the sisters to serve as the
hospitals' anesthetists.

The Sisters of St. Francis traveled north from Illinois to Rochester,
Minnesota, establishing St. Mary's Hospital in 1889, which was operated
by Dr. William Worrell Mayo. Eventually, the
hospital would become the Mayo Clinic. The
hospital became a center point for interested
health professionals to learn the techniques
of the surgeons. The visitors were also privi-
leged to observe the superior administration
of anesthesia by nurse anesthetist Alice McGaw
(**Figure 8-4**) and the other nurse anesthetists
at St. Mary's Hospital. Dr. Mayo bestowed upon
McGaw the title of "mother of anesthesia" for
her many achievements, including mastery of
the "open-drop" technique of anesthesia using
ether and chloroform and her subsequent publication of her findings (Bankert, 1989).

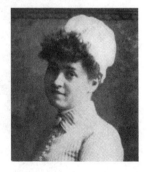

Figure 8-4 Alice McGaw
American Association of
Nurse Anesthetists Archives.
Reproduced with permission.

Hundreds of nurses and physicians from around the world traveled to St. Mary's Hospital to observe Alice McGaw and Dr. Mayo and learn their techniques of anesthesia administration. McGaw documented the anesthesia practice outcomes at St. Mary's and published them in several medical journals between 1899 and 1906. In 1906, McGaw published an article in the medical journal *Surgery, Gynecology and Obstetrics*, "A Review of Over 14,000 Surgical Anesthetics." She noted that during all those anesthetic procedures, not one death was attributed to the anesthetic, an outstanding record for the time.

Sharing the Skill of Anesthesia Administration

Surgeon Dr. George Crile, known for his research in the treatment of surgical shock, followed the Mayo's model of training nurses in the administration of anesthesia. Dr. Crile chose a nurse, Agatha Cobourg Hodgins (**Figures 8-5** and **8-6**), to become his exclusive anesthetist. Dr. Crile taught Miss Hodgins extensively about anesthesia administration, using laboratory animals to become familiar with the symptoms of impending death and to learn how to recognize and treat these symptoms to prevent death. Dr. Crile reported at the Southern Surgical and Gynecological Association that Miss Hodgins had administered thousands of anesthetics without an anesthetic death.

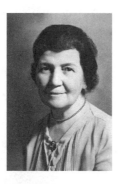

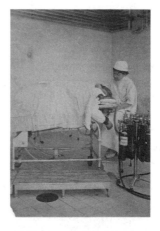

Figure 8-5 Agatha Hodgins
American Association of Nurse Anesthetists Archives. Reproduced with permission.

Figure 8-6 Agatha Hodgins Administers Anesthesia to a Patient, Circa 1914
American Association of Nurse Anesthetists Archives. Reproduced with permission.

Dr. Crile and Agatha Hodgins traveled together to France in 1914 and became instrumental in the creation of hospitals that provided care for the sick and wounded soldiers. It was during this visit that Hodgins had the opportunity to teach nurses and physicians the art of anesthesia administration.

Nurse Anesthetists in World War I and Beyond

Nurse anesthetists have been the primary anesthesia providers to the U.S. military forces since World War I and in some instances the only anesthesia providers. During World War I, hospital administrator Gustaf W. Olson urged that Sophie Gran Winton, a graduate nurse from Swedish Hospital in Minneapolis, Minnesota, be trained as a nurse anesthetist. After administration of more than 10,000 cases without a fatality, she joined the Army Nursing Corps in 1918 and traveled to Chateau-Thierry, France, to serve in Mobile Hospital No. 1. She received the French Croix de Guerre medal, along with six overseas service bars and honors, for her anesthesia service (Bankert, 1989).

"Nurse anesthetists have been held as prisoners of war, suffered combat wounds during wartime service, and have lost their lives serving their country" (American Association of Nurse Anesthetists [AANA], 2009a). The U.S. and foreign governments have recognized the efforts put forth by nurse anesthetists in caring for wounded military men and women and have honored them for their outstanding service (AANA, 2009a). The involvement of certified registered nurse anesthetists (CRNAs) in anesthesia administration during times of war increased the demand for CRNAs, resulting in an increased number of nurse anesthesia educational programs.

American Association of Nurse Anesthetists

In 1931, nurse anesthetist Agatha Hodgins became the founder of the AANA, the first professional organization for nurse anesthetists. It currently represents more than 40,000 CRNAs and student registered nurse anesthetists nationwide. "The AANA promulgates education, and practice standards and guidelines and affords consultation to both private and governmental entities regarding nurse anesthetists and their practice" (AANA, 2009a).

Nurse Anesthesia Education Programs

In 1909, nurse anesthetist Agnes McGee (**Figure 8-7**) established the first-known school of nurse anesthesia at St. Vincent's Hospital in

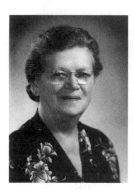

Figure 8-7 Agnes McGee
American Association of Nurse Anesthetists Archives. Reproduced with permission.

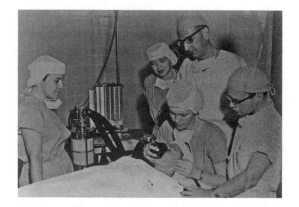

Figure 8-8 Nurse Anesthesia Students Learning How to Administer Inhalation Anesthesia at Easton Hospital, Circa 1964
American Association of Nurse Anesthetists Archives. Reproduced with permission.

Portland, Oregon. The curriculum was 6 months long and included didactic instruction in anatomy and physiology, pharmacology, and the administration of the common anesthetic agents. Following the success of Agnes McGee's program, approximately 19 additional nurse anesthesia schools were opened between 1912 and 1920. All these programs consisted of postgraduate training for nurses in the specialty of anesthesia delivery. A few of these programs included the Mayo Clinic, Johns Hopkins Hospital, Barnes Hospital, New York Post-Graduate Hospital, Presbyterian Hospital in Chicago, Charity Hospital in New Orleans, and Grace Hospital in Detroit.

Currently in the United States, 111 nurse anesthesia educational programs exist, all affiliated with or operated by academic institutions.

Each program awards a degree of either master's or doctorate level, depending on the institution. The programs range from 24 to 36 months in length, determined by the academic requirements of the individual institution. The total number of nurses enrolled in the current nurse anesthesia programs throughout the United States is more than 4,200 graduate students. These graduate nurse anesthesia programs provide the scientific underpinnings of anesthesia practice, including an average of 1,694 hours of clinical anesthesia administration to prepare highly competent nurse anesthesia graduates (**Figure 8-8**).

The future of nurse anesthesia education will require educational institutions to award only a clinical doctorate degree to those seeking a nurse anesthesia education. The AACN introduced the DNP in 2004 and published this statement regarding the DNP: "In many institutions, advanced practice registered nurses (APRNs), including Nurse Practitioners, Clinical Nurse Specialists, Certified Nurse Midwives, and Certified Nurse Anesthetists, are prepared in master's-degree programs that often carry a credit load equivalent to doctoral degrees in the other health professions" (AACN, 2006). The AACN's position statement calls for educating all APRNs and nurses through doctoral education. The organization's decision to move the level of preparation for advanced practice nursing from the master's degree to the doctoral level is suggested to be in place by 2015.

The DNP is a natural progression in CRNA education, which began with the 6-month course at St. Vincent's Hospital in Portland, Oregon; moved to the certificate level and then the bachelor's level; and proceeded to all programs being required to award a master's degree. The DNP continues this advancement in CRNA education. CRNA education is already a two- to three-year postbaccalaureate program. At the completion of law school, a juris doctor is awarded as a recognition of the advanced level of education. The DNP will recognize the advanced level of education involved in CRNA training.

What does the DNP do for nurse anesthetists? The DNP will recognize the continuing advancement of the quality and depth of CRNA education. The DNP recognizes the tremendous responsibility of the CRNA, who literally makes life-and-death decisions and takes lifesaving measures with every anesthetic administered. Many early anesthesia programs were considered apprenticeships. Modern CRNA training programs require extensive didactic instruction, clinical training, and research. This level of academic progress will now result in a DNP. This recognition gives additional credibility to a time-honored advancing profession.

The educational requirements for nurse anesthetists have substantially evolved throughout the 20th century. During most of the 1980s and 1990s, the AANA and the Council on Accreditation evaluated whether there was a need for nurse anesthesia education to move to the practice-oriented doctoral level. After the 2004 release of the AACN's *Position Statement on the Practice Doctorate in Nursing*, the 2005 AANA president, Brian Thorson, appointed a task force (the Doctoral Task Force [DTF]) to develop options related to the doctoral preparation of nurse anesthetists. The DTF presented its final report to the AANA board of directors in April 2007. In June 2007, the AANA board of directors unanimously adopted the position statement in support of the requirement of doctoral education for entry into nurse anesthesia practice by 2025.

Accreditation of Educational Programs: Council on Accreditation

In 1952, the AANA created an accreditation body for nurse anesthesia educational programs in the United States. In 1975, a major revision to the accreditation criteria by the U.S. Office of Education triggered the transfer of the accreditation body from the AANA to a self-governing multidisciplinary body under the AANA's business structure. The newly formed accreditation body became the Council on Accreditation of Nurse Anesthesia Educational Programs/Schools (COA). The COA sets the standards and policies that must be followed by all nurse anesthesia educational programs located in institutions offering a postmaster's certificate or a master's- or doctoral-level nurse anesthesia degree. The standards address administrative policies and procedures, institutional support, curriculum and instruction, faculty, evaluation, and ethics. Each year, the council reviews the standards and presents revisions if warranted (AANA, 2009b).

The council consists of a 12-member assembly who represent the following groups: nurse anesthesia educators and practitioners, nurse anesthesia students, healthcare administrators, university representatives, and the public. The goal of accreditation is to advance the quality of nurse anesthesia education and provide competent practitioners to healthcare consumers and employers (AANA, 2009b).

The U.S. Department of Education and the Council for Higher Education Accreditation recognize the COA as an accrediting agency for the nurse anesthesia profession. Nurse anesthesia students must graduate from an accredited nurse anesthesia program to become eligible to sit for the national certification exam.

Accreditation of nurse anesthesia programs occurs for established as well as new programs desiring accreditation. For a nurse anesthesia program to be accredited, it must be in compliance with each of the standards and policies set forth by the COA. Established programs are required to submit a self-evaluation of their program and welcome a review from the COA's team of reviewers. A summary of the visit is presented to the council for a decision as to the permission of continued accreditation and the time frame of the award, which can be up to 10 years. Possible accreditation actions are as follows (AANA, 2009b):

- *Accreditation:* The program has successfully completed the accreditation process.
- *Probation:* The program has deficiencies that jeopardize the quality of nurse anesthesia education.

- *Revocation:* The program is noncompliant with the standards set forth by the council, or there is evidence of a decrease in quality of the educational program.

Academic institutions seeking consideration for accreditation of a new nurse anesthesia program are required to submit a capability study and welcome an on-site evaluation. If the council deems that the study and on-site evaluation have met the standards, accreditation will be awarded (AANA, 2009b). Each year, the COA publishes a list of current and newly added anesthesia programs to inform the public, other agencies, and prospective students.

Academic Curriculum Requirements

The COA has set forth curriculum requirements for the education of nurse anesthetists. The minimum requirements of a nurse anesthesia program provide the student with the clinical, scientific, and professional foundations to build a safe and sound clinical practice (**Table 8-1**).

Nurse anesthesia students spend many hours gaining clinical experience while being supervised by a nurse anesthetist, allowing them to learn and master the different anesthesia techniques. This intense clinical experience allows the student to apply the knowledge learned in the classroom directly to surgical patients. A 1998 survey of nurse anesthesia

Table 8-1 Coursework and Minimal Contact Hours Required by the Council on Accreditation of Nurse Anesthesia Educational Programs

Coursework	Minimal Contact Hours
Pharmacology of anesthetic agents and adjuvant drugs, including concepts in chemistry and biochemistry	105
Anatomy, physiology, and pathophysiology	135
Professional aspects of nurse anesthesia practice	45
Basic and advanced principles of anesthesia practice, including physics, equipment, technology, and pain management	105
Research	30
Clinical correlation conferences	45

Modified from American Association of Nurse Anesthetists. (2009). Qualifications and capabilities of the registered nurse anesthetist. Retrieved from http://www.aana.com /ceandeducation/becomeacrna/Pages/default.aspx. Modified with permission.

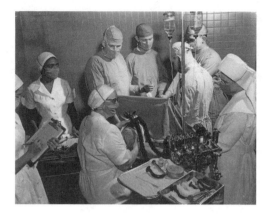

Figure 8-9 Nurse Anesthesia Students Administering Anesthesia at St. Mary of Nazareth Hospital, Date Unknown
American Association of Nurse Anesthetists Archives. Reproduced with permission.

program directors revealed that the nurse anesthesia programs provide an average of 1,595 hours of experience in the clinical area (AANA, 2009c). Nurse anesthesia students are given the opportunity to gain experience with anesthesia administration with patients of all ages in need of medical, surgical, pediatric, dental, and obstetrical surgeries and procedures (**Figure 8-9**).

Certification and Recertification of Nurse Anesthetists

The National Board of Certification and Recertification of Nurse Anesthetists (NBCRNA) is the non-profit corporation that provides the American public assurances that all nurse anesthetists meet objective and predetermined qualifications for providing anesthesia care that are determined by valid and scientifically sound measurements. This voluntary certification is a marker of quality in maintaining the professional standards of anesthesia care. The primary purpose of the NBCRNA is to "seek to ensure that nurse anesthetists have the necessary knowledge and skills to practice safely and effectively. In doing so, it also protects the value of the CRNA credential" (NBCRNA, 2015).

Nurse anesthesia is a leader in certification and recertification. The initial certification program for graduates of nurse anesthesia programs began in 1945. This certification process was administered through the American Association of Nurse Anesthetists (AANA) for 30 years. In 1975, an independent council was formed to make the clear distinction between the interests of the professional advocacy group, the AANA, and the primary role of the Council, which is to protect the public. The Council on Accreditation of Nurse Anesthetists (CCNA) assumed the primary role of administering the National Certification Examination (NCE). It soon became evident that the public also wanted assurances of continued professional development and excellence. In 1976, the membership of the AANA approved a mandatory recertification process that was implemented in 1978 along with establishment of the Council on Recertification (COR). These two Councils functioned independently but had similar goals of protecting the public and the integrity of the CRNA credential. In 2007, the two councils merged, incorporated, and became truly independent of the AANA. The body is now known as the National Board on Certification and Recertification of Nurse Anesthetists (NBCRNA).

The NBCRNA itself is accredited through the National Commission for Certifying Agencies (NCCA), a private non-profit organization. NBCRNA and the Councils that preceded it have been credentialed by the NCCA continuously since 1980 (NBCRNA, 2015). In addition, the NBCRNA programs are accredited by the Accreditation Board for Specialty Nursing Certification (ABSNC). NBCRNA and its predecessors were one of the first national specialty nursing credentialing boards to receive this accreditation (NBCRNA, 2015).

The NBCRNA continues to lead the way in recertification with the introduction of the Continuous Professional Certification Program (CPC) to be implemented over the next eight to ten years. The CPC includes core modules that cover basic anesthesia knowledge. Topics include physiology and pathophysiology, applied clinical pharmacology, airway management, and anesthesia equipment and technology. Knowledge of these topics will be assessed with a pass/fail grade. In addition, each candidate will need some assessed continuing educational units and some that are not assessed but include professional development activities that might include "activities that enhance knowledge of anesthesia practice, support patient safety, or foster an understanding of the healthcare environment" (NBCRNA 2015). As we move forward, the public demand for quality markers will increase the rigor and types of continuous professional certification activities that support the practice of nurse anesthesia and protect the public.

Scope and Standards of Practice for Nurse Anesthetists

In 1974, the AANA created a set of standards to guide the practice of nurse anesthetists according to their amount of experience, state regulations, and the policy at the employed institution. The CRNA's scope of practice provides the responsibilities that must be maintained during the practice of anesthesia performed in collaboration with other healthcare providers.

Anesthesia care delivered by CRNAs consists of four general categories:

- Preanesthetic preparation and evaluation
- Anesthesia induction, maintenance, and emergence
- Postanesthesia care
- Perianesthetic and clinical support function

A nurse earning certification as a nurse anesthetist holds the qualifications to provide the functions of the CRNA's scope of practice shown in **Table 8-2**.

Standards for Nurse Anesthesia Practice

The standards for nurse anesthesia practice are designed to guide the practice of a nurse anesthetist. The intention of the standards is to:

1. Assist the profession in evaluating the quality of care provided by its practitioners.
2. Provide a common base for practitioners to use in their development of a quality practice.
3. Assist the public in understanding what to expect from the practitioner.
4. Support and preserve the basic rights of the patient. (AANA, 2013, p. 3)

Each standard applies to all anesthetizing locations. **Table 8-3** outlines the standards that are intended to encourage the nurse anesthetist to provide the highest quality of patient care.

Clinical Practice Outside the Operating Room

A majority of nurse anesthetists provide anesthesia in the operating room, but there is also opportunity for CRNAs to administer anesthesia outside the operating room. Anesthesia services have expanded to areas such as cardiac catheterization labs, magnetic resonance imaging units, and lithotripsy suites. Anesthetists are also contacted by referrals outside the anesthesia department to provide consultation for respiratory concerns, including intubation, to participate in emergency situations such as cardiopulmonary resuscitation, and to manage blood, fluid, electrolyte, and acid–base balance.

CRNAs also perform administrative activities for the department of anesthesia. The overall function of an anesthesia department depends on services provided by the directors and managers of the anesthesia division to ensure the efficiency and quality of the provided anesthesia

Table 8-2 Scope of Practice for Certified Registered Nurse Anesthetists

1. Performing and documenting a preanesthetic assessment and evaluation of the patient, including requesting consultations and diagnostic studies; selecting, obtaining, ordering, or administering preanesthetic medications and fluids; and obtaining informed consent for anesthesia

2. Developing and implementing an anesthetic plan

3. Selecting and initiating the planned anesthetic technique, which may include general, regional, and local anesthesia and intravenous sedation

4. Selecting, obtaining, or administering the anesthetics, adjuvant drugs, accessory drugs, and fluids necessary to manage the anesthetic, to maintain the patient's physiologic homeostasis, and to correct abnormal responses to the anesthesia or surgery

5. Selecting, applying, or inserting appropriate noninvasive and invasive monitoring modalities for collecting and interpreting patient physiological data

6. Managing a patient's airway and pulmonary status using endotracheal intubation, mechanical ventilation, pharmacological support, respiratory therapy, or extubation

7. Managing emergence and recovery from anesthesia by selecting, obtaining, ordering, or administering medications, fluids, or ventilatory support in order to maintain homeostasis, to provide relief from pain and anesthesia side effects, or to prevent or manage complications

8. Releasing or discharging patients from a postanesthesia care area and providing postanesthesia follow-up evaluation and care related to anesthesia side effects or complications

9. Ordering, initiating, or modifying pain relief therapy through the utilization of drugs, regional anesthetic techniques, or other accepted pain relief modalities, including labor epidural analgesia

10. Responding to emergency situations by providing airway management, administration of emergency fluids or drugs, or using basic or advanced cardiac life support techniques

11. Additional nurse anesthesia responsibilities that are within the expertise of the individual CRNA, including administrative and management, quality assessment, education, research, committee assignments, and interdepartmental liaison efforts

American Association of Nurse Anesthetists. Modified with permission.

services. Functions include, but are not limited to, continuing education, financial management, personnel and resource management, quality assurance, and risk management.

CRNA Scholarship

Nurse anesthetists participate on healthcare centers' committees and are involved as educators for both professional and nonprofessional staff. CRNAs serve on committees within their state and governmental

Table 8-3 Standards for Nurse Anesthesia Practice	
Standard I	Perform a thorough and complete preanesthesia assessment.
Standard II	Obtain informed consent for the planned anesthetic.
Standard III	Formulate a patient-specific plan for anesthesia care.
Standard IV	Implement and adjust the anesthesia care plan based on the patient's physiologic response.
Standard V	Monitor the patient's physiologic condition as appropriate for the type of anesthesia and specific patient needs.
	1. Monitor ventilation continuously.
	2. Monitor oxygenation continuously.
	3. Monitor cardiovascular status continuously.
	4. Monitor body temperature continuously.
	5. Monitor neuromuscular function and status.
	6. Monitor and assess the patient positioning.
Standard VI	Document pertinent information on the patient's medical record completely, accurately, and in a timely manner.
Standard VII	Transfer the responsibility for care of the patient to other qualified providers in a manner that ensures continuity of care and patient safety.
Standard VIII	Adhere to appropriate safety precautions, as established within the institution, to minimize the risks of fire, explosion, electrical shock, and equipment malfunction. Document on the patient's medical record that the anesthesia machine and equipment were checked.
Standard IX	Take precautions to minimize the risk of infarction to the patient, the CRNA, and other healthcare providers.
Standard X	Assess anesthesia care to ensure its quality and contribution to positive patient outcomes.
Standard XI	Respect and maintain the basic rights of patients.

Council on Certification of Nurse Anesthetists. Modified with permission.

agencies, including the state boards of nursing and the U.S. Food and Drug Administration. Nurse anesthetists are also directly involved in professional and standard-setting organizations such as the National Fire Protection Association and the American Society for Testing and Materials.

Research is a fundamental component of anesthetic administration. Nurse anesthetists have served in multiple roles related to research as early as the beginning of the 20th century. Nurse anesthetists' involvement in research has included roles as principal investigators, as holders of consultative and collaborator positions, and as users of the research findings. Nurse anesthesia programs include research as part of the standard curriculum, providing the graduate student with the basic skills necessary for conducting research. The AANA Foundation promotes nurse anesthetists' involvement with research, focusing on the quality of anesthesia care and outcome-based research. Funding for research by CRNAs and nurse anesthesia students has been provided by private and governmental grants and by the AANA Education and Research Foundation. Students and CRNAs are given the opportunity to present and disseminate their research findings at the AANA annual meetings.

Nurse anesthetists have been involved in authoring or contributing to anesthesia textbooks and clinical, educational, and research topics published in peer-reviewed journals. Some of these professional publications include the *AANA Journal, CRNA: The Clinical Forum for Nurse Anesthetists, Nurse Anesthesia, Anesthesiology, Anesthesia and Analgesia, Journal of the American Society of Regional Anesthesia, Journal of the American Medical Association, Nursing Research*, and *Hospitals and Nursing Forum*.

The needs of the healthcare environment are in constant change. The DNP degree will provide nurse anesthetists with an education that is comparable with other practice-focused professional degrees such as the doctor of pharmacy, the doctor of physical therapy, and the doctor of occupational therapy. Research conducted by Linda Aiken in 2003 revealed that in hospitals with higher proportions of nurses educated at the baccalaureate level or higher, surgical patients experienced lower mortality and failure-to-rescue rates. This shows a clear link between higher levels of nursing education and better patient outcomes. The DNP degree will prepare tomorrow's nurse anesthetists at the highest education level and will provide them with the capability to transform healthcare delivery by designing, evaluating, and continuously improving the framework within which care is delivered. Also, CRNAs educated within a doctoral framework will have the capability to influence local and national health care by demonstrating effective leadership and political advocacy.

Nurse-Midwife

Deborah Ringdahl
Melissa Saftner

Nurse-midwives represent a vital part of advanced practice nursing, with a long history of patient advocacy, leadership, service to underserved populations, development of new models of healthcare delivery, and commitment to the provision of high-quality health care for women and families. In many important ways, nurse-midwives have broken ground for all APNs, leading the way in APN outcome-based research, the development of educational programs, and access to healthcare systems through legislative reform. From the time nurse-midwifery was first introduced into this country in 1925 to the present, the midwifery profession has demonstrated many of the attributes that are now associated with the doctorally prepared NP. Awareness and understanding of a larger practice context is required for the midwifery profession to remain strong and viable. The formal integration of midwifery clinical practice skills with a DNP education will serve to further strengthen the midwifery profession and ultimately improve the health of women and families. This section provides an overview of midwifery practice, followed by a discussion of the role of the DNP-prepared midwife.

Nurse-Midwifery Practice

As an organized profession, nurse-midwives have worked hard to define who they are, maintain high standards of education and practice, and interact with other professional organizations. The professional documents of the American College of Nurse-Midwives (ACNM) define the standards of midwifery practice (ACNM, 2009a) and also serve to educate the public about the roles and responsibilities of the nurse-midwife. *Philosophy of the American College of Nurse-Midwives* affirms the entitlement of basic human rights in health care and the value of the midwifery model of health care, which includes supporting normalcy in women's life cycle events (ACNM, 2004). The majority of practicing midwives in this country are certified nurse-midwives (CNMs), individuals "educated in the two disciplines of nursing and midwifery, who possess evidence of certification according to the requirements of ACNM" (ACNM, 2011a). In 1994, the ACNM approved adding a nonnurse-midwifery option to its educational programs, resulting in the addition of the title certified midwife (CM), "an individual educated in the discipline of midwifery, who possesses evidence of certification according to the requirements of ACNM" (ACNM, 2011a). The decision to include nonnurses in ACNM-accredited education programs and the certification process was made to set uniform standards for midwifery education and practice, leading to the development of direct-entry educational programs. Not surprisingly, developing one midwifery standard for nurses and nonnurses has presented many challenges, including consumer awareness, institutional credentialing, legislative practice regulations, and policy development. Legal recognition of midwifery practice exists primarily through nursing boards, requiring licensure in nursing as a prerequisite to practice.

Midwives have made significant progress toward gaining legitimacy within the healthcare system even though their numbers are small (11,546 CNMs/CMs), and they have encountered legislative and institutional barriers to practice. Certified nurse-midwifery practice is legal in all 50 states, and CMs can practice in New Jersey, New York, Rhode Island, Delaware, and Missouri. Medicaid reimbursement for CNM/CM care is mandatory in all states, and in 2010, legislation was passed for nurse-midwives to receive 100% of the physician fee schedule under Medicare Part B. CNMs have prescription-writing authority in all 50 states, and CMs have prescription-writing authority in New York (ACNM, 2011b).

Many important professional issues affect access to clients and the financial viability of CNM/CM practice, among them direct access; liability insurance; reimbursement, including Medicare and Medicaid; antitrust laws; and midwifery admitting privileges. These issues require development of legislative and policy strategies. The ACNM has provided leadership by developing resources on the politics and business of midwifery practice, allocating more resources for legislative work, and forming Midwives-PAC (political action committee) in 2000.

Midwives work primarily in hospitals, and the number of women choosing midwives as their birth attendants continues to increase. In 2008, 11.1% of all vaginal births were attended by CNMs in the United States, which represents more than a doubling of the 1990 rate (Declercq, 2009). Of these CNM/CM-attended births, 96.1% occurred in hospitals, 2.1% occurred in freestanding birth centers, and 1.7% occurred in homes. More than 50% of CNMs/CMs list physician practices or hospitals/medical centers as their principal employers. Midwives also provide primary care: 86% of visits to CNMs/CMs are for primary, preventive care, including annual exams and reproductive health visits (ACNM, 2011b).

There are currently 39 accredited midwifery educational programs in the United States, mostly housed in nursing schools as graduate programs. Nine of these programs offer a DNP option, mostly after master's programs. The majority (82%) of CNMs have a master's degree, and 4.8% hold a doctoral degree (ACNM, 2011b). For the remainder of this section, the term *midwife* will be reserved for the CNM because CMs are not currently eligible for DNP educational programs.

History

Midwives have moved from serving as home birth attendants within their communities during the 1800s and 1900s to an organized group of healthcare professionals who now meet the primary healthcare needs of women in a variety of healthcare settings. These changes have been influenced by social trends and the shifting healthcare landscape. Understanding the history of midwifery in this country provides perspective on two of the recurring themes that accompany midwifery practice: recognition of midwifery as a legitimate profession and access by midwives to the healthcare system. It is particularly noteworthy that a vital connection was made between the practice of midwifery and the nursing profession when midwifery was formally introduced into this country. Although there is ongoing debate about whether midwifery practice requires a nursing background, it is clear that midwifery's connection to nursing has been instrumental in establishing professional legitimacy in midwifery practice (Burst, 2005).

The informal origins of midwifery practice in the United States can be traced to the immigrant midwives who arrived during the late 1800s and early 1900s and the African American midwives who provided care to women in the South. At the beginning of the 20th century, 50% of births occurred at home with a midwife (Dawley, 2003). During this same time period, studies revealed alarmingly high infant and maternal mortality rates, resulting in a chain of events that dramatically affected midwifery practice. Health officials were concerned that midwives did not have adequate education or training, and several strategies were developed to resolve this "midwife problem," including training public health nurses to provide maternity care (Varney, Kriebs, & Gegor, 2004). The Sheppard-Towner Act was passed in 1921 and funded through 1929, providing training of midwives by public health nurses. During this same time, medical schools started to include obstetrics in their curricula; obstetrics became a medical specialty in 1930, and birth began moving out of the home and into the hospital (Varney et al., 2004).

Mary Breckinridge introduced the nurse-midwifery model of care to the United States when she brought British-trained nurse-midwives to rural Kentucky in 1925. The Frontier Nursing Service (FNS) was a carefully crafted program that used nurse-midwives as birth attendants and provided a comprehensive scope of healthcare services; it yielded dramatic improvements in both maternal and infant mortality rates, which were lower than the national rates from 1931 to 1950 (Varney et al., 2004). These outcomes were particularly significant given that most births occurred in homes with primitive living conditions, and further advanced the credibility of nurse-midwives as competent healthcare providers.

The first educational nurse-midwife program opened in 1931, and by the end of the 1950s, there were seven nurse-midwifery educational programs nationwide. Practice opportunities remained limited until the 1970s, with the majority of nurse-midwifery practices providing care to low-income women who lived in underserved areas of the country. Many events occurred during the 1960s and 1970s that led to greater acceptance of the nurse-midwifery model of care and extended nurse-midwifery care into the middle-class population. Social movements promoting more autonomy for women, federally funded projects that included nurse-midwives, a 1971 joint statement between the nurse-midwife and obstetrician/gynecologist professions, the need for more birth attendants to provide care to the baby boomer generation, the inclusion of family planning and gynecologic care in clinical competencies, and the demonstration of the safety and efficacy of nurse-midwives all converged to create a more favorable climate for the proliferation of nurse-midwifery educational programs and clinical practice opportunities (Varney et al., 2004).

Midwifery history is rich with examples of leadership "in the areas of clinical excellence, educational strategies, business savvy, and policy development" (Ament, 2006, p. 328), contributing to increased access to the healthcare system. By the 1980s, nurse-midwives were practicing in a variety of settings, providing a wide range of services and providing care to all classes of women. Physicians became aware that nurse-midwives were now competing for their middle- and upper-class clients, and some efforts were made to restrict midwifery practice (Varney et al., 2004). Nonetheless, midwifery education and practice experienced more growth in the 1990s, in part as a response to managed care and the focus on providing high-quality and cost-effective care.

Professional Organization

The ACNM, incorporated in 1955, provides a foundation for the growth and development of nurse-midwifery education and practice. The mission of the ACNM is to "promote the health and well-being of women and infants within their families and communities through the development and support of the profession of midwifery as practiced by certified nurse-midwives (CNMs) and certified midwives (CMs)" (ACNM, 2003). The ACNM has developed position statements, political and legislative resources, and executive staff positions that reflect a strong commitment to professional involvement in local, state, and national politics. At the national level, the ACNM provides leadership through the board of directors, divisions, and committees that work to address clinical practice issues, health policy, and educational standards. The ACNM conducts research, administers and promotes continuing education programs, establishes clinical practice standards, and creates liaisons with state and federal agencies and members of Congress.

The International Confederation of Midwives (ICM) confers membership to ACNM members, promoting professional relationships with midwives throughout the world. The ACNM website (www.midwife.org) has become a particularly useful vehicle for keeping its membership up to date with current issues affecting nurse-midwifery practice.

Education and Certification

The education of midwives is central to professional credibility and viability. Midwifery education has undergone many changes since the first program was introduced in 1931. Requirement of a baccalaureate degree on entrance to or completion of the program was initiated in 1996, and in 2006, the ACNM issued a position statement requiring a graduate degree by 2010 for entry into midwifery practice (ACNM, 2009b). Although the ACNM supports a graduate degree, it does not require the DNP degree for entry into midwifery practice (ACNM, 2012). "At the present time, evidence points to the fact that current education requirements produce safe, knowledgeable, competent midwives. Because data are lacking regarding the potential impact of the proposed Doctor of Nursing Practice on the cost of education to both the institution and the student, on the applicant pool, and the health care system, the Directors of Midwifery Education (DOME) endorse a statement affirming support for multiple routes of midwifery education based on the ACNM Core Competencies, and does not endorse a mandatory requirement for the clinical doctorate for entry into practice" (Avery & Howe, 2007, p. 14).

The Accreditation Commission for Midwifery Education (ACME) has been the accrediting agency for nurse-midwifery education since 1988. All programs accredited by ACME provide curricula as defined by ACNM's *Core Competencies for Basic Midwifery Practice* (ACNM, 2008). *The Knowledge, Skills, and Behaviors Prerequisite to Midwifery Clinical Coursework*

(ACME, 2005) was developed for direct-entry (CM) midwifery programs to ensure that all graduates emerge with the foundational knowledge that nursing education provides for nurse-midwife graduates. Since 1996, all accredited educational programs have required affiliation with a university, college, or other institution of higher learning accredited by a U.S. Department of Education–recognized accrediting agency (ACNM, 2009d). The ACNM, ACME, and the American Midwifery Certification Board (AMCB) have endorsed the Consensus Model for APRN Regulation (APRN Consensus Work Group & National Council of State Boards of Nursing APRN Advisory Committee, 2008).

CNM and CM candidates must sit for the national certification exam (NCE), which was first offered in 1971 by the ACNM. The ACNM Certification Council became the certifying body in 1991, changing its name to the American Midwifery Certification Board in 2005. Since 1995, all candidates passing the NCE have received an 8-year time-limited certificate, with two options for renewal through the Certificate Maintenance Program. In 2011, the AMCB initiated time-limited certification for all CNMs in active practice.

Scope of Practice

Midwifery practice has changed over time, reflecting the need for expanding the scope of practice beyond pregnancy and childbirth. Midwifery practice now includes providing reproductive and primary health care to women from menarche to menopause. The ACNM's position statement *Definition of Midwifery Practice and Scope of Practice of Certified Nurse-Midwives and Certified Midwives* (2012b) outlines the parameters of clinical practice:

> *Midwifery as practiced by certified nurse-midwives (CNMs®) and certified midwives (CMs®) encompasses a full range of primary health care services for women from adolescence beyond menopause. These services include the independent provision of primary care, gynecologic and family planning services, preconception care, care during pregnancy, childbirth and the postpartum period, care of the normal newborn during the first 28 days of life, and treatment of male partners for sexually transmitted infections. Midwives provide initial and ongoing comprehensive assessment, diagnosis and treatment. They conduct physical examinations; prescribe medications including controlled substances and contraceptive*

> *methods; admit, manage and discharge patients; order and interpret laboratory and diagnostic tests and order the use of medical devices. Midwifery care also includes health promotion, disease prevention, and individualized wellness education and counseling. These services are provided in partnership with women and families in diverse settings such as ambulatory care clinics, private offices, community and public health systems, homes, hospitals and birth centers.*

Core Competencies for Basic Midwifery Practice (ACNM, 2008) provides the practice and educational template for CNMs and CMs and applies to all midwifery settings, including hospitals, ambulatory care settings, birth centers, and home. These competencies were first developed in 1978 to provide a set of uniform standards for clinical practice and nurse-midwifery education and have been revised five times, illustrating the evolving nature of midwifery practice. Some of the major points of revision have been delineation of the role of midwives in collaborative management; expansion of the components of midwifery care outside the maternity cycle; description of professional responsibilities; identification of the hallmarks of midwifery; inclusion of primary care; and addition of business competencies (Avery, 2005). The changes made to this document provide evidence of the professional growth of midwifery practice, the changing healthcare environment, and the need for expanding the scope of practice beyond maternity care and the development of nonclinical skills. The AACN's essentials of doctoral education for advanced nursing practice (AACN, 2006) and the NONPF's practice doctorate NP entry-level competencies (2006) are reflected in several of the nonclinical components of the core competencies, such as leadership, business, research, and policy development (**Table 8-4**).

Table 8-4 Congruency of ACNM Core Competencies for Basic Midwifery Practice with DNP Competencies

ACNM Core Competencies for Basic Midwifery Practice	Essentials of Doctoral Education for Advanced Nursing Practice: AACN	DNP Entry-Level Competencies: NONPF
Incorporation of scientific evidence into clinical practice	Scientific underpinnings for practice	Scientific foundation

Table 8-4 (*continued*)

Participation in evaluation, peer review, other activities that ensure and validate quality practice, understanding of bioethics related to women, newborns, families	Organizational and systems leadership for quality improvement and systems thinking	Quality, ethics
Ability to evaluate, apply, interpret, and collaborate in research	Clinical scholarship and analytical methods for evidence-based practice	Practice inquiry
Standards for Practice of Midwifery (VI): accessible and complete documentation	Information systems/ technology and patient care technology for the improvement and transformation of health care	Technology and information literacy
Support of legislation and policy initiatives that promote quality health care, knowledge of issues and trends in healthcare policy and systems	Healthcare policy for advocacy in health care	Policy
Development of leadership skills, collaboration with other members of the healthcare team	Interprofessional collaboration for improving patient and population health outcomes	Leadership
Health promotion, disease prevention, and health education, cultural competence, promotion of a public health perspective, care to vulnerable populations	Clinical prevention and population health for improving the nation's health	Health delivery system
Midwifery management process, fundamentals, primary care, childbearing family, knowledge of legal basis for practice, knowledge of licensure, clinical privileges, credentialing	Advanced nursing practice	Independent practice

Data from ACNM. (2008). *Core competencies for basic midwifery practice.* Retrieved from http://www.midwife.org/siteFiles/descriptive/Core_Competencies_6_07.pdf; ACNM. (2003). *Standards for the practice of midwifery.* Silver Spring, MD: ACNM; AACN. (2006). *The essentials of doctoral education for advanced nursing practice.* Washington, DC: AACN; NONPF. (2006). *Practice doctorate nurse practitioner entry-level competencies.* Retrieved from http://c.ymcdn.com/sites/www.nonpf.org/resource/resmgr/competencies/dnp%20np%20competenciesapril2006.pdf?hhSearchTerms=%22Practice+and+doctorate+and+nurse+and+practitioner+and+entry-level%22

Federal and state laws, institutional regulations, and practice guidelines also play a role in determining scope of practice. Federal and state laws affect scope of practice primarily through federal regulations and state regulatory boards, such as boards of medicine or nursing. Institutional regulations, typically hospital bylaws, can restrict scope of practice by preventing midwives from obtaining hospital or admitting privileges. "Practice guidelines define the legal basis for a clinician's practice, describe parameters or scope of practice, and describe situations in which a physician should be consulted" (Slager, 2004, p. 38). Supervisory language in practice guidelines is strongly discouraged because it implies a dependent relationship with the physician consultant rather than supporting independent clinical decision making within a defined scope of practice. It is generally recommended that practice guidelines not be overly proscriptive and leave room for clinical judgment and the experience level of the midwife. Practice guidelines are typically updated on a yearly basis to include new research and professional standards.

The DNP-Prepared Midwife

The DNP-prepared midwife learns knowledge and skills that further support autonomy, leadership, and the role of change agent in an increasingly complex healthcare system. Advancing knowledge of leadership, educational and change theories, health policy, economics, and epidemiology add depth and breadth to midwifery education and practice. As change agents, midwives need to develop skills that promote evidence-based practice, evaluation of clinical practice, integration of nursing theory into practice, and effective use of information systems to document outcomes. Educational programs leading to the master's degree for midwives include some of this content in their coursework, but the primary focus is the development of clinical competencies, leaving little time for in-depth study of less clinically based practice competencies.

Table 8-4 provides an overview of the congruency between the ACNM's *Core Competencies for Basic Midwifery Practice* (ACNM, 2008) and the DNP competencies developed by the AACN and the NONPF. Within the ACNM core competencies, the majority of the DNP competencies are found in the "Hallmarks of Midwifery" and "Professional Responsibilities" (ACNM, 2008). These ACNM core competencies are incorporated into all CNM and CM educational programs and must be present in the curriculum for programs to achieve accreditation. DNP course content that addresses healthcare economics, policy, evidence-based practice, leadership and change theories, and program evaluation will further develop these midwifery core competencies. "Although the focus of the practice doctorate is not on basic research, the potential exists for the development of much needed evaluation and systems research in the practice and business of midwifery" (Avery & Howe, 2007, p. 17).

Midwives have provided leadership in many healthcare arenas, from safeguarding normal pregnancy and childbirth to advocating for high-quality, affordable, and accessible health care for all women. DNP-prepared midwives should retain strong leadership in their primary area of expertise, namely, providing high-quality health care to women. Midwives have long advocated for the healthcare needs of all women by building alliances with other professional organizations, using public health and business strategies, creating new models of health care, developing international programs, and remaining committed to the normalcy of women's life cycle events. DNP-prepared midwives can further advance women's health by assuming leadership in the following areas: development of maternal–child health public policy; development of quality measures and data collection tools that promote maternal–child health; creation of a healthcare model that safeguards the normalcy of women's life cycle events and promotes cultural competency; development of standards for midwifery that promote safe motherhood; development of programs that teach healthcare business acumen; and active engagement in healthcare reform. These areas are discussed in more detail in the following sections.

Maternal–Child Health Public Policy

The roots of midwifery practice lie in providing care to disadvantaged and vulnerable women and children. Research on the socioeconomic component of health status has informed the public health perspective and provided a better understanding of how poverty directly and indirectly affects health. The Healthy People Initiative provides a framework for addressing health disparities, examining both healthcare access and healthcare delivery. The midwife's expert clinical skills and experience in working effectively with vulnerable populations and commitment to reducing health disparities provide a strong foundation for improving maternal–child health outcomes and achieving the public health goals outlined in this initiative (Jesse & Blue, 2004). The DNP-prepared midwife can further advance the public policy agenda for maternal–child health by integrating epidemiologic and evidence-based research into the development of community health programs and engaging in legislative work that informs public policy.

Quality Measures and Data Collection

Midwives have achieved recognition as healthcare providers who provide high-quality care. The first midwifery service in this country maintained careful records that demonstrated improved outcomes with nurse-midwifery care; a statistical analysis of the first 30 years of FNS practice (1925–1954) estimated that national adoption of their processes would prevent 60,000 perinatal deaths every year (Metropolitan Life Insurance Company, 1960). Since then, numerous studies have documented highly favorable outcomes in births attended by nurse-midwives (ACNM, 2005).

The value of accurate record keeping cannot be underestimated: midwifery statistics lead to both recognition of high standards of care and credibility within the healthcare system. Data collection should be integrated into every clinical practice, selecting quality measures that reflect the high standard of care that is provided. Intrapartal and antepartal data sets have been developed by the ACNM that provide a template for midwifery data collection. The ACNM recently initiated a benchmarking project aimed at collecting data from midwifery practices across the country, and 5 years of data on best practices have been collected to date. The DNP-prepared midwife has the knowledge and resources to further develop quality management skills, including development of clinically relevant data sets, consolidation and organization of data through information technology, and developing partnerships with other organizations invested in providing high-quality care.

Safeguarding the Normalcy of Women's Life Cycle Events

Midwives have maintained a philosophy of birth as normal and incorporated this model of health care into a variety of healthcare settings.

According to Barger (2005), "The midwifery model of care emanates from the belief that pregnancy, birth, and menopause are normal processes of life and that it is, therefore, part of the role of the midwife to help protect the normalcy of these events from a culture or society that might believe otherwise" (p. 88). Safeguarding the normalcy of birth is no small feat in the current climate of rising cesarean sections, representing 32.9% of all births in 2009 (Hamilton, Martin, & Ventura, 2010). The ACNM supports the normalcy of birth by using research to demonstrate the safety of out-of-hospital births, developing position statements supporting nonintervention in normal processes, and supporting evidence-based research as the gold standard in providing health care.

The DNP-prepared midwife can move this agenda further forward by maintaining currency with clinical research and educating consumers, healthcare providers, and policy makers about the risks associated with intervening unnecessarily in normal processes.

Cultural Competency

A long history of providing health care to women who are uninsured; immigrant; adolescent; and ethnically, racially, and socioeconomically diverse (Declercq et al., 2001) has given midwives many avenues for cultivating cultural competency. According to Varney et al. (2004), "Midwives must be at the forefront in the implementation of cultural competence training programs, which are now considered key interventions in reducing the health care disparities that disproportionately affect women of color" (p. 56). Although there is no specific DNP competency that addresses cultural competency (see Table 8-4), development of effective healthcare policy requires cultural understanding and research on health outcomes among different cultural groups. The DNP-prepared midwife has a more comprehensive understanding of health policy and epidemiologic trends, contributing to a wider application of cultural competency, including clinical practice, research, and policy development.

Midwifery Standards and Safe Motherhood

Midwives exist in all cultures and countries, and although educational backgrounds may differ, all midwives are part of the global community. Midwives carry the international torch for safe motherhood, playing a central role in "global efforts to make pregnancy and birth safe throughout the world and promote the health and well-being of girls and women wherever they reside" (Varney et al., 2004, p. 60). The ACNM has a long history of active involvement in the International Confederation of Midwives and developing international programs to support safe motherhood. The ACNM Division of Global Health has undertaken projects to support the education of traditional birth attendants (TBAs) and the development of *The Lifesaving Skills Manual for Midwives* (Varney et al., 2004). In 1997 the ACNM spearheaded the Safe Motherhood Initiative, leading to partnership with other professional organizations in developing priorities for improving maternity care in the United States. More recently, the ACNM formed the Ad Hoc Committee on Disaster Preparedness, providing leadership in managing the needs of mothers and infants during disasters (ACNM, 2009c; Al Gasseer, Dresden, Keeney, & Warren, 2004).

As a birth attendant, the midwife assumes a unique position among APNs in the care of women during labor and birth, demonstrating commitment and leadership in preserving the health of mothers and babies. The word *vivant*, or *let them live*, takes center stage on the ACNM seal, representing midwives' "unremitting dedication to safeguarding and promoting the health and wellbeing of family life, particularly the mother and infant" (Varney et al., 2004, p. 22). Evidence-based practice needs to be recognized as an international standard and applied to improving maternal and child outcomes in all countries (Miller, Sloan, Winikoff, Langer, & Fikree, 2003). In addition to improving maternal outcomes by providing excellent clinical care, the DNP-prepared midwife has access to knowledge and resources that will activate leadership in health policy, education, and program evaluation.

Healthcare Business Acumen

Most healthcare providers do not learn business skills in conjunction with their healthcare education. Midwives learned about the business aspects of clinical practice as a survival strategy. Viability meant learning the nuts and bolts of marketing and financial management as well as developing skills to influence legislative and institutional barriers to practice. Educational programs responded by adding more professional issues into their curricula, and the ACNM developed guidelines for starting a practice and resources on marketing and managed care. The Nurse-Midwifery Service Director's Network (SDN) published editions of *An Administrative Manual for Nurse-Midwifery Services* in 1994, 1996, and 2005 (Slager), focusing on the administrative and business aspects of midwifery practice. The Midwifery Business Institute has sponsored annual conferences since 1996, and the ACNM publishes handbooks on specific aspects of business practice, such as billing and coding.

According to Joan Slager, author of *Business Concepts for Healthcare Providers* (2004), "[Business] ignorance has resulted in inadequate compensation, inappropriate restriction, and unfair representation of the non-physician provider" (p. ix). Although each nursing specialty may have some unique business needs, the business knowledge and resources culled through the experience of midwives can serve as a template for all APNs. This template, combined with coursework in health economics, informatics, and policy, will generate APNs with healthcare business acumen.

Healthcare Reform

The unique role that midwives play in healthcare reform needs to be framed within the context of quality and cost-effectiveness. The concepts of high-quality and cost-effective care are embedded in midwifery philosophy, making the midwifery model of care useful as a healthcare exemplar. The Pew Health Professions Committee convened a task force in 1998 that concluded that "the midwifery model of care should be incorporated into the health care system in order to make it available to all women and their families" (Paine, Dower, & O'Neil, 1999). A 2008 Cochrane review by Hatem, Sandall, Devane, Soltani, and Gates showed that midwifery care is associated with many positive outcomes, including shorter hospital stays and increased probability of vaginal birth. The overuse of costly interventions and underuse of evidence-based care were recently outlined in *Evidence-Based Maternity Care*, emphasizing the need to use a low-intervention model of maternity care (Sakala & Corry, 2008). Additionally, the midwifery model of care places a strong emphasis on health promotion and disease prevention, positioning midwives as effective primary care providers (Shah & King, 2006).

The ACNM issued a set of seven key principles for healthcare reform that highlight the need for improved access to women's healthcare services, including primary, gynecologic, family planning, and maternity care, and the urgency of removing barriers to midwifery practice in these vital areas of health care (ACNM, 2009d). These principles intersect well with the IOM report, *The Future of Nursing* (2010), identifying the importance of utilizing APNs to the full extent of their education and training and as full partners in redesigning health care. The ACNM Government Affairs Committee assists in the development of a federal legislative and regulatory agenda that advocates for healthcare reform in women's health services, professional liability, third-party reimbursement, and access to midwifery care.

The DNP-prepared midwife is prepared to assume leadership in advocating for healthcare reform that provides accessible, high-quality, and cost-effective care for all citizens, integrating information from leadership and change theory, health policy, the economics of health care, evidence-based practice, and epidemiology. Successful development and implementation of healthcare reform requires the expertise of healthcare providers who understand the complexity of our healthcare system and have the necessary skills to develop solutions.

Conclusion

Midwives are an innovative and tenacious lot, functioning as leaders and change agents within our healthcare system. In spite of many barriers to practice, midwives have persisted in making inroads into mainstream health care. The vision of the early nurse-midwife leaders, development of a strong professional organization, and strategic educational and practice changes have greatly contributed to professional recognition and access to the healthcare system. It is also clear that visibility and viability in the healthcare system require cultivation of business acumen and legislative engagement. In addition to maintaining high clinical practice standards, gaining recognition and access to the healthcare system requires an understanding of business, politics, data collection, public health, and quality improvement. Successful completion of a DNP degree prepares graduates to provide leadership in the clinical practice arena.

The DNP-prepared midwife is especially well suited to assume leadership roles in the clinical arena. He or she will enter the healthcare system with additional knowledge and skills that will strengthen his or her capacity to interact effectively with the healthcare system. Strong clinical expertise in maternal–child health, combined with an understanding of healthcare economics and policy, will increase the effectiveness of midwives as they practice within an increasingly complex healthcare system. Utilization of information systems, program evaluation, and evidence-based research will enhance clinical practice and serve to reinforce the merits of the midwifery model of care. The DNP-prepared midwife will have new tools for promoting high-quality care for women and children, adding value to the role of the midwife as a woman's healthcare provider.

References

Accreditation Commission for Midwifery Education. (2005). *The knowledge, skills, and behaviors prerequisite to midwifery clinical coursework.* Silver Spring, MD: Author.

Aiken, L. H. (2003). Educational levels of hospital nurses and surgical patient mortality. *Journal of the American Medical Association, 290,* 1617–1623.

Al Gasseer, N., Dresden, E., Keeney, G., & Warren, N. (2004). Status of women and infants in complex humanitarian emergencies. *Journal of Midwifery and Women's Health, 49*(4 Suppl. 1), 7–13.

Ament, L. (2006). *Professional issues in midwifery.* Sudbury, MA: Jones and Bartlett.

American Association of Colleges of Nursing. (2004). *Position statement on the practice doctorate in nursing.* Retrieved from http://www.aacn.nche.edu/DNP/pdf/DNP.pdf

American Association of Colleges of Nursing. (2006). *The essentials of doctoral education for advanced nursing practice.* Washington, DC: Author.

American Association of Colleges of Nursing. (2008). *Doctor of nursing practice (DNP) talking points.* Retrieved from http://www.aacn.nche.edu/DNP/talkingpoints.htm

American Association of Colleges of Nursing. (2009). *Doctor of nursing practice programs.* Retrieved from http://www.aacn.nche.edu/dnp/DNPProgramList.htm

American Association of Colleges of Nursing. (2010). *Adult-gerontology clinical nurse specialist competencies.* Retrieved from http://www.aacn.nche.edu/geriatric-nursing/adultgeroCNScomp.pdf

American Association of Nurse Anesthetists. (2007). *Scope and standards for nurse anesthesia practice.* Park Ridge, IL: Author.

American Association of Nurse Anesthetists. (2009a). *History of nurse anesthesia practice.* Retrieved from http://www.aana.com/crnahistory.aspx

American Association of Nurse Anesthetists. (2009b). *Council on Accreditation of Nurse Anesthesia Educational Programs: Overview.* Retrieved from http://www.aana.com/councilaccreditation.aspx

American Association of Nurse Anesthetists. (2009c). *Qualifications and capabilities of the certified registered nurse anesthetist.* Retrieved from http://www.aana.com/qualifications.aspx

American Association of Nurse Anesthetists. (2009d). *Council on Certification of Nurse Anesthetists (CCNA) overview.* Retrieved from http://www.aana.com/Credentialing.aspx?id=138

American Association of Nurse Anesthetists. (2013). *Standards for nurse anesthesia practice.* Retrieved from: http://www.aana.com/resources2/professionalpractice/Documents/PPM%20Standards%20for%20Nurse%20Anesthesia%20Practice.pdf

American Association of Nurse Practitioners. (2015a). *Affordable Care Act.* Retrieved from http://www.aanp.org/legislation-regulation/federal-legislation/affordable-care-act-aca/19-legislation-regulation/federal-legislation/1336-aca-general-information

American Association of Nurse Practitioners. (2015b). *NP fact sheet.* Retrieved from http://www.aanp.org/all-about-nps/np-fact-sheet

American Association of Nurse Practitioners. (2015c). *Scope of practice for nurse practitioners.* Retrieved from http://www.aanp.org/images/documents/publications/scopeofpractice.pdf

American College of Nurse-Midwives. (2003). *ACNM mission statement.* Silver Spring, MD: Author.

American College of Nurse-Midwives. (2004). *Philosophy of the American College of Nurse-Midwives.* Silver Spring, MD: Author.

American College of Nurse-Midwives. (2005). *QuickInfo: Quality and effectiveness of nurse-midwifery practice.* Silver Spring, MD: Author.

American College of Nurse-Midwives. (2008). *Core competencies for basic midwifery practice.* Retrieved from http://www.midwife.org/siteFiles/descriptive/Core_Competencies_6_07.pdf

American College of Nurse-Midwives. (2009a). *Standards for the practice of midwifery.* Silver Spring, MD: Author.

American College of Nurse-Midwives. (2009b). *Position statement: Mandatory degree requirements for entry into midwifery practice.* Silver Spring, MD: Author.

American College of Nurse-Midwives. (2009c). *ACNM Ad Hoc Committee on Disaster Preparedness.* Retrieved from http://www.midwife.org/disaster_preparedness.cfm

American College of Nurse-Midwives. (2009d). *Healthcare reform: Seven key principles.* Retrieved from http://www.midwife.org/ACNM/files/ccLibraryFiles /Filename/000000000308/ACNMHealthReformPrinciples_000.pdf

American College of Nurse-Midwives. (2011a). *Essential facts about midwives.* Silver Spring, MD: Author.

American College of Nurse-Midwives. (2011b). *Position statement: Definition of midwifery practice, certified nurse-midwife, and certified midwife.* Silver Spring, MD: Author.

American College of Nurse-Midwives. (2012). *Position statement: Midwifery education and the doctor of nursing practice (DNP).* Silver Spring, MD: Author.

American College of Nurse-Midwives. (2012b). *Definition of Midwifery and Scope of Practice of Certified Nurse-Midwives and Certified Midwives.* Silver Spring, MD: ACNM. The Preamble from the Definition and Scope of Practice. Reprinted by permission of ACNM.

American Nurses Association. (2009). *More about RNs and advanced practice RNs.* Retrieved from http://www.nursingworld.org/EspeciallyForYou/Advanced PracticeNurses

American Nurses Association. (2010). *Nursing: Scope and standards of practice* (2nd ed.). Silver Spring, MD: Author.

American Nurses Credentialing Center. (2012a). *ANCC Certification Center—Choose your specialty.* Retrieved from http://www.nursecredentialing.org/Certification .aspx

American Nurses Credentialing Center. (2012b). *APRN News—new and retiring APRN certifications.* Retrieved from http://replyonline.org/CLIENTS/ANCC/3744/

APRN Consensus Work Group & National Council of State Boards of Nursing APRN Advisory Committee. (2008). *Consensus model for APRN regulation: Licensure, accreditation, certification, and education.* Retrieved from http://www.aacn .nche.edu/education-resources/APRNReport.pdf

APRN Joint Dialogue Group. (2008). *Consensus model for APRN regulation: Licensure, accreditation, certification and education.* Retrieved from http://www .aacn.nche.edu/Education/pdf/APRNReport.pdf

Auerbach, D. I., Martsolf, G., Pearson, M. L., Taylor, E. A., Zaydman, M., Muchow, A., . . . Dower, C. (2014). *The DNP by 2015: A study of the institutional, political, and professional issues that facilitate or impede establishing a post-baccalaureate doctor of nursing practice program.* Retrieved from http://www.aacn.nche.edu/dnp /DNP-Study.pdf

Avery, M. (2005). The history and evolution of the core competencies for basic midwifery practice. *Journal of Midwifery and Women's Health, 50*(2), 102–107.

Avery, M., & Howe, C. (2007). The DNP and entry into midwifery practice: An analysis. *Journal of Midwifery and Women's Health, 52*(1), 14–22.

Baldwin, K. M., Clark, A. P., Fulton, J., & Mayo, A. (2009). National validation of the NACNS clinical nurse specialist core competencies. *Journal of Nursing Scholarship, 41*(2), 193–201.

Baldwin, K. M., Lyon, B. L., Clark, A. P., Fulton, J., & Dayhoff, N. (2007). Developing clinical nurse specialist practice competencies. *Clinical Nurse Specialist, 21*(6), 297–302.

Bankert, M. (1989). *Watchful care: A history of America's nurse anesthetists.* New York, NY: Continuum.

Barger, M. (2005). Midwifery practice: Where have we been and where are we going? *Journal of Midwifery and Women's Health, 50*(2), 87–90.

Bedroussian, A., & DeVol, R. (2007). *An unhealthy America: The economic burden of chronic disease.* Santa Monica, CA: The Milken Institute.

Bullough, B. (1995). Professionalization of nurse practitioners. *Annual Review of Nursing Research, 13,* 239–265.

Burst, H. V. (2005). The history of nurse-midwifery education. *Journal of Midwifery and Women's Health, 50*(2), 129–137.

Centers for Medicare and Medicaid Services. (2012). *National healthcare data projected.* Retrieved from http://www.cms.hhs.gov

Chase, S. K., & Pruitt, R. H. (2006). The practice doctorate: Innovation or disruption? *Journal of Nursing Education, 45*(5), 155–161.

Chism, L. (2009, January 12). *Understanding the DNP: Advance for nurse practitioners.* Retrieved from http://nurse-practitioners.advanceweb.com/Editorial/Content/Editorial.aspx?CC=191812

Critchley, D. L. (1985). Evolution of the role. In D. L. Critchley & J. T. Maurin (Eds.), *The clinical specialist in psychiatric mental health nursing* (pp. 5–22). New York, NY: Wiley.

Dawley, K. (2003). Origins of nurse-midwifery in the United States and its expansion in the 1940s. *Journal of Midwifery and Women's Health, 48*(2), 86–95.

Declercq, E. (2009). Births attended by certified nurse-midwives in the United States reach an all-time high: Trends from 1989 to 2006. *Journal of Midwifery and Women's Health, 54*(3), 263–265.

Declercq, E. R., Williams, D. R., Koontz, A. M., Paine, L. L., Streit, E. L., & McClosky, L. (2001). Serving women in need: Nurse-midwifery practice in the United States. *Journal of Midwifery and Women's Health, 46*(1), 11–16.

Denzler, S. (2011). Urgent measures for an old problem. *Health Affairs, 30*(9), 1626.

Goudreau, K. A., Baldwin, K., Clark, A., Fulton, J., Lyon, B., Murray, T., . . . Sendelbach, S. (2007, July). *A vision of the future for clinical nurse specialists.* Harrisburg, PA: National Association of Clinical Nurse Specialists.

Hamilton, B., Martin, J., & Ventura, S. (2010). Births: Preliminary data for 2009. *National Vital Statistic Reports, 59*(3), 1–19.

Hamric, A. B. (2009). A definition of advanced nursing practice. In A. B. Hamric, J. A. Spross, & C. M. Hanson (Eds.), *Advanced nursing practice: An integrative approach* (pp. 75–94). Philadelphia, PA: Saunders.

Hamric, A. B., Spross, J. A., & Hanson, C. M. (Eds.). (2009). *Advanced practice nursing: An integrative approach* (4th ed.). St. Louis, MO: Saunders Elsevier.

Hanson, C. M. (2009). Understanding regulatory, legal, and credentialing requirements. In A. B. Hamric, J. A. Spross, & C. M. Hanson (Eds.), *Advanced practice nursing:
An integrative approach* (4th ed., pp. 605–624). St. Louis, MO: Saunders Elsevier.

Hatem, M., Sandall, J., Devane, D., Soltani, H., & Gates, S. (2008). Midwife-led
versus other models of care for childbearing women. *Cochrane Database of
Systematic Reviews, 4.*

Hathaway, D., Jacob, S., Stegbauer, C., Thompson, C., & Graff, C. (2006). The
practice doctorate: Perspectives of early adopters. *Journal of Nursing Education,
45*(12), 487–496.

Institute of Medicine. (1999). *To err is human: Building a safer health system.*
Washington, DC: National Academy Press.

Institute of Medicine. (2001). *Crossing the quality chasm: A new health system for
the 21st century.* Washington, DC: National Academies Press.

Institute of Medicine. (2003a). *Health professions education: A bridge to quality.*
Washington, DC: National Academies Press.

Institute of Medicine. (2003b). *Keeping patients safe: Transforming the work environment of nurses.* Washington, DC: National Academies Press.

Institute of Medicine. (2010). *The future of nursing: Leading change, advancing
health. Report recommendations.* Retrieved from http://www.iom.edu/nursing

Jesse, D., & Blue, C. (2004). Mary Breckinridge meets Healthy People 2010: A
teaching strategy for visioning and building healthy communities. *Journal of
Midwifery and Women's Health, 49*(2), 126.

Kaiser Family Foundation. (2009). *Trends in health care costs and spending.* Retrieved
from http//www.kff.org

Keeling, A. W. (2009). A brief history of advanced practice nursing in the United
States. In A. B. Hamric, J. A. Spross, & C. H. Hanson (Eds.), *Advanced practice nursing: An integrative approach* (4th ed., pp. 3–32). St. Louis, MO: Saunders Elsevier.

Komnenich, P. (2005). The evolution of advanced practice in nursing. In
J. M. Stanley (Ed.), *Advanced practice nursing: Emphasizing common roles*
(pp. 3–32). Philadelphia, PA: F. A. Davis.

Magaw, A. (1906). *A review of over 14,000 surgical anesthetics.* In Surgery, Gynecology and Obstetrics. Retrieved from: https://www.aana.com/newsandjournal
/Documents/imagining_0299_p33-38.pdf

McKinley, M. G. (2007). *Acute and critical care clinical nurse specialists: Synergy for
best practices.* Wheeling, MO: Saunders Elsevier.

Metropolitan Life Insurance Company. (1960). Summary of the ten thousand
confinement records of the Frontier Nursing Service. *Bulletin of the American
College of Nurse Midwifery, 5,* 1–9.

Miller, S., Sloan, N. L., Winikoff, B., Langer, A., & Fikree, F. F. (2003). Where is the
"e" in MCH? The need for an evidence-based approach in safe motherhood.
Journal of Midwifery and Women's Health, 48(1), 10–18.

National Association of Clinical Nurse Specialists. (1998). *Statement on clinical
nurse specialist practice and education.* Glenview, IL: Author.

National Association of Clinical Nurse Specialists. (2004). *Statement on clinical
nurse specialist practice and education.* Harrisburg, PA: Author.

National Association of Clinical Nurse Specialists. (2005). *White paper on the nursing practice doctorate.* Retrieved from http://www.nacns.org/docs/PaperOnNPDoctorate.pdf

National Association of Clinical Nurse Specialists. (2007). A *vision of the future for clinical nurse specialists.* Retrieved from http://www.nacns.org/docs/AVisionCNS.pdf

National Association of Clinical Nurse Specialists. (2009a). *Clinical nurse specialist meeting the new demands of a reformed health care system.* Retrieved from http://journals.lww.com/cns-journal/Documents/CNS%20Statement%202004.pdf

National Association of Clinical Nurse Specialists. (2009b). *Core practice doctorate clinical nurse specialist (CNS) competencies.* Retrieved from http://www.nacns.org/docs/CorePracticeDoctorate.pdf

National Association of Clinical Nurse Specialists. (2012). *APRN fact sheet.* Retrieved from http://www.nacns.org

National Association of Clinical Nurse Specialists. (2015). *National Association of Clinical Nurse Specialists endorses requiring doctor of nursing practice degree for clinical nurse specialists.* Retrieved from: http://www.nacns.org/docs/PR-DNP-Statement1507.pdf

National Council of State Boards of Nursing. (2009). *NCSBN Model Nursing Practice Act and model nursing administrative rules.* Retrieved from http://hawaii.gov/dcca/pvl/news-releases/nursing_announcements/Model_Nursing_Practice_Act_Dec09.pdf

National Organization of Nurse Practitioner Faculties. (2006). *Practice doctorate nurse practitioner entry-level competencies.* Retrieved from http://c.ymcdn.com/sites/www.nonpf.org/resource/resmgr/competencies/dnp%20np%20competenciesapril2006.pdf

National Organization of Nurse Practitioner Faculties. (2011). *Nurse practitioner core competencies.* Retrieved from http://www.aacn.nche.edu/dnp/program-schools

NBCRNA (2015). *National Certification Handbook.* NBCRNA, Chicago, IL

NBCRNA (2015). *The Continued Professional Certification (CPC) Program of the National Board of Certification & Recertification for Nurse Anesthetists.* NBCRNA, Chicago, IL.

Nurse-Midwifery Service Director's Network. (1994). *An administrative manual for nurse-midwifery services.* Dubuque, IA: Kendall/Hunt.

Nurse-Midwifery Service Director's Network. (1996). *An administrative manual for nurse-midwifery services* (2nd ed.). Dubuque, IA: Kendall/Hunt.

Paine, L., Dower, C., & O'Neil, E. (1999). Midwifery in the 21st century: Recommendations from the Pew Health Professions Commission/UCSF Center for the Health Professions 1998 Taskforce on Midwifery. *Journal of Midwifery and Women's Health, 44*(4), 341–348.

Phillips, S. J. (2015). 27th annual legislative update: Advancements continue for APRN practice. *Nurse Practitioner, 40*(1), 16–42.

Pulcini, J., & Wagner, M. (2001). *Perspectives on education and practice issues for nurse practitioners and advanced practice nursing.* Retrieved from http://onlinelibrary.wiley.com/doi/10.1111/j.1365-2648.2004.03234.x/abstract

Robb, I. (1893). *Nursing: Its principles and practice; for hospital and private use.* Philadelphia, PA: Saunders.

Safriet, B. (2002). Closing the gap between can and may in health care providers' scopes of practice: A primer for policymakers. *Yale Journal of Regulation, 19,* 301–334.

Sakala, C., & Corry, M. (2008). *Evidence-based maternity care: What it is and what it can achieve.* New York, NY: Milbank Memorial Fund.

Shah, M., & King, T. (2006). Primary health care by midwives: Comprehensive and competent health services for women. *Journal of Midwifery and Women's Health, 51*(3), 139–140.

Slager, J. (2004). *Business concepts for healthcare providers.* Sudbury, MA: Jones and Bartlett.

Slager, J. (Ed.). (2005). *An administrative manual for nurse-midwifery services* (3rd ed.). Greenwood Village, CO: Midwifery Business Network.

Sparacino, P. S., & Cartwright, C. (2009). In A. B. Hamric, J. A. Spross, & C. H. Hanson (Eds.), *The clinical nurse specialist* (4th ed., pp. 349–379). St. Louis, MO: Saunders.

U.S. Census Bureau. (2009). *Income, poverty, and health insurance coverage in the United States: 2008.* Retrieved from http://www.census.gov/prod/2009pubs/p60-236.pdf

Varney, H., Kriebs, J., & Gegor, C. (2004). *Varney's midwifery* (4th ed.). Sudbury, MA: Jones and Bartlett.

Chapter 9

Emerging Roles for the DNP

Nurse Educator

Kathryn Waud White

As the nursing profession moves toward implementation of the American Association of Colleges of Nursing's (AACN's) recommendation that all advanced practice nurses (APNs) be educated in a doctor of nursing practice (DNP) framework (AACN, 2006), the DNP-prepared nurse educator is certain to emerge as a clear and vital component of advanced practice nursing education. The education of APNs focuses on the development of the knowledge and skills to care for patients at the highest level possible and implies the infusion of clinical scholarship into the care of all patients, at all times, and in all practice settings. The role of APNs in health care is receiving national attention (Institute of Medicine [IOM], 2010). The DNP-prepared nurse educator is well suited to teach clinical scholarship in the context of a practice doctorate to help advanced practice nursing students achieve this level of practice.

The notion of advanced practice nursing faculty with practice doctorates versus research degrees is supported by several professional organizations. In 2005, the National Organization of Nurse Practitioner Faculties (NONPF) issued a statement on faculty practice (NONPF, 2005). In this statement, they asserted that "faculty practice is necessary to maintain competence, a forum for scholarship, and the expectation of professionalism." NONPF has also proposed that the competence of faculty should be evaluated in both the teaching arena and the clinical arena (NONPF, 2000). The board of governors of the National League for Nursing (NLN) issued a position statement in 2002 that states in part that "nurse educators practice in both academic and clinical settings and they must be competent clinicians." It also goes on to state that "while being a good clinician is essential, it is not sufficient for the educator role" (NLN, 2002).

The American Nurses Credentialing Center (ANCC) and the American Academy of Nurse Practitioners (AANP) require APNs to document a minimum of 1,000 hours of nursing practice in the specialty and population for which they are prepared every 5 years in order to renew certification (AANP, 2015; ANCC, 2012). The Commission on Collegiate Nursing Education's (CCNE's) National Task Force on Quality Nurse Practitioner Education's report from 2008 states in Standard I.C that "institutional support ensures that NP faculty teaching in clinical courses maintain currency in clinical practice" (CCNE, 2008). This again supports the role of the educator who is prepared as a content expert with a practice doctorate rather than a research doctorate.

Neither traditional research doctorates nor practice doctorates are adequate preparation for the role of a nurse educator (AACN, 2006). Both the NLN and the AACN have suggested that advanced practice nursing faculty should have additional course work in curriculum design and evaluation and teaching methodologies. The Council on Accreditation of Nurse Anesthesia Educational Programs (COA) requires that nurse anesthesia faculty have "formal instruction" in curriculum, evaluation, and instruction (COA, 2014). The nursing educator who is prepared with both formal instruction in these topics and a practice doctorate brings some unique skills to the educational practice.

In examining *Essentials of Doctoral Education for Advanced Nursing Practice*, as delineated by the AACN in 2006, it is clear that the DNP-prepared educator who has mastered these essentials has a unique skill set that enhances the education of APNs (AACN, 2006). The first essential, *scientific underpinnings for practice*, reveals the complexities of nursing practice and the many ways that DNP graduates will be able to quickly integrate science and theory from nursing and other disciplines into practice. As a DNP-prepared educator, this faculty member will bring the scholarship of integration into the academic setting and use many different concepts from other disciplines to educate APNs, integrating these concepts into the discipline of nursing and making the discipline richer.

Mastery of the second essential, *organizational and systems leadership for quality improvement and systems thinking*, also brings a unique perspective to the education of advanced practice students. Many APN programs exist within large, complex educational organizations. It could be said that there is an analogous situation between the large educational institution and a large healthcare organization. The DNP-prepared nurse educator will have the skills to work effectively within the organization to evaluate education delivery and make evidence-based educational recommendations for systems change within these large university settings. The DNP-prepared educator will be able to use the principles of business, finance, economics, and health policy to improve the delivery of the education, and he or she will have the advanced communications skills to lead such changes.

Diers (1995) asserted that scholarship is a habit of the mind that begins with observations of the phenomena of health and illness but then applies the "disciplined habits of analysis and analogy," which brings new comprehension to the phenomena. The DNP-prepared nurse educator who has mastered the third essential, *clinical scholarship and analytical methods for evidence-based practice*, will bring those skills and habits of mind into the academic setting. The DNP educator is also a scholar who is in the habit of seeking evidence to support the practice of education and integrating evidence from many fields of study into the solutions to problems in education. In 1984, Jeroslav Pelikan described the difference between good scholarship and great scholarship: "The difference between good scholarship and great scholarship is, as often as not, the general preparation of the scholar in fields other than the field of preparation. It is the general preparation that makes possible that extra leap of imagination and analogy by which scholarship moves ahead." The broad preparation of the DNP in the areas of foundational science, theory, economics, informatics, advocacy, epidemiology, leadership, and collaboration across professions places this educator in a unique place to use the scholarship of integration in an educational setting.

Technology in education is an emerging tool for teaching and learning, and educators are rapidly learning how to leverage technology to improve education. The DNP-prepared educator who has mastered the fourth essential, *information systems/technology and patient care technology for the improvement and transformation of care*, will not only be proficient in the use of technology for patient care but will also bring that expertise into the academic environment. Distance education and online teaching are the accepted norms. Simulation experiences for advanced practice students are burgeoning as well, and these simulation environments can be very technologically sophisticated. The DNP-prepared nurse educator will not only be able to navigate in this technological environment but also will model the use of technology to improve systems and outcomes in the educational setting.

The fifth essential, *health care policy for advocacy in health care*, is another area in which the DNP-prepared nurse educator will have valuable skills for providing a secure place for nursing in the future. Health policy includes not only healthcare system reform but also those issues that are relevant to the education of APNs. Advocacy for significant federal money to support nursing education is only one area where efforts are needed to secure the future of nursing. This educator will also have the skills to effectively advocate for resources within the academic institutions that are experiencing budget cuts from donors and state sources. The DNP educator will have the ability to analyze internal and external policy processes and competently influence policy within and outside academic institutions. He or she will serve as a role model of advocacy for the advanced practice students.

Interprofessional collaboration is an area where the DNP-prepared educator brings unique skills to the academic setting. What better, richer environment for interprofessional collaboration is there than an academic health center? The DNP-prepared educator will have the skills to value, model, and implement interprofessional teams in the clinical area as well as the academic area beginning with the interprofessional education of all providers. Team leadership and collaboration are the skills recommended by the IOM report of 2001, *Crossing the Quality Chasm*. The DNP-prepared nurse educator who has mastered the sixth essential, *interprofessional collaboration for improving patient and population health outcomes*, will be ready to bring team leadership and collaboration to the academic arena.

The DNP-prepared nurse educator will readily recognize that the student body is a population with its own unique characteristics. Students who are taking classes on a doctoral level—going to clinical rotations, managing personal relationships, trying to remain engaged in family activities, and perhaps working part time—are prone to fatigue and are certainly functioning in a stressful environment. The DNP educator who has mastered the seventh essential, *clinical prevention and population health for improving the nation's health*, will seek evidence-based solutions to monitor student stress and interventions to assist students in adopting healthy behaviors.

It is in the last essential, *advanced practice nursing*, that the DNP-prepared nurse educator's skills will be most valuable as he or she seeks out specific competencies, formulates a plan for students to become proficient in those areas, and implements evaluation programs to measure progress toward competency. Although clinical competency is the last competency, nursing is a clinical profession that synthesizes evidence from all these essentials into competent evidence-based clinical practice of the highest quality for patient safety and improved outcomes. The measurement of clinical ability and continuous process improvement for the educational program are key to maintaining this high level of performance in the complex, rapidly changing healthcare environment.

The notion of the DNP graduate as a nurse educator has come into its own, but challenges remain. It appears that DNP graduates are no more likely to accept the low salaries in academia than their PhD faculty colleagues (Kelly, 2010). Kelly refuted the notion that the DNP degree is the solution to the nursing faculty shortage. Kelly cited the paucity of evidence that DNP graduates who work in advanced practice roles will choose a career in academics and thus advocated for a comprehensive approach to the faculty shortages. In addition, the ability of DNP faculty members to attain tenure is a controversial subject. In many large universities, this is not likely at this time because of concerns about the DNP's ability to produce research and secure grants (Nicholes & Dyer, 2012). Although Nicholes and Dyer found positive attitudes toward DNP-prepared faculty being eligible for tenure among the deans of colleges of nursing and the PhD-prepared nursing faculty they surveyed, these concerns reflect the continued undervaluing of the scholarship of application and integration articulated by Boyer in 1990. Boyer's definition of the scholarship of practice as it relates to nursing has been a catalyst for change except in the academy. Nicholes and Dyer advocate for an attitudinal expansion of the definition of scholarship, as Boyer suggested in 1990, to embrace the scholarship of practice and thus the work of the DNP. Most recently, the UniSCOPE Learning Community at Pennsylvania State University articulated a multifaceted model of scholarship with the underlying principle that all forms and functions of scholarship should be equally valued, not just the scholarship of discovery (Hyman et al., 2002). Whether these thought streams will change the culture of the academy is still very much in question.

The DNP course of study confers a set of unique skills that are highly valuable and add to the academic preparation of APNs. These skills support the education of APNs to the highest level and help to fulfill the promise of the IOM report for improvements in the education of advanced practice nursing (2010). However, challenges remain for acceptance of the role of the DNP-prepared educator in academia.

The Nurse Administrator

Mary Jean Vickers

The DNP educational program prepares nurses to lead health care in a tremendously challenging reform atmosphere that demands better access and quality while reducing the costs. During this period of rapid change, it is critical for the administrator to have an appreciation of the many governmental and private influences on healthcare programming. Among these agencies are The Joint Commission, the Centers for Medicare and Medicaid Services (CMS), the National Quality Forum (NQF), the Agency for Healthcare Research and Quality (AHRQ), insurance companies, private businesses, and, specifically for nursing, the American Nurses Association Magnet Certification program and the National Database for Nursing Quality Indicators (NDNQI). These groups are developing certification programs and/ or quality improvement measures in which hospitals are encouraged and rewarded for participation. Sometimes the improvement projects are educational in nature, but often the projects are redesigns of past processes intended to embrace technology in order to improve efficiency and the metrics related to care delivery. Specific best practices are embedded into the care requirements of common diagnoses to promote standardized care and reduce readmissions. Embracing these best practices is often rewarded with higher reimbursement fees, also understood as pay-for-performance strategies. A DNP-prepared administrator has an appreciation of the delicate balance between cost and quality. He or she has a keen understanding of the interdependencies between providing high-quality patient-centered care and achieving the highest reimbursement rates available.

Change Theory

An administrator is well served by the study of the concepts explored in change theories and the knowledge gained through DNP coursework. There are many change models to explore, and each can be helpful in guiding our decisions and facilitating change assimilation into practice. As a novice nurse, this author was educated about Lewin's change theory (Smith, 2001). The early work of social psychology researcher Kurt Lewin is seminal in understanding how groups process change (Smith, 2001). Kurt Lewin developed a simple theory with three phases: unfreezing, change, and freezing. This theory, in its simplest form, suggests that first you need to prepare those who will change through a process of unfreezing their current view of the issue. Next, you must implement the change and, finally, freeze the new process into place. Current business literature abounds with books on the subject of leading change and managing change for large organizations. These publications offer a more comprehensive model from which to design project plans. The works of Kotter (1996) and Taylor (2006) are helpful to DNP graduates in administrative positions. These authors provide a useful approach to leading change and managing large projects effectively. A change theory that this administrator has found helpful is the model developed by Kotter (1996). John Kotter is a professor at the Harvard Business School and published *Leading Change* in 1996. His model consists of eight steps:

1. Establishing a sense of urgency
2. Creating a guiding coalition
3. Developing a vision and strategy
4. Communicating the change vision
5. Empowering employees for broad-based action
6. Generating short-term wins
7. Consolidating gains and producing more change
8. Anchoring new approaches in the culture

This model was an excellent guide in leading our nursing education department through several large projects. Establishing the sense of urgency required nurse managers, clinical nurse specialists, staff nurses, and preceptors to become engaged in each project. Nursing executive leadership must also become engaged to help build a guiding coalition for each project. Developing the vision and a strategy is best served by having a collaborative effort among those involved. Ultimately, creating the vision for the implementation of any project often becomes the sole responsibility of the administrator. Empowering the team to follow the plan and implement the change is motivated by this vision.

Communication is constant in any change project. Repeating, reinforcing, and reviewing messages previously delivered are necessary. Refining the process during implementation is critical to the ultimate success of all projects. This refining process merges into the next step, empowering employees for broad-based action. One of the most difficult tasks of the project leader is relinquishing control over every element of the project. Letting others take ownership of the project and empowering them to help guide the decisions during implementation will serve the DNP-educated nurse leader well during the implementation phase of each project undertaken. Measuring and reporting short-term gains and consolidating those gains is motivational for those employees involved in the project and fuels their enthusiasm. Consolidating gains, producing more change, and ultimately anchoring the change into practice require continued vigilance.

Each model that a leader explores will have some areas of weakness. The one area in which Kotter's (1996) theory is weak is the evaluation phase of the program. Exploring program evaluation methods is a skill found in DNP programs. A review of the literature to find the right tool of evaluation for each project may be time consuming. Many projects undertaken by this administrator have been educational in nature, so alignment of these training projects with the Bersin (2008) model of training measurement and evaluation promotes consistency in how each project outcome is measured. Kotter's theory of change and Bersin's model of training measurement provide useful theoretical frameworks to guide projects in the real world, with real people to motivate and lead.

Leadership Style

Exploring leadership models is another skill that the DNP-prepared administrator gains in the course of study. Throughout this administrator's academic career, leadership models have often been a part of the curriculum. The first leadership styles explored were limited to authoritarian, laissez-faire, or democratic (Cherry, 2011). As a staff nurse, this author often experienced the authoritarian style, which was frequently unsatisfying. Nurses experience the decisions of nursing leaders and other administrators daily. They often express the need to be involved in these decisions. Authoritarian leadership styles are autocratic and do not involve other participants in making the decision. This style of leadership can be useful in emergency situations but is limited in relationship building and staff development of those who report to us.

The Magnet certification program encourages more decision-making control by the staffs that are served by administrators. Participative management is a form of democratic leadership. This style of leading has always held an attraction for this author. Democratic leaders will allow for group discussion of a problem and the selection of an acceptable solution. This participative leadership style promotes shared responsibility and greater involvement of those who are charged with implementation of the solution. We should not underestimate the importance of dialogue in the workplace. The ability of staff to openly share their concerns, offer ideas for resolving problems, and participate in both the discussion and the selection of resolutions empowers staff toward greater personal and professional satisfaction. This approach is also likely to improve the adoption of implementing change. The goal of all change is to ultimately improve patient outcomes and patient satisfaction.

In the past, when in an academic role as clinical faculty, the desire to intellectually stimulate students, mentor them toward the acquisition of knowledge and skills, and develop their abilities improved this author's leadership competencies. Developing a transformational and transactional leadership style, as suggested by Failla (2008), is a worthy professional goal for all administrators. This article effectively describes the importance of more contemporary leadership models. The five critical strategies of transformational leaders described by Failla (2008) are useful:

- Instill employee pride in the leader's vision and mission.
- Use leader behaviors to demonstrate the values and mission to employees.
- Increase staff awareness and acceptance of the desired mission.
- Intellectually stimulate employees and others to think in new ways.
- Individualize consideration by mentoring and expressing appreciation when the mission and related goals are accomplished. (Failla, 2008)

A publication related to improving the nursing work environment, *Keeping Patients Safe: Transforming the Work Environment of Nurses* (IOM, 2003), supports transformational nursing leadership style for nursing leaders.

The accountabilities of leaders discussed in Stefl (2008) are: "communication and relationship management, professionalism, leadership, knowledge of the healthcare system, and business skills and knowledge" (p. 360). Missing from this model are the skills needed to evaluate and improve the competency of followers. Holding others accountable and maintaining the clinical discipline required for the delivery of safe care is an important competency of managers in a healthcare environment. One area for skills growth among many administrators and managers is holding people accountable and motivating them to improved clinical performance. It is beneficial as an administrator to have strong values and high expectations of those you lead and those with whom you need to collaborate. Many times, communicating your expectations clearly will lead to accomplishing these goals. Many employees have a strong desire to meet their manager's expectations and even to exceed them. However, if the goals are not clearly communicated, it is not unusual to be disappointed when one's team fails to meet expectations. Being a good coach by spending time with all employees to train them and facilitate their performance at the level expected is a valuable approach. However, it is also wise to understand that the learning curve is steeper for some, and this can create some tension for both the leader and the team.

Evidence-Based Management Practices

The DNP program will prepare graduates to embrace evidence-based practice (EBP). An administrator also needs to adopt evidence-based management practices. This is accomplished through exploring the literature or delegating this task to those working on projects with the administrator. A review of executive summaries and formal literature reviews, as well as local programs and processes, will provide the administrator with the clearest picture of the current situation. Discussions with the team regarding these findings and selection of the best management approaches to achieve the organization's goals will result in improved outcomes. It is not unusual for administrators to set goals that might not be achievable and then try to force the team to achieve an unrealistic goal. This can be costly and should be avoided unless urgent situations require quick solutions. Consider setting short-term achievable goals that will build momentum toward the larger goal desired.

Balancing the objectives of many healthcare disciplines can often challenge the administrator. Physicians' need for adequate bed capacity to provide for the care of patients in their specialty and those receiving specialized treatments can challenge the skills and abilities of the available nursing staff. Working in a collaborative manner with the physicians, educators, nurses, and specialists in other disciplines to promote the care needs of patients and provide for the education that nurses or others need requires patience and commitment. Approaching these situations in a manner that does not address the educational needs of the nurses may result in less than optimal outcomes for patients.

Collaboration

One of the most important skills the DNP-prepared administrator needs is that of collaboration. In its simplest form, collaboration "implies collective action toward a common goal in a spirit of trust and harmony" (D'Amour, Ferrada-Videla, San Martin-Rodriguez, & Beaulieu, 2005, p. 116). Working well in teams to achieve the goals of the organization requires this level of collaboration. In the experience of this administrator, barriers to achieving good collaborative relationships can be work-related boundary concerns ("it's not my job") and competition. Healthcare reform requires healthy work relationships that use limited resources to provide the best care possible. Working together in healthy teams that put the patient and organizational goals ahead of our own will serve us in reducing costs, managing limited resources, and reforming in an efficient and effective manner. Deliberate collaboration can strengthen colleagues of the same discipline and interdisciplinary teams. This approach can lead to improved patient safety and staff satisfaction.

Conclusion

DNP preparation provides an opportunity to explore leadership theories, project management and evaluation techniques, EBPs, and change theories. Lifelong learning and exploring the literature to improve leadership skills must be embraced. The challenge for the administrator is to integrate this academic preparation and lifelong learning into practice to promote innovative approaches to problems in our highly complex healthcare environments. Thinking outside the box, exploring technologies that allow for more efficiency, and embracing new ideas while consistently paying attention to patient safety, patient and staff satisfaction, and cost will promote both better patient care and the role of DNP-prepared administrators.

Public Health Nurse

Carol Flaten and Jeanne Pfeiffer

Dramatic effects on the health of populations have been the work of public health nurses (PHNs) who consider population-level assessment, intervention, and evaluation to impact the health of the communities they serve. This work has improved the quality and quantity of life of individuals and communities. In the 20th century, life expectancy increased from 47.3 years in 1900 to 78.7 years in 2010 (National Center for Health Statistics, 2013). The 10 great public health achievements of the 20th century ("Ten Great Public Health Achievements," 2011) can be credited with this dramatic change in life expectancy. These 10 achievements are: (1) immunizations, (2) motor vehicle safety, (3) workplace safety, (4) control of infectious disease, (5) decline in deaths from heart disease and stroke, (6) safer and healthier foods, (7) healthier mothers and babies, (8) family planning, (9) fluoridation of water, and (10) identifying tobacco as a health hazard. PHNs have played a part in all these areas. DNP-prepared PHNs bring a depth of knowledge and an advanced skill set to the healthcare arena, which is becoming ever more complex. These nurses focus their practice and expertise at the community and systems levels. The DNP-prepared PHN is pivotal in this multifaceted, interprofessional work to protect and promote health and prevent disease and disability in our communities. National initiatives such as the Affordable Care Act, which emphasizes prevention and wellness, and the Institute for Healthcare Improvement (2015), which clearly identifies *population health* as one component of its framework known as the "triple aim" to improve health care, are areas where the PHN excels. These shifts in perspective at a national level over the past decade speak to the core principles that embody public health nursing practice.

Public Health Nurse: A Definition

Public health nursing practice is grounded in knowledge from nursing and social and public health sciences. Public health nursing practice is focused on the health of populations rather than the specific health needs of individuals. PHNs are involved in interventions that promote health, prevent disease and disability, and create conditions in which all people can be healthy (Quad Council of Public Health Nursing Organizations, 2005; Stanhope & Lancaster, 2012). According to the American

Public Health Association's definition, a PHN has "preparation in public health and nursing science with a primary focus on population-level outcomes" (American Public Health Association, 1996). The population may be based on geographical boundaries or characteristics of interest—such as the elderly or children receiving cancer treatment—or a combination of the two. The underlying ethical principle of public health nursing practice is the theory of utilitarianism, which states, "the greatest good for the greatest number" (Bayer, Gostin, Jennings, & Steinbock, 2007). In addition, the concept of social justice is considered a foundation of public health nursing (Stanhope & Lancaster, 2012).

The terms *community health nursing* and *public health nursing* have historically caused confusion. *Community based* tends to focus on nursing care of individuals and families in the community, typically managing acute or chronic conditions in the community. The terms *community health nurse* and *public health nurse* have been used interchangeably. In this discussion, the term *public health nurse* will be used. The primary focus of care is on the population, with the goal of preventing disease and promoting health (Stanhope & Lancaster, 2012).

The IOM published a report that defined public health as "what we, as a society, do collectively to assure the conditions in which people can be healthy" (IOM, 1988, p. 1). This definition demonstrates the broad scope of practice and interprofessional nature of public health work, within which PHNs play an important role based on scientific principles of public health and public health nursing. Along with these central definitions, the PHN is also a master at developing and maintaining relationships with individuals, communities, and systems. The ability to establish and maintain caring relationships is one of the cornerstones of public health nursing identified by the Minnesota Department of Health (2007).

History of Public Health Nursing

Many nursing leaders have influenced the practice of public health nursing. Florence Nightingale (1820–1910) improved health outcomes of soldiers in Europe during the Crimean War by being aware of environmental conditions that affected health and using basic principles of epidemiology to document outcomes such as mortality rate (Nightingale, 1946). Epidemiology is a foundational science for public health nursing. Understanding this notion of population-based nursing and systematically collecting data to inform practice was a new methodology and provided nursing with another dimension to assess the health of a population.

The life and work of Lillian Wald (1867–1940) carried the concept of population-based nursing even further in the late 1800s in the United States. Wald is credited with coining the term *public health nursing*. Wald's impact on nursing and the community in which she practiced was revolutionary for the time. Wald noticed the impoverished conditions and lack of basic necessities among the residents on the Lower East Side of New York City. After seeing firsthand the poor living and health conditions of recent immigrants and their families, Wald, along with several colleagues, established the Visiting Nurse Service. The Visiting Nurse Service provided the beginning model for PHNs interacting with families in their homes and communities. The Henry Street Settlement followed a short time later, which provided a variety of services to this population. It is important to note that Wald believed in meeting the individual in the home or on the street and emphasized the importance of the environment surrounding the individual. However, it was Wald's capacity to notice and act on behalf of individuals and families at the community and system levels, as well as at the individual level, that has left a legacy of work that many still attempt to achieve today. Wald was very effective as a community organizer, advocate, and leader and effected dramatic changes in the quality of life in the community. In public health nursing, a single intervention at the community or systems level has the potential to affect large numbers of individuals (Jewish Women's Archive, n.d.).

At the population level, Wald's work provides a variety of examples of population-based public health nursing interventions, including: (1) developing safe playground spaces for neighborhood children; (2) advocating for the role of school nurses to ensure that children had adequate nutrition and health care; (3) advocating for decent working conditions for women; (4) partnering with the Metropolitan Life Insurance Company to provide health care to policy holders; (5) advocating for safe industrial working conditions; (6) campaigning for the first federal Children's Bureau to abolish child labor; (7) promoting children's health; and (8) supporting children who had dropped out of school. All these examples addressed individual needs, yet the interventions were aimed at the systems level or at the community level to affect programs and develop policy. That the entire population benefited from these interventions ultimately improved the lives of individuals. These accomplishments at the state and federal levels were all made before women had a voice through voting in the United States. Lillian Wald was a reformer of her day who has greatly influenced public health nursing as it is practiced today

(Jewish Women's Archive, n.d.). Other PHNs include Margaret Sanger, who advocated for birth control and women's health and started the first birth control clinic in 1916.

Foundational Principles of Public Health Nursing

In light of the preceding definition and examples of public health and public health nursing, the core functions of public health in which the PHN practices are assessment, policy development, and assurance, along with the 10 essential services of public health (Public Health Functions Steering Committee, 1998). This is illustrated in **Figure 9-1**.

The three core functions that drive public health practice are (IOM, 1988; Stanhope & Lancaster, 2012, p. 7):

> Assessment: *Refers to systematically collecting data on the population, monitoring the population's health status, and making information available about the health of the community.*
>
> Policy Development: *Refers to the need to provide leadership in developing policies that support the health of the population, including the use of the scientific knowledge base in making decisions about policy.*

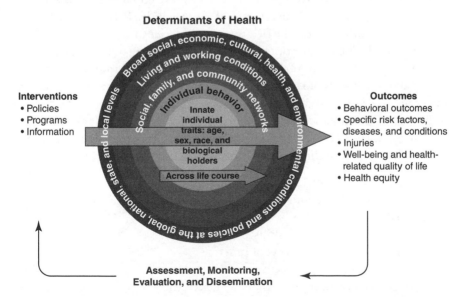

Figure 9-1 Action Model to Achieve Healthy People 2020's Overarching Goals
Reproduced from U.S. Department of Health and Human Services, Secretary's Advisory Committee on Health Promotion and Disease Prevention Objectives for 2010. (2008). Phase I report: Recommendations for the framework and format of *Healthy People 2020* (p. 7). Retrieved from http://www.healthypeople.gov/sites/default/files/PhaseI_0.pdf

> Assurance: *Refers to the role of the public health nurse in ensuring that essential community-oriented health services are available, which may include providing essential personal health services for those who would not otherwise receive them. Assurance also refers to making sure that a competent public health and personal health care workforce is available.*

Specific to public health nursing practice, the *intervention wheel* is a model that identifies specific PHN interventions that support the work toward these core functions and 10 essential services (Keller & Strohschein, 2012).

Public Health Nursing National Organizational Framework

The Quad Council of Public Health Nursing is the overarching entity that includes four national nursing organizations that address public health nursing issues: (1) the Association of Community Health Nurse Educators (ACHNE), (2) the American Nurses Association's Congress on Nursing Practice and Economics (ANA), (3) the American Public Health Association-Public Health Nursing Section (APHA), and (4) the Association of State and Territorial Directors of Nursing (ASTDN). The purpose of the Quad Council is to promote and stimulate collaboration among the member groups. The Quad Council also includes PHN experts who advance the work of public health nursing practice and education at the national level. The Quad Council posted a document, "Quad Council PHN Competencies," in April 2003. This document distinguishes between characteristics of the "generalist/staff PHN" and the PHN in a manager/specialist/consultant role. These competencies were intended to be a guide for practice and academic settings in order to facilitate the education of the PHN. The competencies were grouped in eight domains (Quad Council of Public Health Nursing Organizations, 2011):

1. Analytic assessment skills
2. Policy development and program planning skills
3. Communication skills
4. Cultural competency skills
5. Community dimensions of practice
6. Basic public health sciences
7. Financial planning and management skills
8. Leadership and systems thinking skills

At the advanced level of practice, for the most part, the PHN is expected to be "proficient" (rather than knowledgeable or aware) in each of the domains. Each domain has specific criteria listed. The AACN supports doctoral education for community/public health nursing. This is noted in Essential VII of doctoral education (AACN, 2006). The Quad Council Competencies and the AACN document complement each other. Both documents recognize the advanced level of practice that is needed in the PHN role and the complexities that this role embraces. Doctoral education is imperative to meet these demanding components of PHN practice in the context of an ever-changing healthcare environment; the PHN must seek doctoral education to practice to the fullest extent of his or her ability and license (Quad Council of Public Health Nursing Organizations, 2009).

National Public Health Performance Standards Program

The office of the Chief of Public Health Practice, Centers for Disease Control and Prevention (CDC), has led a partnership with national public health organizations to develop a program to "improve the practice of public health, the performance of public health systems, and the infrastructure supporting public health actions" (CDC, n.d.). These performance standards are key components of an accreditation process for government public health agencies similar to that used in acute care settings. The accreditation process is currently being carried out by the Public Health Accreditation Board (PHAB), and state and local boards of health are in the process of submitting applications (PHAB, 2013).

As the practice of public health moves toward standards for accreditation, the PHN must be educated at an appropriate level and be able to practice in an environment with high expectations to serve the population in an era of growing concern aimed at population-level assessment, interventions, and outcome measures. There is a need for DNP-prepared PHNs to fill roles in this type of environment. The vision, mission, and goals put forth by the National Public Health Performance Standards Program align with the education and practice of a PHN with a DNP degree. This initiative indicates the high standards expected of public health practitioners. The convergence of the PHAB accreditation standards and the emergence of DNP-prepared PHNs speaks to the importance of the level of education needed for PHNs to provide leadership and to guide public health nursing practice.

Theoretical Framework for Nursing Practice in Public Health

There are multiple issues to consider in providing good quality care to populations. A strategy that encompasses the multifaceted nature of public health work is the ecological approach (Stanhope & Lancaster, 2012). As noted in the example of Wald's work, multiple factors impact the health of individuals and populations. These multiple factors are termed "determinants of health" and include (1) health, social, economic, cultural, and environmental conditions; (2) family, social, and living conditions; and (3) individual traits and biological factors. It is the linkages between all these factors that are important to consider as interventions are developed to affect the health of populations. The ecological model provides a structure that incorporates these linkages (Quad Council of Public Health Nursing Organizations, 2011).

The diagram in **Figure 9-2** incorporates the ecological approach at the center. This approach illustrates how the goals of the action model for *Healthy People 2020* initiative converge with the work of PHNs (U.S. Department of Health and Human Services, 2008, p. 7).

Two initiatives, one at the global level and one at the national level, highlight these concepts as PHNs work in population-based programs that incorporate the principles of the ecological approach. The Millennium Development Goals (MDGs) were established in 2002 from the Millennium Project commissioned by the United Nations Secretary-General. The charge of this project was to develop a concrete action plan to "reverse the grinding poverty, hunger, and disease affecting billions of people" (United Nations, 2002). There are eight MDGs, which range from reducing extreme poverty by 50% to enhancing environmental stability. All eight goals are associated with the determinants of health described earlier and operationalize the definitions of public health and public health nursing.

Vision
A society in which all people live long, healthy lives.

Mission
To improve health through strengthening policy and practice,

Healthy People will:

- Identify nationwide health improvement priorities;
- Increase public awareness and understanding of the determinants of health, disease, and disability and the opportunities for progress;
- Provide measurable objectives and goals that can be used at the national, state, and local levels;
- Engage multiple sectors to take actions that are driven by the best available evidence and knowledge;
- Identify critical research and data collection needs.

Figure 9-2 *Healthy People 2020* Vision and Mission Statement
Secretary's Advisory Committee on National Health Promotion and Disease Prevention Objectives for 2020. (2008). Phase 1 report: Recommendations for the framework and format of *Healthy People 2020*, p. 5. Retrieved from https://www.healthypeople.gov/sites/default/files/PhaseI_0.pdf

On a national level in the United States, the Healthy People initiative has driven public health programs and awareness over the past 40 years. There have been four previous initiatives, in 1979, 1990, 2000, and 2010. *Healthy People 2020* is now providing goals and objectives to guide national health promotion and disease prevention strategies to improve the health of all people over the next decade. The overarching goals of this initiative for 2020 are to (U.S. Department of Health and Human Services, 2008):

1. Attain high quality, longer lives, free from preventable disease, disability, injury, and premature death
2. Achieve health equity, eliminate disparities, and improve the health of all groups
3. Create social and physical environments that promote good health for all
4. Promote quality of life, healthy development, and healthy behaviors across all life stages

Educational Preparation and Credentialing

In today's nursing education environment, baccalaureate programs that prepare beginning practitioners typically include public health nursing content, theory, and clinical practice. This allows the new nurse to practice as a beginning staff-level PHN. This is similar to the new graduate beginning a medical-surgical position in an acute care setting. Additional orientation time is likely required as the new graduate transitions from the student role to practice. Some states (e.g., Minnesota, California) also have PHN certification for baccalaureate graduates who apply to the state board of nursing. This certification acknowledges the PHN content in the curriculum and allows the individual to use the PHN credentials with his or her title.

Specializing in public health nursing requires an advanced degree. Currently, a master's degree in nursing is required to sit for a certification exam administered by the ANCC (2012). In the future, it is likely that the DNP will be the required prerequisite for taking this certification exam. The 1984 Consensus Conference on the Essentials of Public Health Nursing Practice and Education sponsored by the U.S. Department of Health and Human Services Division of Nursing identified that minimal qualifications for a PHN include a baccalaureate degree in nursing and that specialists in the field hold either a master's or doctorate degree that focuses on public health sciences and have the ability to work with populations to assess and intervene at the aggregate level (U.S. Department of Health and Human Services, Health Resources and Services Administration, Bureau of Health Professionals, Division of Nursing, 1984). ACHNE has affirmed this position, and the ANA has also supported this position in *Public Health Nursing: Scope and Standards of Practice* (ANA, 2013; Quad Council of Public Health Nursing Organizations, 2011).

Roles of Advanced Practice PHNs

The roles of advanced practice public and community health nurses have evolved over time. States have the authority to determine the scope of practice of a PHN. For instance, in Virginia, PHN roles reflect the essential elements of the National Association of County Health Officials contained within the *Blueprint for a Healthy Community*. The nine essential elements are: (1) conducting community assessments; (2) preventing and controlling epidemics; (3) providing a safe and healthy environment; (4) measuring performance, effectiveness, and outcome of health services; (5) promoting healthy lifestyles; (6) providing targeted outreach and forming partnerships; (7) providing personal healthcare services; (8) conducting research and innovation; and (9) mobilizing the community for action. Within each of these essential elements, public health nursing specialists contribute their expertise and leadership to develop programs to promote health and prevent disease; tools to standardize case definitions, data collection, and analysis; indicators to monitor the health status of the population; regulatory guidelines for the prevention of targeted diseases; community partnerships and resources to promote informed decision making for the health of its citizens; direct services to patients for targeted diseases that threaten the health of a community; leadership and advocacy strategies through collaboration, coalition building, and public relations; and healthy community research projects with measurable outcomes (National Association of County Health Officials, 1994).

PHNs with expertise in the field have traditionally been promoted to lead agency-related, population-based health programs as funding is allocated to administer and implement them. PHNs who take on administrative responsibilities write program proposals and testify for the support of these programs at federal and state legislative committees and jurisdictional board meetings. Programs routinely led by PHNs include immunizations; family, maternal, and child health; disease prevention and control; family planning; health promotion; emergency preparedness; school health; senior services; home care refugee health; healthcare services; children with disabilities; women, infants, and children (WIC); chronic disease; adults with disabilities; and environmental health (ASTDN, 2008). Furthermore, advanced practice PHNs who work in the public policy and advocacy arenas serve as executive nurse leaders at departments of health in each state to: (1) represent nursing issues within the health department; (2) ensure effectiveness, efficiency, and quality of programs and services delivered; (3) ensure a workforce prepared for the nursing needs of the state; and (4) collaborate with educational systems to ensure the quality of the future public health nursing workforce (ASTDN, 2008). The roles of advanced practice PHNs, who will benefit from the DNP preparation, continue to develop as the complexity of health care increases in proportion to the growth of the population, particularly in relation to the rate of growth of the senior citizen population in the United States.

Practice Sites

PHNs commonly enter practice within a local public health agency that may be governed by a city or county. Proficient public health nursing leaders discover satisfying careers in diverse practice settings. PHNs with expertise in the field are employed in jurisdictional levels that encompass federal, state, regional, county, and city public health agencies. The federal employer may be the U.S. Public Health Service, the CDC, or the American Public Health Association. Advanced PHN expertise is critical to the planning, piloting, and implementation of evidence-based population health programs initiated at the state or federal jurisdiction level. DNP-prepared PHNs will support these leaders with the needed skill sets to perform in the complex socioeconomic environment of health promotion and disease prevention in this country. Advanced practice PhD- and DNP-prepared PHNs are employed in academic settings to teach, direct programs, and conduct research. They are also working in acute and long-term care systems to manage population-based infection prevention, safety, quality improvement, occupational health, and emergency preparedness programs (Stanhope & Lancaster, 2012). Within the last decade, public health nursing leaders have been hired by health systems that provide a continuum of care to their chronically ill or rehabilitating patients in the community to direct hospice, home care, palliative care, complex medical care, and advanced care directive programs. Insurance companies have also benefited from the skills of DNP-prepared PHNs (Stanhope & Lancaster, 2012). These health-integrated organizations are complex, and their operations (Melnyk & Fineout-Overholt, 2011) need to be informed by practice-based evidence related to client outcomes within each specialty program. The DNP-prepared PHN has the academic preparation to address these growing multifaceted demands in the marketplace.

Evidence-Based Practice in Population-Based Public Health Nursing

EBP was introduced into medicine initially to guide professionals' decision making using the best available evidence (Guyatt & Rennie, 2002). Sackett, Straus, and Richardson (2000) later developed the definition for evidence-based medicine that has become an industry standard. This approach seeks to answer a clinical question about an individual patient condition (Guyatt & Rennie, 2002; Sackett et al., 2000). EBP was a 7-step process initiated to make an accurate diagnosis and to prescribe the most appropriate treatment or outcome. When nursing began implementing EBP, the concentration tended to be related to a collection of patients (Leven, Keefe, & Marren, 2010; Melnyk & Fineout-Overholt, 2011). The application of EBP started in acute care and primary care. There is little in the literature about its application to community settings. Examples of EBP that surface in public health nursing when the literature is searched include: (1) the Family Nurse Partnership program, which is designed to help teen mothers make healthy life choices, complete their education, and space future pregnancies (Olds et al., 1997); (2) public health nursing interventions with individuals, families, and the community, and the systems that impact them as modeled by the public health "wheel" (Keller & Strohschein, 2012); (3) survey of the tasks and frequencies performed by PHN participants from local and state health departments in the United States (ASTDN, 2008); (4) mining aggregate electronic data in the public health record for health outcomes and indicators to inform practice (Monsen, 2005); and (5) public health nursing competencies as developed by the Quad Council of Public Health Nursing Organizations (2011). These examples are instrumental in guiding and informing practice and form the basis for further PHN research, which is a key action of the Quad Council of Public Health Nursing Organizations. PHN-initiated research has traditionally been funded by government agencies, such as the National Institutes of Health and the Health Resources and Services Administration, and private foundations, including the Robert Wood Johnson Foundation and the Bill and Melinda Gates Foundation.

The Doctor of Nursing Practice–Prepared Public Health Nurse as Leader

The Association of Community Health Educators (formerly the Association of Graduate Faculty in Community Health Nursing/ Public Health Nursing), established in 1978, has promoted the increase in graduate-level programs to prepare the public health nursing leaders of the future. In addition to holding traditional responsibilities, PHNs are assuming high-functioning roles in the complex planning and implementation of health promotion and maintenance programs in the community.

The skill sets that DNP-prepared nurses bring to the multiagency planning groups involve knowledge about EBP related to population health programs, the science of nursing intervention, policy development, financial astuteness, informatics, patient-centered care, quality improvement, safety, and interprofessional teamwork and collaboration. DNP-prepared public health leaders will be influenced daily by information generated by professional associations and government and nongovernment agencies. These leaders will be expected to access and evaluate this information in relation to its role in advocacy for population-based health programs. DNP-prepared nurses will advocate for population health initiatives in writing, in public testimony, and within interdepartmental and interagency planning groups. PHN nurses are customarily respected in the community by the clients they serve, but a DNP-prepared PHN is better equipped to articulate strategic population health positions effectively with nonnursing professionals, policy planners, and legislative bodies. The public recognizes the nurse as a trusted professional who is now publicly advocating with confidence for the health of the nation (ANA, 2013).

Nurse Entrepreneur

Timothy F. Gardner

Definitions

To aid in the comprehension of how the DNP prepares APNs to become entrepreneurs, one must begin by understanding the definition of what entrepreneurship is; what an entrepreneur does; what the DNP course of study covers; and what all of these have in common. Entrepreneurship by definition "is a process through which individuals identify opportunities, allocate resources, and create value. This creation of value is often through the identification of unmet needs or through the identification of opportunities for change. Entrepreneurs see 'problems' as 'opportunities,' then take action to identify the solutions to those problems and the customers who will pay to have those problems solved. Entrepreneurial success is simply a function of the ability of an entrepreneur to see these opportunities in the marketplace, initiate change (or take advantage of change) and create value through solutions" (Watson, 2011).

An entrepreneur is "one who undertakes innovations, finance and business acumen in an effort to transform innovations into economic goods" (Shane, 2004, p. 205). The attributes and abilities of a successful entrepreneur are self-motivation, autonomy, problem solving, leadership, decision making, risk taking, self-confidence, determination, and being ethical (Dayhoff & Moore, 2003).

Comparatively, the DNP is the highest clinical degree that exists in the profession of nursing, and it is the terminal practice degree for the profession. The DNP is a practice-focused degree and is designed to prepare experts in a specialized advanced practice role (AACN, 2006). The DNP educational course of study builds on the generalist foundation of the core knowledge and competencies of the professional nursing undergraduate bachelor of science in nursing (BSN) and the graduate master's of science in nursing (MSN) degrees for post-MSN DNP programs (AACN, 2006). When envisioning the DNP, the AACN (2006) identified and developed eight core competencies that the DNP graduate will have mastered upon completing the doctoral course of study. These core competencies are in addition to those attained at the BSN and MSN levels of educational preparation. To address these competencies, programs typically have coursework that covers the fields of epidemiology, economics, business management, organizational systems analysis, health policy, EBP, healthcare information technology, and leadership. The majority of programs require students to plan, develop, implement, and evaluate a scholarly project. The purpose of the scholarly project is for students to synthesize, apply, and demonstrate learned concepts (Sperhac & Clinton, 2008). Students are required to complete advanced didactic and clinical coursework in physiology, pathophysiology, pharmacology, health/ physical assessment, and the student's area of specialization, such as acute care, family primary care, midwifery, clinical nurse specialist, nurse anesthetist, and so on (AACN, 2006). Throughout this section, these core essential competencies will be identified as they relate to doctoral educational preparation and entrepreneurship.

It should be noted that the DNP-prepared APN is an independently licensed healthcare professional who performs as an independent and interdependent member of an interdisciplinary healthcare team. As a result of professional licensure and educational preparation, the DNP APN is well positioned to independently own and operate a private business venture.

Background

Embedded throughout the nursing educational process is a combination of the three fundamental specialized skills of problem solving, critical thinking, and decision making. This combination is known in the profession as the nursing process. This trifecta of fundamental skills forms the core entrepreneurial skill essentials of the DNP. Because of their educational underpinnings, DNP entrepreneurs are prepared to perform a needs assessment, identify a problem, develop a plan of action, implement evidence-based interventions, evaluate the plan, and start over if needed. These concepts are not unique to the nursing profession. Critical thinking, problem solving, and decision making are also core concepts of, and basic critical skills in, the business world. The procedural steps of the nursing process are very similar to those actions outlined in the business definition of entrepreneurship.

Nursing today is, and has always been, an eclectic profession with a scope of practice that overlaps with other professional disciplines such as medicine, pharmacology, public health, psychology, sociology, and business in the effort to provide optimal health care. For example, advanced practice nursing combines the holistic perspective of nursing science with specialized knowledge and skill sets obtained from the biomedical sciences, medicine, and pharmacology to provide healthcare services (AACN Essentials I and II; AACN, 2006). Because of this acquired expanded knowledge, APNs are able to use clinical thinking and skills traditionally associated with medicine to obtain a health history, perform a physical examination, and formulate a diagnosis gleaned from the patient's signs, symptoms, and results of ordered diagnostic/laboratory tests in order to develop a treatment plan, including prescribing pharmaceuticals. It should be noted that the expanded knowledge and skills needed to provide these services are now fundamental to the APN educational process and should no longer require medical delegation, protocols, supervision, or mandatory written collaboration (Wisconsin Nurses Association, 2015). Similarly, nursing has incorporated other expanded knowledge and specialized skills from the business profession, such as principles of management, elements of accounting, budgeting, and contract negotiation. Given these overlapping scopes of practice, the DNP-prepared APN possesses great entrepreneurial potential.

The Relationship of Entrepreneurship and the DNP Degree

Doctoral-level education provides the nurse entrepreneur with expanded knowledge and specialized skill sets necessary to navigate and thrive in today's complex healthcare environment, not simply to become a clinician with "the ability to design and deliver effective care to patients" (Hanson & Bennett, 2005, p. 543). In addition, the "enhanced leadership, policy making and collaboration skills" obtained during the course of study positions the DNP entrepreneur to "make changes at the system and practice setting level" (Hanson & Bennett, 2005, p. 543). This enables the DNP-prepared entrepreneur to function as an administrator, educator, consultant, and community leader and to operate as an agent of change in legislation and policy making (depending on his or her area of expertise). Doctoral-level education enhances the entrepreneur's ability to analyze and bring evidence-based research from the laboratory and scientific literature to the clinical arena. This area addresses AACN Essential III (AACN, 2006). This is in line with the AACN's position that requires the DNP educational process to be designed to prepare the graduate APN to gain competence in the application of research to practice, to be able to evaluate evidence and research findings for decision making, and to implement potential innovations to change current clinical practice. It is also the AACN's position that during the course of study, significant consideration should be given to programmatic decision making and program evaluation using assessment data collected at the population or cohort level (AACN, 2006, p. 2).

However, in the call for healthcare restructuring by institutions such as the IOM and the National Research Council of the National Academies (NRCNA), the consistent mantra has been "patient-centered care." By definition, patient-centered care is "healthcare that establishes a partnership among practitioners, patients, and their families (when appropriate) to ensure that decisions respect patients' wants, needs, and preferences and that patients have the education and support they need to make decisions and participate in their own care" (American Academy of Family Physicians, American Academy of Pediatrics, American College of Physicians, & American Osteopathic Association, 2010). In patient-centered care, the central theme is that a healthcare provider can provide care for only one individual at a time, and therefore, the tenets of population-based care belong in the public health domain and should not be the guiding principles of an individual healthcare practitioner (Peraino, 2011).

Herein lies a conundrum. How can a doctoral education process that focuses on the tenets of EBP with data obtained from population-based research studies effectively support the call for patient-centered care? The appropriate answer would be through individualizing the findings. However, EBP, as it is currently implemented in health care, does not individualize care; rather, it standardizes care through clinical guidelines, protocols, and best practices. It must be remembered that all research findings are not generalizable. Is it prudent for all healthcare decisions to be based on the cultural health beliefs, values, and behaviors of an individual patient's racial and ethnic background? Isn't this racial profiling and cultural stereotyping? Consequently, this does not constitute patient-centered care; it is providing care based on the patient's culture and ethnicity (Hasnain-Wynia, 2006).

In answering these questions, the doctoral educational process prepares the DNP graduate to obtain population-based information, individualize the findings based on the individual patient's risk assessment, and use this information to provide high-quality, evidence-based, patient-centered care (AACN Essential VII; AACN, 2006). Other provisions of the call for restructuring include providing care that is "safe, effective . . . timely, efficient, and equitable . . . as members of an interdisciplinary team, emphasizing evidence-based practice, quality improvement, and informatics," and the report calls for nursing to have "the best prepared senior level nurses in key leadership positions and participating in executive decisions" (AACN, 2006, p. 6). Again, the doctoral education process prepares the DNP graduate to meet these needs and provide care that addresses all these provisions. DNP-prepared entrepreneurs must have these added competencies to enhance the development of their personal professional business and practice management.

Business and Practice Management

Doctoral education will prepare the nurse entrepreneur to plan, organize, finance, and operate his or her own business venture. DNP programs typically offer courses that address practice management, economics, and management of the client in the healthcare system, healthcare information technology, and project planning and evaluation in order to strengthen business acumen and performance. The DNP core courses and advanced practice specialization provide the nurse entrepreneur with the scientific underpinning for practice, and expert advanced clinical knowledge and skills to provide direct and indirect care in an area of role specialization (AACN Essentials I and VIII; AACN, 2006). Knowledge of direct and indirect care processes is vital for the successful management of healthcare systems, regardless of the organization's size or capacity (Hanson & Bennett, 2005).

Doctoral-level education enables the APN to participate in both direct and indirect care processes within the scope of the role. It prepares the nurse entrepreneur to design and develop healthcare services provided to clients. Providing direct care to clients/patients is a central competency of an APN regardless of the specific specialized role of the practitioner (Tracy, 2005). However, many tasks performed are the same across various specialty APN roles (Tracy, 2005). For example, role specialization prepares the DNP-educated primary care nurse to participate in direct care processes, such as obtaining comprehensive medical histories; performing physical examinations; diagnosing, treating, and managing acute and chronic illnesses and diseases; and performing minor procedures such as suturing, incision and drainage, and intrauterine device insertion. Direct care processes also include providing services such as wound management, pain management, counseling, and education; providing health promotion and disease prevention services (AACN Essential VII; AACN, 2006); and using electronic medical records and e-prescribing (AACN Essential IV; AACN, 2006). Some of these tasks may fall under the role of clinical nurse specialist and other advanced practice nursing roles (Hanson & Bennett, 2005; Tracy, 2005).

Indirect processes of care include organizational, administrative, and operational systems. The DNP-educated entrepreneur, regardless of area of specialization, will incur control over, and responsibility for, an increased proportion of indirect processes of care within the specialty role. These may include administration, budgeting, management, inventory and purchasing, quality control, risk management, development of office policies and procedures, supervision of staff, mentoring, medical coding and billing, and reimbursement issues. Other important indirect processes include the assessment and acquisition of appropriate office computer systems and information technology software that requires knowledge of Certification Commission for Health Information Technology-certified electronic health record (EHR) programs (AACN Essential IV; AACN, 2006; Hanson & Bennett, 2005).

The scholarly project that is undertaken and completed during the course of DNP study prepares the entrepreneurial nurse with the specialized knowledge and skills of project management and evaluation. Knowledge of these principles enables the nurse to (1) identify a systems-based problem; (2) perform a scholarly literature review; (3) develop process and outcome objectives; (4) develop, plan, and implement evidence-based interventions to address the problem; and (5) develop, implement, manage, and evaluate program outcomes. This again demonstrates the eclectic nature of nursing and its overlapping scope of practice with other professional disciplines such as engineering and project management.

Practice Start-Up, Closure, and Credentialing

Given that this is a discussion on nursing entrepreneurship, it is appropriate to highlight basic tenets of business, including start-up, merger, and closure procedures, and credentialing with commercial insurance carriers. Although specific rules and regulations for establishing a business may vary by state, these general guidelines are essential for nursing entrepreneurs. Independence in practice is the cornerstone of nursing entrepreneurship. In contemplation of the start of a new practice, it is necessary to review the state board of nursing statutes and the state medical association guidelines applicable to the location where the practice is to open. This review will provide thorough detail of regulatory requirements and outline scope of practice guidelines, licensure, and other necessary credentialing requirements, such as a collaborative agreement (in some states). Additionally, local rules and requirements pertaining to licensing and liability must be reviewed thoroughly before the start of practice. This portion of the review may include business name search.

Another essential area for entrepreneurs deciding to open a new practice is a review of the business regulations set forth by the Internal Revenue Service (IRS), which can be accessed at www.irs.gov or by contacting your local IRS agency. This information is critical in establishing the new business as a federally recognized entity through obtaining a federal identification number (FIN), which is separate from an individual taxpayer identification number (TIN) and used for annual tax reporting purposes. Here, the expertise of an IRS business professional or certified public accountant (CPA) is a sound investment in the future of your new practice.

To begin the process of starting a new practice, start at the prospective state's medical association. For example, the Indiana State Medical Association (ISMA) provides prospective business owners with basic information on starting a practice. The ISMA has a packet of information on starting a practice that includes setting up the legal entity, obtaining licensure, National Provider Identifier numbers, payer contracts, and malpractice insurance. The prospective owner is advised to contact ISMA's legal department for the full packet (ISMA, 2015).

Additionally, ISMA provides information concerning provider retirement, closing a practice, and leaving a practice. The information available on this site will answer specific questions pertaining to practice terminations, including standard processes for giving patient notice, credentials management, and handling of medical records. This information may be used in conjunction with existing practice policies of the independent or group practice to ensure proper termination actions.

Another area of concern for APNs or nurse practitioners (NPs) is credentialing. This is because each insurance company may reserve the right to adhere to its own business policies as they reflect current laws and practice guidelines. What this means is that in any given state, each insurance company within that state can have a different set of policies and operate under those policies so long as operations do not violate the law. So why credential?

Although credentialing does not guarantee insurance company contracting with APNs or NPs as primary care providers (PCPs), whether individually, as specialists, or part of a group, credentialing is vital to independent practice recognition and most essential to enrollment with many health insurance companies for reimbursement purposes. This is often a tedious and time-consuming process because each individual insurance or health organization may require different information for credentialing considerations. Many health insurance providers, such as Anthem, United Healthcare, and Tricare, require credentialing with Medicaid and Medicare for participation.

To circumvent this dilemma, credentialing is best accomplished through completion of the online enrollment form from the Council for Affordable Quality Healthcare (CAQH) Universal Provider Datasource (UPD) service. The UPD is the industry standard for collecting provider data used in credentialing: "The UPD is a unique streamlined electronic data collection system that enables physicians and other health professionals, participating health plans, hospitals, and healthcare organizations the ability to access, manage, revise, and verify professional credentials" (CAQH, 2015). Further, "the UPD online form meets the data-collection requirements of URAC, the National Committee for Quality Assurance (NCQA) and the Joint Commission standards. Indiana, Kansas, Kentucky, Louisiana, Maryland, Missouri, New Jersey, New Mexico, Ohio, Rhode Island, Tennessee, Vermont, and the District of Columbia have adopted the CAQH standard form as their mandated or designated provider credentialing application" (CAQH, 2015).

In addition, a resource to assist the DNP entrepreneur in obtaining insurance credentialing can be found through the National Nursing Centers Consortium (NNCC), a premier organization for the advocacy and support of nurse-managed clinics. The NNCC offers nurse entrepreneurs a managed care contracting toolkit with a "7-step process specifically designed to walk the APN through the insurance credentialing process for reimbursement and proper recognition as a primary care provider (PCP)," following its mission statement of "advancing nurse-led health care through policy, consultation, programs and applied research to reduce health disparities and to meet people's primary care and wellness needs" (NNCC, 2015). It should be noted here that although there are many layers and levels of credentialing, the nurse entrepreneur must be cognizant of the distinct requirements for proper licensure, liability, and reimbursement and be prepared to take necessary actions to comply with federal, state, and local laws.

Organizational Systems Leadership and Collaboration

Doctoral education prepares the nurse entrepreneur to assume leadership positions and understand the basic principles of strategic planning, organizational management, systems thinking, and interprofessional collaboration. The DNP-educated entrepreneur will have the knowledge necessary to develop the skills to become a successful and effective leader. As a leader, the entrepreneur must be visionary and creative. Doctoral education includes coursework on strategic planning that involves exercises on developing vision and vision statements. Consequently, these exercises instill in the nurse entrepreneur the concept that "any success achieved in life must begin with a vision" (Love, 2005). A vision is defined as forming a detailed mental picture of exactly what you intend to accomplish or produce. "The visionary entrepreneur is able to see exactly what his or her business is going to look like in every detail when it is finished . . . a visionary entrepreneur constantly thinks in terms of innovation, and continually searches for opportunities for innovation and implementation" (Love, 2005).

Potential opportunities for "innovation come through the creation of a new process" (direct or indirect) or with the redesigning of an existing process to render it more cost effective, efficient, and profitable (Hanson & Bennett, 2005, p. 544). In the effort to be successful and maintain success, it is essential that DNP-educated entrepreneurs "develop, implement, and continuously analyze direct and indirect processes of care" they may use to meet healthcare outcomes for their clients (Hanson & Bennett, 2005, p. 543). More often than not, this will occur when "working within the constraints of available resources and reimbursement" (Hanson & Bennett, 2005, p. 543), especially during these unsettled economic times when healthcare dollars are very sparse.

The DNP-educated entrepreneur exhibits transformational leadership and will be capable of clearly conveying the corporate vision to tap into the creativity of other members of the organization as potential sources of new ideas. This entrepreneur uses systems thinking and has an understanding of the principles of systems theory, chaos theory, and the butterfly effect as they apply to an organization. The DNP-educated entrepreneur is apt in utilizing other principles of organizational systems thinking and leadership styles, such as team, situational, and participative leadership. Of the three, team leadership is most pertinent in health care today. This is in line with the AACN's position stating that DNP graduates will "have preparation in methods of effective team leadership and are prepared to play a central role in establishing interprofessional teams, participating in the work of the team, and assuming leadership of the team when appropriate" (2006, p. 14).

The entrepreneur is often the major risk taker in a business venture and at times may need to employ alternative leadership styles. The DNP-prepared nurse entrepreneur understands that leadership is about accomplishing critical tasks for the organization, and in some business situations, an autocratic or paternalistic style of decision making may be required. On the other hand, DNP-educated nurse entrepreneurs understand that interprofessional collaboration is essential to practicing effectively (AACN Essential VI; AACN, 2006). According to the AACN's position, "today's highly complex multi-tiered health care environment depends on the contribution of highly skilled and knowledgeable individuals from multiple professions," and "healthcare professionals must function as highly collaborative teams" (AACN, IOM, & O'Neil, as cited in AACN, 2006, p. 14). Doctoral education prepares the entrepreneur to understand both the clinical microcosm and the macrocosm of health care, which define practice and directly influence their ability to provide care (AACN Essential II; AACN, 2006).

The DNP-prepared nurse entrepreneur understands healthcare policies and legislative issues that "facilitate or impede the delivery of health care services or the ability of the provider to engage in practice to address health care needs" (AACN, 2006, p. 13).

Healthcare Policy and Legislative Issues

Doctoral education provides the nurse entrepreneur with the essential skills to function in the arena of political activism. Courses and class activities provide the student with learning experiences that deal with healthcare policy and legislative issues. This addresses AACN Essential V of the DNP educational process, which states that the graduate should possess the ability to "analyze the policy process and . . . to engage in politically competent action" (O'Grady, as cited in AACN, 2006, p. 13) and "design, influence, and implement health care policies that frame health care financing, practice regulation, access, safety, quality, and efficacy" (IOM, as cited in AACN, 2006, p. 13). Now more than ever, it is imperative that nurses, especially nurse entrepreneurs, be able to function competently in the political arena during these very volatile times in health care as critical decisions concerning nursing's scope of practice are being pondered by legislative and judicial systems.

Current and Future Trends

In the current healthcare environment, DNP-prepared entrepreneurs are standing on the threshold of playing key roles as leaders and agents of change at the decision-making tables and in the clinical setting as primary care providers. As stated in the IOM's landmark report on the future of nursing, the DNP-prepared nurse must be capable of functioning "from the bedside to the board room" (IOM, 2010, p. 6). All of this is a result of a perfect storm playing out in health care today as fewer medical students pursue careers in general practice, thus increasing the shortage in available primary care physicians. These factors, combined with the soaring costs of health care, an aging population that is living longer, chronic health problems, and the implementation of the Affordable Care Act, indicate a growing need for high-quality, affordable, and available health services. As a result, there is an increased demand for primary care services such as those provided by the healthcare professional created to address this problem over 40 years ago: the APN (Robert Wood Johnson Foundation, 2011). These circumstances position the DNP-prepared APN entrepreneur to be a viable complement to the traditional physician internist or primary care provider for the health care–seeking consumer. Other precipitating factors, such as lack of appreciation, subordination to physicians, role diminution, low wages, short staffing, poor working conditions, inflexible schedules, frequent schedule changes, and burn-out, have reduced the number of experienced professional nurses in the United States, further ripening the field of opportunity for nurse entre-preneurs ("Nurse Practitioners as Entrepreneurs," 2008; Wood, 2009).

Commercial opportunities abound for DNP-prepared entrepreneurs in private practice, foundations, retail clinics, legal and business consulting, journalism, education, information technology development, pharmaceu-ticals, and organizational management and administration ("Nurse Prac-titioners as Entrepreneurs," 2008). As barriers to practice are eliminated and the national move for true autonomous APN practice progresses, the future is very promising for DNP-prepared entrepreneurs in the business world. This effort has been greatly bolstered by the findings of the IOM's landmark report (IOM, 2010, p. 4), which calls for restructuring of the current healthcare system to allow "nurses to practice to the full extent of their education and training" by removing the scope of practice barri-ers that currently exist in the system. At present, the regulations defining APN scope of practice vary widely from state to state (IOM, 2010, p. 4). This is one major hurdle that must be addressed. Another is the recogni-tion and impaneling of APNs as primary care providers by government agencies, insurance companies, and third-party payers, whether APNs are part of a physicians group or in independent practice. These changes are destined to happen; there is no turning back at this point. Nursing at all levels will play significant supporting and defining roles in the restruc-turing of the healthcare system that is under way in the United States.

The nursing profession must learn to speak in one voice to address pro-fessional issues. By speaking in one voice, the nursing profession, which includes over 3.1 million nurses (Health Resources and Services Adminis-tration, 2010), becomes a very formidable presence in the political arena and at the decision-making tables. The doctorally educated nurse entrepreneur is prepared to accept the challenge of leading change. During the restruc-turing, it is imperative that the profession learn to speak in one strong voice. The profession must not sit idly at the sidelines and allow other pro-fessions, agencies, and entities to decide and define what these roles will be.

Biosketches of Select Successful DNP Entrepreneurs

Margaret A. Fitzgerald

Margaret A. Fitzgerald, DNP, FNP-BC, NP-C, FAANP, CSP, FAAN, DCC, is the founder, president, and principal lecturer of Fitzgerald Health Education Associates, Inc. (FHEA), an international provider of NP certification preparation and continuing education for healthcare providers. More than 60,000 NPs have used the Fitzgerald review course to successfully prepare for certification.

An internationally recognized presenter, Dr. Fitzgerald has provided thousands of programs for numerous professional organizations, universities, and national and state healthcare associations on a wide variety of topics, including clinical pharmacology, assessment, laboratory diagnosis, and health care and NP practice. For more than 20 years, she has provided graduate-level pharmacology courses for NP students at a number of universities, including Simmons College (Boston, MA), Husson College (Bangor, ME), University of Massachusetts Worcester, Pennsylvania State University, La Salle University (Philadelphia, PA), and Samford University (Birmingham, AL). She is a family NP at the Greater Lawrence Family Health Center, Lawrence, Massachusetts, and adjunct faculty for the Greater Lawrence Family Health Center Family Practice Residency Program. She holds a DNP degree from Case Western Reserve University, Cleveland, Ohio, where she received the Alumni Association Award for Clinical Excellence. She is also certified by the American Board of Comprehensive Care as a Diplomate of Comprehensive Care (DCC), a designation available to DNP graduates who are licensed advanced practice registered nurses (APRNs) and nationally certified in an APRN specialty.

Dr. Fitzgerald is the recipient of the NONPF's Lifetime Achievement Award, given in recognition of vision and accomplishments in successfully developing and promoting the NP role; the American College of Nurse Practitioners Sharp Cutting Edge Award; and the Outstanding Nurse Award for Clinical Practice by the Merrimack Valley Area Health Education Council. She is also a fellow of the American Academy of Nursing and a charter fellow in the Fellows of the AANP. Dr. Fitzgerald is a Professional Member of the National Speakers Association and is the first NP to earn the Certified Speaking Professional (CSP) designation in recognition of excellence and integrity as a speaker.

Dr. Fitzgerald is an editorial board member for the *Nurse Practitioner Journal*, *Medscape Nurses*, Lexi-Comp, Inc., *American Nurse Today*, and *Prescriber's Letter*. She is widely published, with more than 100 articles, book chapters, monographs, and audio and video programs to her credit. Her book, *Nurse Practitioner Certification Examination and Practice Preparation* (2nd edition), received the *American Journal of Nursing* Book of the Year Award for Advanced Practice Nursing and has been published in English and Korean. She has provided consultation to nursing organizations in the United States, Canada, the Dominican Republic, Japan, South Korea, Hong Kong, and the United Kingdom. Dr. Fitzgerald is an active member of numerous professional organizations at national and local levels.

Providing a description of her business, Dr. Fitzgerald stated, "Fitzgerald Health Education Associates, Inc. (FHEA), an NP-owned company, is the industry leader in NP certification review, as well as a major provider of ongoing NP education and university courseware. FHEA delivers the most up-to-date, evidence-based NP certification exam preparation available, while also providing practicing nurse practitioners and other healthcare providers with the continuing education and resources needed to maintain professional competence." In regard to her perspective on how the DNP degree has enhanced her current practice and/or business, Dr. Fitzgerald stated,

> *The purpose of the Doctor of Nursing Practice study is to provide rigorous education to prepare clinical scholars who translate science to improve population health through expert leadership that powers innovation in health care. I serve my profession in a number of roles; entrepreneur, scholar, and clinician. As part of my DNP studies at Case Western Reserve University, I developed a business plan for the expansion of Fitzgerald Health Education Associates, Inc., with the project's focus being the NP certification preparation course. The process of developing the business plan afforded the opportunity to delve into areas that would be critical to the company's success and helped me to realize the significant possibilities in this niche market. My capstone project focused on the NP certification marketplace. These products of my DNP studies directly have influenced my business's success. I also practice as a family NP and Adjunct Faculty to the Family Practice Residency at the Greater Lawrence (MA) Family Health Center. As a result of my DNP, my ability*

*to critique healthcare literature has been further enhanced,
reinforcing my role as a clinical scholar and teacher.*

In sharing her thoughts on nurse entrepreneurship, Dr. Fitzgerald
further stated,

> *As a nurse entrepreneur, I quickly realized that nursing
> practice is business practice. The strong clinical assessment
> skills of the advanced practice nurse, the ability to analyze
> a problem, study options to work towards the problem's
> resolution, develop a plan to address the problem, perform
> ongoing evaluation, and adjust intervention to ensure the
> desired outcome, serve the entrepreneur well. In addition,
> DNP prepares the nurse leader; leadership is critical to
> entrepreneurship. The successful entrepreneur must have
> expert intrapersonal skills, possess initiative, and be risk
> tolerant; again, these are skills that are developed as part of
> nursing education and critical to nursing practice. While not
> all nurses aspire to be entrepreneurs, nurse trailblazers can
> fulfill the role of the intra-preneur, applying the entrepreneur's
> skill set within an organization. The nurse intra-preneur
> [sic] provides the forward-thinking mind set needed,
> focusing on creativity, innovation, and leadership. (Personal
> communication, December 16, 2011)*

David O'Dell

Dr. David O'Dell is a professor in the Chamberlain College of Nursing DNP program, with a part-time faculty practice in neurology with a special interest in neurocognitive disorders and coordinating family dynamics. Outside of these roles, Dr. O'Dell is the lead member of Doctors of Nursing Practice, Inc., an organization founded by a small group of students at the University of Tennessee Health Science Center in 2006, which today has grown from a small website that shared static information about the DNP role to a robust site with many components, features, and benefits. The site has several databases describing DNP scholarly projects, DNP programs, and their characteristics, as well as a bibliography and a careers page. The online networking feature specifically aims to build the DNP community and has approximately 6,000 current members and a mailing list of approximately 9,000 nurses from a wide background to include advanced practice, administration, informatics, students, faculty, and those interested in the growth and development of the DNP degree. The site encourages open discussions through forums, blogs, a listing of events, and specialty groups as a result of participant interests that have helped to form an identifiable and consequential community. The site has been instrumental in building a community of DNP-prepared nursing professionals bolstering the strength and reach of the nursing profession. Another important function of the organization is the development and management of an annual national DNP conference. Dr. O'Dell is also a site evaluator for the CCNE. The CCNE, the nation's top nursing school review body, evaluates baccalaureate, graduate, and residency programs in nursing to ensure that they meet the standards set forth by the AACN. Dr. O'Dell purports that the DNP degree has afforded him the opportunity to enhance his clinical, academic, and professional life. The DNP degree and past professional experiences have allowed him to assume his academic role to continue to enhance efforts to grow the profession while bolstering an organization with the mission of DNP growth and development. He believes these efforts would not have been possible if not for the DNP degree. Dr. O'Dell believes that, as a result of the DNP degree and the dynamics caused by the growth in DNP graduates, the DNP, Inc. website and online community continue to grow, and the need for community development continues. The need for educational venues and platforms to evaluate the contributions of DNP-prepared professionals also continues and no doubt will expand in the future. He believes these are exciting times to be a nurse and a DNP. Dr. O'Dell surmises that entrepreneurship has been a natural phenomenon for him. He states that he incorporated his professional life many years ago with the recognition that a business entity has more opportunities to augment and grow than an individual. He further stated, "I've maintained and plan to always work within my self-created corporate structure." Similarly, the business entity of DNP, Inc. affords many opportunities for growth and development in the profession that individuals could not appreciate in isolation. The opportunities for growth and development of the profession of the discipline as a result of the collective contributions of professional colleagues cannot be underestimated. The creation of the DNP, Inc. organization has evolved into the generation of other areas of service, to include continuing education, a foundation, and plans for an online journal. These efforts are in keeping with the mission of professional growth and development for the DNP-prepared professional.

Dr. O'Dell believes that an alternate perspective on nurse entrepreneurship is that "We are all business people in our own way. All professionals, regardless of the discipline, have something to contribute in whatever environment we choose to flourish. No matter where we are in our professional lives, we all contribute and attempt to enhance the flow and outcomes as a result of our individual and collective efforts. This is an entrepreneurial spirit that can be satisfied within and outside of [an] existing organization. Therefore, we are all *in the same boat* trying to move it up stream." On a personal note, Dr. O'Dell believes that his own entrepreneurial spirit has allowed him to experience great satisfaction as a business owner and as a developer of an organization designed to enhance the discipline of nursing through the facilitation of the growth of the professional DNP degree (personal communication, October 10, 2011).

Carol Lisa Alexander

Dr. Carol Lisa Alexander is cofounder, president, and CAO of CAAN Academy of Nursing. Over the past 34 years, Dr. Alexander has committed herself to caring for the medically underserved, vulnerable, economically disadvantaged, and at-risk populations. During this period, she actively advanced her educational background to more effectively accomplish her goals. Those goals are to promote and improve healthcare services within the minority community, thereby decreasing the existing healthcare disparity. Dr. Alexander is a postmaster's DNP-prepared board-certified clinical nurse specialist presently serving in the role of NP and providing medical healthcare services for the Aunt Martha's Healthcare Network in Illinois.

Dr. Alexander is the visionary for the Coalition of African American Nurses (CAAN), founded in 2002 in an effort to decrease the existing healthcare disparities in her inner-city community. With the realization that nurses are critical in keeping people healthy and safe, Dr. Alexander cofounded CAAN Academy of Nursing with Rose M. Murray, RN, MS, ACNS-BC, in 2007. Dr. Alexander's vision for CAAN is "to inspire, motivate, cultivate, and educate nurses woven in the moral fibers of care and compassion."

Dr. Alexander serves as the administrator for CAAN and an educator for the CAAN Academy of Nursing. She is an active member of Rotary International and serves on the board of directors for the Illinois

Nurses Association (INA) District 20 and the board of directors for the Governors State University (GSU) Alumni Association. Dr. Alexander serves on the advisory board of Southland Healthcare Career Forum and is an active lifetime member of the Chicago Chapter of the National Black Nurses Association (CCNBNA). She is a member of Sigma Theta Tau Nursing Honor Society—Lambda Lambda Chapter GSU, and the Meadow-lake Homeowners Association, to mention a few.

In regard to the synergy of possessing the DNP degree and entrepreneurship, Dr. Alexander stated,

> *I found the course content from my DNP program an essential aid in the strategic plan in developing our business plan. The program also influenced the building of my character in my assuming the leadership role. The ongoing conceptualization of leadership throughout my DNP program actually gave me a more in-depth initiation to translate evidence-based research into practice "right here" and "right now." The courses guided me in refining my leadership skills most specifically in communicating the vision, the ideas and the needs of the organization, which proved indispensable in contract negotiations. The concept of communication infiltrated every course, redefining the essentials in negotiating, delegating, planning, and managing financial resources effectively and efficiently.*
>
> *The structure of my administrative courses allowed me to recognize that it is acceptable to operate at various levels of competencies in the role of leadership. I acknowledge that I have developed many leadership role competencies demonstrated within the following: identifying and meeting my customers/partners' needs and expectations expeditiously. In conducting my business, I have learned the significance in having a strong ethical value system which provides for obtaining mutual respectable outcomes in negotiations. CAAN is partnered with two other major community organizations. Our company has received grant funding that is supporting*

our adult students. One of those partners is Governors State University, the institution where I received my DNP. My DNP program has not only afforded me the academic tools that I need in order to be successful but has extended itself beyond to aid in the financial support of the vision and success of the program. To date, we have 74 students in our adult program and 29 in our high school program. (Personal communication, December 10, 2011)

Integrative Practitioner

Joy Elwell, Kathryn Waud White, and Mary E. Zaccagnini

According to Dr. Andrew Weil, integrative medicine "is healing-oriented medicine that takes account of the whole person (body, mind, and spirit), including all aspects of lifestyle. It emphasizes the therapeutic relationship and makes use of appropriate therapies, both conventional and alternative" (Lemley, 2015). An example would be the use of ginger or peppermint to prevent nausea in oncology patients undergoing chemotherapy.

Integrative health care continues to be a choice for Americans. The CDC's National Health Statistics Report on Complementary and Alternative Medicine (CAM) Use Among Adults and Children (Barnes, Bloom, & Nahin, 2008) revealed that 38% of American adults and 12% of children use alternative or complementary therapies of some type. The skills gained in the DNP program will enhance the APN in integrative therapy in accordance with *The Essentials of Doctoral Education for Advanced Nursing Practice*. Essential III, for instance, states that the DNP program prepares APNs to "critically appraise existing literature and other evidence to implement the best evidence for practice" (AACN, 2006). Essential VI speaks to interprofessional collaboration, which is truly an essential for the practice of this specialty that reaches across many different healthcare fields (AACN, 2006). Essential VII describes clinical prevention and population health, all facilitated through integrative health care (AACN, 2006). The DNP-prepared integrative health practitioner will have much to offer patients.

To address the DNP-prepared APN as an integrative practitioner, it is essential to explore integrative health as a specialty within health care. Integrative health, also known as holistic health, is described as "treating the whole person, helping the person to bring the mental, emotional, physical, social, and spiritual dimensions of his or her being into greater harmony, using the basic principles and elements of holistic healing and, as much as possible, placing reliance on treatment modalities that foster the self-regenerative and self-reparatory processes of natural healing" (Otto & Knight, 1979, p. 3). Nursing is an approach to wellness from a holistic perspective and therefore makes nursing and integrative health perfect partners for the APN.

Nurses as Integrative Practitioners

Historically, Florence Nightingale may be considered one of the first professional integrative health practitioners in nursing. Nightingale "was a mystic, visionary, healer, reformer, environmentalist, feminist, practitioner, scientist, politician and global citizen" (Dossey, Selanders, Beck, & Attewell, 2005). She looked beyond the era's traditional medical and surgical treatment of disease and injury to include nutrition, sanitation, lighting, and activity. She addressed the mind, body, and spirit connection that would pave the way for modern professional integrative practitioners.

Since Nightingale's death in 1910, professional nursing has evolved in numerous ways, including the development of advanced practice nursing roles. Numerous nursing pioneers have explored integrative modalities to assist clients in achieving optimum levels of wellness, alleviating suffering, and facilitating healing. Founded in 1980, the American Holistic Nurses Association (AHNA) focuses on holistic nursing as "all nursing practice that has healing the whole person as its goal" (AHNA, n.d.). That nurses practice integrative health is not a novel concept. Major nursing theorists incorporate holism into their theories. Dr. Jean Watson's theory of human caring is one example. She identifies caring beliefs and behaviors that benefit not only the client but the nurse as well.

New York University established the first holistic NP program, and others have followed. Within the United States, certain states (e.g., New York) identify holistic health as a specialty (New York State Office of the Professions, n.d.). There are also clinical nurse specialists in integrative health. The ANA now recognizes holistic nursing as a specialty, and certification can be obtained through the American Holistic Nurses Credentialing Corporation (AHNCC, 2015). In addition, the AHNA has articulated standards of practice, core values, a certification curriculum, and requirements for endorsement of holistic nursing programs. It also is a provider of continuing education in holistic nursing, which now includes a section specific to advanced geriatric education and resources. A current listing of nursing programs endorsed by the AHNCC can be found at http://ahncc.org/home/endorsedschools.html.

Nurses can pursue educational programs for integrative or holistic modalities at all levels of postlicensure preparation. Certification through the AHNCC reflects the level of academic study in the board certification test administered and the credential conferred on the successful applicant. The general requirements for certification include active practice as a holistic nurse for one year (full time) or 2,000 hours in the past 5 years (part time) and 48 contact hours of continuing education in holistic nursing over the preceding 2 years (AHNCC, 2012). APNs who hold a master's or doctoral degree may sit for the Advanced Holistic Nurse Board Certification (APHN-BC) (AHNCC, 2015). Certain roles within the realm of integrative practitioners, such as chiropractors, acupuncturists, and massage therapists, are licensed and have educational requirements. Nurses who pursue these roles must fulfill those requirements in addition to any nursing curriculum.

Types of Integrative Healing Modalities

Integrative health care includes many healing modalities. There are five different approaches to care as organized by the National Center for Complementary and Alternative Medicine (NCCAM): whole medical systems, manipulative and body-based practices, mind–body medicine, biologically based practices, and energy medicine (NCCAM, 2007). The modalities described here are not intended to be an exhaustive list of every integrative healing modality known. **Table 9-1** lists websites where further information can be found.

Whole Medical Systems

- *Homeopathy:* A medical discipline that facilitates healing through the administration of substances prescribed according to three principles: (1) like cures like, also known as the "law of similars"; (2) the more a remedy is diluted, the greater the potency; and (3) illness is specific to the individual. Homeopathy is based on

---

Table 9-1 Websites for Further Information on Integrative Health

American Holistic Nurses Credentialing Corporation
http://www.ahncc.org

Center for Spirituality & Healing at the University of Minnesota
http://www.csh.umn.edu

Life Science Foundation
http://lifesciencesfoundation.org

National Center for Complementary and Alternative Medicine (NCCAM)
http://nccam.nih.gov/health/whatiscam

Academy of Integrative Health & Medicine (AIHM)
https://www.aihm.org

the belief that symptoms are signs of the body's effort to get rid of disease; treatment is based on the whole person rather than on the symptoms (NCCAM, 2009).

- *Osteopathic medicine:* A form of medicine focusing on the relationship between the structure of the body and its function, identifying that both structure and function are subject to a range of illnesses. In treating the client, osteopathic practitioners use various types of physical manipulation to stimulate the body's self-healing ability, as well as traditional allopathic medical modalities. Osteopathic physicians are licensed to diagnose, treat, and prescribe nationally.

Manipulative Modalities

- *Acupressure:* Pressure, by fingers and hands, over specific areas of the body, is used to alleviate pain and discomfort and to positively influence the function of internal organs and body systems. Various approaches are used to release tension and restore the natural flow of energy in the body.
- *Acupuncture:* Use of fine-gauged needles inserted into specific points on the body to stimulate or disperse the flow of energy. This ancient Oriental technique is used to alleviate pain or increase immunity by balancing energy flow. Massage, herbal medicine, and nutritional counseling are often used in conjunction with acupuncture.
- *Alexander technique:* This technique, developed by Australian actor Frederick Matthias Alexander, involves learning a series of lessons in rebalancing the body through awareness, movement, and touch. As the student explores new ways of reorganizing neuromuscular function, the body is reintroduced to healthy posture and direct, efficient movement (Trivieri & Anderson, 2002).
- *AMMA therapy:* AMMA therapy is a form of Oriental massage that focuses on the balance and movement of energy within the body.
- *Applied kinesiology:* Originated by chiropractic physician George Goodheart Jr. in the 1960s, applied kinesiology incorporates the principles of a number of holistic therapies, "including chiropractic, osteopathic medicine and acupuncture, and involves manual manipulation of the spine, extremities, and cranial bones in performing its procedures" (Trivieri & Anderson, 2002, p. 71).
- *Aromatherapy:* Aromatherapy incorporates the use of essential oils extracted from plants and herbs to treat physical imbalances and to achieve psychological and spiritual well-being. The oils

are inhaled, applied externally, or ingested. According to Dr. Kurt Schnaubelt, "the chemical makeup of essential oils gives them a host of desirable pharmacological properties, ranging from antibacterial, antiviral, and antispasmodic, to uses as diuretics, vasodilators, and vasoconstrictors. Essential oils also act on the adrenals, ovaries, and thyroid, and can energize, pacify or detoxify, and facilitate the digestive process" (Trivieri & Anderson, 2002, p. 76).

- *Breema bodywork:* Breema bodywork incorporates simple, playful bodywork sequences along with stretch and movement exercises that help create greater flexibility, a relaxed body, a clear mind, and calm, supportive feelings. Developed by chiropractic physician Jon Schraiber, Breema bodywork is based on nine principles: body comfortable, no extra, firmness and gentleness, full participation, mutual support, no judgment, single moment/single activity, no hurry/no pause, and no force (Mann, 2009).

- *Chiropractic medicine:* A healthcare system emphasizing structural alignment of the spine. Adjustments involve the manipulation of the spine and joints to reestablish and maintain normal nervous system functioning. Some chiropractors employ additional therapies, such as massage, nutrition, and specialized kinesiology.

- *Cranial osteopathy:* Gentle and almost imperceptible manipulation of the skull to reestablish its natural configuration and movement. Such correction can have a positive influence on disorders manifested throughout the body.

- *Craniosacral therapy:* Diagnosis and treatment of imbalances in the craniosacral system. Subtle adjustments are made to the system through light touch and gentle manipulations.

- *Dance therapy:* Dance therapy is a modality in which dance and music combine to allow the body, mind, soul, and spirit to be refreshed and uplifted and to experience the freedom that natural bodily movement allows.

- *Feldenkrais method:* The Feldenkrais method is a method of instruction, through movement and gentle manipulation, to enhance self-image and restore mobility. Students are taught to notice how they are using their bodies and how to improve their posture and move more freely.

- *Jin shin jyutsu:* This is a bodywork technique that balances body energy as it travels along specific pathways. Specific combinations of healing points are held with the fingertips to restore balance and harmony.

- *Lymphatic therapy:* Lymphatic therapy is a vigorous form of massage that helps the body release toxins stored in the lymphatic system— excellent for the immune system and rebuilding the body.

- *Massage:* Massage involves the use of strokes and pressure on the body to dispel tension, increase circulation, and relieve muscular pain. Massage can provide comfort and increased body awareness and can facilitate the release of emotional as well as bodily tension.
- *Movement therapy:* This modality involves a guided series of movements and body work to open energy pathways and facilitate healing.
- *Neuromuscular therapy:* Neuromuscular therapy is a massage therapy in which moderate pressure over muscles and nerves, as well as on trigger points, is used to decrease pain and tension.
- *Physical therapy:* Physical therapy includes the treatment of physical conditions of body malfunction, damage, or injury using procedures designed to reduce swelling, relieve pain, strengthen muscles, restore range of motion, and return functioning to the patient.
- *Shiatsu:* Shiatsu is an energy-based system of bodywork that uses a firm sequence of rhythmic pressure held on specific pressure points on the body, designed to awaken acupressure meridians.
- *Trigger point therapy:* This is a method of compression of sensitive points in the muscle tissue, along with massage and passive stretches, for the relief of pain and tension. Treatment decreases swelling and stiffness and increases range of motion. Exercises may be assigned.

Mind–Body Medicine

- *Art therapy:* Art therapy incorporates the use of basic art materials to discover how to restore, maintain, or improve physical and mental health. Through observation and analysis, the art therapist is able to formulate treatment plans specific to the individual.
- *Color therapy:* Color therapy involves the use of electronic instrumentation and color receptivity, according to the work of Jacob Lieberman (1993), to integrate the nervous system and body–mind. It increases well-being and can be helpful for many acute and chronic ailments.
- *Counseling/psychotherapy:* A broad category of therapies that treat individuals as a whole. Treatments and sessions are focused on integrated care on all levels for individuals, families, or groups.
- *Eye movement desensitization and reprocessing (EMDR):* EMDR is an accelerated information-processing method that uses alternating stimuli—either eye movements or sounds—to desensitize and reprocess emotional wounds and install a healthier belief system. EMDR is effective with posttraumatic stress syndrome, childhood trauma, depression, addictions, compulsions, unhealthy patterns, and future-oriented solutions.

- *Guided imagery:* A holistic modality that assists clients in connecting with their inner knowledge at the thinking, feeling, and sensing levels, thus promoting their innate healing abilities. Together, guide and client cocreate an effective way to work with pain, symptoms, grief, and stress management; conflict resolution; and self-empowerment issues; and to prepare for medical or surgical interventions.

- *Hypnotherapy:* A state of focused attention, achieved through guided relaxation, hypnotherapy is used to access the unconscious mind. Hypnosis is used for memory recall, medical treatment, and skill enhancement or personal growth.

- *Interactive imagery:* Fostering active participation, disease prevention, and health promotion, interactive imagery returns the focus of wellness to the individual.

- *Meditation:* A method of relaxing and quieting the mind to relieve muscle tension and facilitate inner peace. There are numerous forms of meditation, taught individually or in group settings, and it is thought that prayer for the self might have an effect similar to meditation. The nonsectarian form of prayer, which is akin to meditation and used for stress reduction, has long been recognized by clinicians to improve one's sense of well-being.

- *Music therapy:* An expressive art form designed to help the individual move into harmony and balance. Through the use of music, individuals explore emotional, spiritual, and behavioral issues. Musical skill is not necessary because the process, rather than technique, is emphasized.

- *Neurolinguistic programming:* A systematic approach to changing behavior through changing patterns of thinking. Its originators, Dilts, Grinder, Delozier, and Bandler (1980), proposed theoretical connections between neurological processes (neuro), language (linguistic), and behavioral patterns that have been learned through experience (programming), which can be organized to achieve specific goals in life.

- *Stress management:* Any therapy or educational practice with the objective of decreasing stress and enhancing one's response to the elements of life that cannot be changed. This broad category may include bodywork, energy work, visualization, and counseling.

- *Tai chi (chuan):* A movement practice and Chinese martial art that enhances coordination, balance, and breathing and promotes physical, emotional, and spiritual well-being. Tai chi is taught in classes or as private lessons and requires home practice to be effective.

- *Yoga therapy:* The use of yoga postures, controlled breathing, relaxation, meditation, and nutrition facilitates the release of muscular and emotional tension, improves concentration, increases oxygen levels in the blood, and assists the body in healing itself.

Biologically Based Practices

- *Biofeedback:* A relaxation technique involving careful monitoring of vital functions (such as breathing, heart rate, and blood pressure) to improve health. By conscious thought, visualization, movement, or relaxation, one can learn which actions result in desirable changes in these vital functions. Biofeedback is used for medical problems related to stress and for management of many health problems, including pain syndrome, migraine, and irritable bowel syndrome.

- *Herbal therapy:* The use of herbs and their chemical properties to alleviate specific conditions or to support the function of various body systems. Herbal formulas have three basic functions: elimination and detoxification, health management and maintenance, and health building. The scope of herbal medicine is sometimes extended to include fungal and bee products, as well as minerals, shells, and certain animal parts (Acharya & Shrivastava, 2008).

- *Hydrotherapy:* The use of water, ice, steam, and hot and cold temperatures to relieve pain, fever, and inflammation and to maintain and restore health. Treatments include full-body immersion, steam baths, saunas, and the application of hot and/or cold compresses.

- *Nutritional counseling:* Nutritional counseling is performed by a practitioner who uses diet and supplementation therapeutically as the primary or adjunctive treatment for illness and for maintaining good health. Nutritionists employ a variety of approaches, including food combining, macrobiotics, and orthomolecular theory.

Energy Medicine

- *Chi kung healing touch:* An Eastern method of healing involving breath and gentle movements that follows the Chinese five-element theory and works with the meridian system.

- *Energy work:* A broad category of healing influencing the seven major energy centers (chakras) and the flow of energy around and through this field.
- *Healing touch:* A therapeutic approach in which touch is used to influence energy systems. Healing touch is employed to affect physical, emotional, mental, and spiritual health and healing.
- *Magnetic therapy:* A modality using magnets to generate controlled magnetic fields. Magnetic therapy is used to improve the functioning of bodily systems and facilitate healing.
- *Reiki:* Using the hands and visualization, the Reiki practitioner directs energy to affected areas of the client's body to facilitate healing and relaxation.
- *Therapeutic touch:* A technique for balancing energy flow in the body through human energy transfer.

The DNP as Integrative Practitioner: Unique Aspects of DNP Preparation

The question will be asked, what advantage is there to having DNP preparation for an APN specializing in integrative health? Any professional registered nurse (RN) who takes a course in holistic nursing at the post-RN level should be able to function competently and therapeutically as an integrative practitioner. What, then, does the DNP bring to integrative health? And what is the advantage to seeking DNP preparation for this role?

The AACN addresses the competencies of the doctorally prepared APN (AACN, 2006). The DNP, a practice-focused terminal degree, prepares the APN to serve as an expert in nursing practice. Compared with the PhD and DNS degrees, which are research-focused degrees, the DNP is unique in providing education in those components of advanced nursing practice that are essential to practice at the highest clinical level. The skills gained in the DNP course of study will not only prepare the nurse for clinical competence but also prepare him or her for establishing a successful practice or business. As DNP programs proliferate in colleges and universities across the nation, certain states (e.g., Alabama and New York) are mandating that the curricula include a significant percentage of clinical content; indeed, some DNP programs (e.g., Columbia University, University of Wisconsin, University of Washington) include a clinical residency in the curriculum. The AACN *Essentials of Doctoral Education for Advanced Nursing Practice* states that

DNP programs should require a minimum of 1,000 supervised clinical hours of practice for the baccalaureate-to-DNP degree course of study in any specialty (AACN, 2006). Including clinical components in the DNP curriculum strengthens the DNP-prepared APN as a clinician. The University of Minnesota's Doctor of Nursing Practice Integrative Health and Healing area of concentration "prepares graduates with skills necessary for working with individuals, families, communities and health systems in developing holistic approaches to health promotion, disease prevention and chronic disease management, with a special emphasis on managing lifestyle changes and incorporating the use of complementary therapies" (University of Minnesota, n.d.). This program fully integrates the specialty courses relevant to integrative practice with those courses designed to meet the requirements of the AACN's Essentials competencies. These courses uniquely position the DNP graduate to succeed on many different fronts of integrative health.

DNP curricula are unique in other areas, in that they include coursework in business finance, health policy, human resource management, change, and leadership (Rush University, n.d.). The APN engaging in integrative health practice benefits from understanding past, current, and future trends in health policy. Healthcare legislation and regulation undergo frequent change, affecting the right to practice; scope of practice; definition of specialty; and related rights, privileges, and responsibilities. Legislation and regulation are influenced by many factors, including political, socioeconomic, and cultural. Advanced coursework in public policy provides the DNP with a firm foundation to clearly view the nuanced political landscape.

The number of APNs owning or directing solo practices remains small, due in part to the expensive and adventurous nature of being an entrepreneur. Because of the lack of research on APNs in private practice, it is not possible to quantify with any specificity the number of APNs who own their own businesses. However, one survey on NPs indicated that 3% are engaged in private practice (Rollet & Lebo, 2007/2008). Given the nature and challenges of integrative health care (e.g., that health insurers do not consistently pay for holistic health services, that clients may be more inclined to pay for these services with disposable income, and that educated healthcare consumers are becoming increasingly interested in modalities that are more wellness oriented), it is reasonable to speculate that the number of APNs starting integrative health practices will increase. DNP programs provide the APN with education in health economics, financial management, budget creation and management, human resources, practice management, and business models.

In the case of the DNP as integrative or holistic practitioner, earning the DNP degree provides advantages in the areas of direct delivery of health care, practice development and management, and interpreting and synthesizing research. Although some will posit that enough is learned at the baccalaureate or master's levels, the competencies needed to provide health care to increasingly complex populations while managing a practice autonomously, using research for evidence-based care, and advocating for patient access to all relevant forms of interventions that promote wellness are all presented comprehensively in a DNP curriculum and provide the APN with the most optimal level of preparation for practice.

Nursing Informaticist

Sandra L. McPherson

Nursing informatics is defined by the ANA (2008, p. 1) as "a specialty that integrates nursing science, computer science and information science to manage community data, information, and knowledge in nursing practice." The APN informaticist can guide practice in both hospitals and private practice settings to meet *meaningful use* criteria and contribute to the delivery of safer patient care.

Recent developments in American health care have promoted the role of the nurse informaticist. Chief among those developments is the meaningful use incentive program developed by the CMS. This CMS program provides incentive payments to eligible professionals, eligible hospitals, and critical access hospitals (CAHs) as they adopt, implement, upgrade, or demonstrate meaningful use of certified EHR technology. The certification ensures "purchasers and other users that an EHR system or module offers the necessary technological capability, functionality, and security to help them meet the meaningful use criteria. Certification also helps providers and patients be confident that the electronic health IT products and systems they use are secure, can maintain data confidentially, and can work with other systems to share information" (CMS, 2015). The DNP-prepared nurse informaticist can help practitioners and facilities achieve meaningful use incentives from the CMS.

The meaningful use criteria were developed and written by physicians, for physicians. Scherger (2010) mentioned that these physicians knew that criteria placed into certain software applications could help prevent some medical errors and possibly save lives. One motivator for this development was the IOM publication *To Err Is Human* (IOM, 1999). This IOM report brought to light that many deaths in the United States are due to medical errors. In fact, it states that more Americans die from preventable medical errors than from motor vehicle accidents, breast cancer, and AIDS (IOM, 1999). It encouraged development of systems to reduce errors and improve communication between healthcare providers. In addition to the medical influence on meaningful use, nurses and other members of the interdisciplinary health team have made contributions to improve safety and reduce errors.

Despite the good intent of the meaningful use criteria, many hospitals are struggling to meet the criteria and with the impact of an EHR. Many physicians and providers struggle with EHR entries because the output of the electronic record does not resemble a progress note (Baron, 2010), and it is difficult to submit for reimbursement. Another struggle that hospitals are experiencing in meeting the meaningful use criteria involves achieving provider proficiency in navigating the EHR and making accurate, timely entries into the EHR across all specialties. Training of providers is crucial for the success of any software implementation such as the EHR. As clinical practice changes to an electronic, digital workflow, the manual, analog workflow is quickly departing from clinical care areas. Technology is appearing in the basic functions of the nursing role.

In the past, supplies were stored on wire racks or in closets that were open to all providers—and visitors. Now they are stored in electronic cabinets that track utilization and control access. These computerized cabinets associate the patient name with the supplies being accessed. An additional interface sends charges to the patient account once the provider clicks on a button that decrements the inventory. Only authorized providers are allowed to access the cabinet. Intravenous (IV) pumps are another example of emerging technology. Newer IV pumps have a database that allows maximum drug doses to be programmed in order to prevent overdosing. Many of the pumps also have an interface that allows the data collected at the bedside to be automatically entered into the EHR. In addition, the clinical documentation of assessments, flow sheets, care plans, and orders is all electronic, and the hard copy patient paper record is becoming a part of history.

The emerging *informatics DNP* specialty role is a result of the changing demands in our health care. The complexity of patient care and the concern from the public about quality and safety of care are catalysts for the rapid enrollment in these advanced degree programs. Nationwide, enrollment into DNP programs at both the postmaster's and postbaccalaureate level has been steady and competitive (Kirschling, 2014), including the DNP specialty focused on informatics.

Curriculum/Preparation

The curriculum for the DNP degree builds on the master's-level program and encompasses many areas of practice. Chism (2010, p. 23) stated that the "DNP degree builds upon the advanced nursing specialization that one has and provides additional preparation in formulation, interpretation and utilization of evidence-based practices, health policy, information technology and leadership."

Generally, the curriculum has a core set of courses that all DNP-level students, regardless of their nursing specialty, are required to complete. The specialty classes are based on the student's field of practice. Colleges vary greatly with what specialties they offer, and this must be researched before enrollment. Additional courses for a DNP degree focused on informatics can include classes on project management, system development life cycle, nursing terminologies, database and technology, knowledge management, decision support systems, and other related technology courses, depending on the institution. These courses fulfill the requirements for the AACN's Essential IV, Information Systems/Technology and Patient Care Technology for the Improvement and Transformation of Health Care, and expand the practitioner's knowledge beyond the basics.

Certification

One can obtain many certifications within the field of informatics that complement the education received in the DNP degree course of study. The American Health Information Management Association (AHIMA), the ANCC, and the Health Information Management System Society (HIMSS) offer these specialty certifications. Certificate programs can be found through many colleges both on site and online. The Project Management Professional (PMP) is another certification that may be obtained through the doctoral study of informatics.

Project Management

Project management is often part of the nursing informatics role. The informaticist may work on or manage a range of projects, from simple customizations of a computer screen or minor upgrades, to an EHR, to full systems implementation. Most of these projects include a needs assessment and the full system development life cycle (SDLC). The SDLC includes planning, analysis, design, implementation, and evaluation (Dennis & Wixom, 2003). The DNP program in informatics allows for a deep immersion in all phases of the project life cycle to achieve an organized method of delivering the project.

Work plans, work breakdown structures, project schedules, and project reporting tools can all be part of the project management role for the nursing informaticist. Process improvement activities such as flow mapping can be beneficial to the overall project success when workflows are changed. Project reporting tools can vary depending on the project. The DNP-prepared nurse informaticist will use many tracking tools to facilitate delivery of projects on time and within budget. Pert and Gantt charts are the most commonly used visual charts in project management to display a visual representation of the milestones for the project and the date associated with each milestone.

The Gantt chart represents the timeline of the project with estimated task durations and sequences. At a quick glance, it displays the project status and the overall anticipated project duration. A disadvantage of Gantt charts is the inability to show relationships between items or display items that are on the critical path (Luecke, 2004). The critical path items determine the entire project length. Failure to complete critical path items will delay overall implementation of the project. The PERT chart shows both the critical path items and the relationships between tasks. This type of chart has a great amount of information. The disadvantage of this chart is that it is not as simplified as the Gantt. The chart does not lend itself to a quick, at-a-glance assessment of the status of the project.

Hybrid Health Records

Because of the rapid pace of technology enhancements and rapidly changing requirements, the literature for EHRs can become out of date within a short period. A common theme that this author found is that many facilities were in a hybrid status with health records; some portions of the record were electronic, whereas others were on paper or possibly in a different electronic system, and the data were not shared. Studies identified the value of sharing documentation as much as possible and removing hybrid systems if feasible, though results of the search and path varied. Some authors have stated that hybrid systems do not work well (Borycki, Lemieux-Charles, Nagle, & Eysenbach, 2009; Dimick, 2008; Hall, 2008), whereas others have claimed that hybrid systems do work well (Hamilton, Round, Sharp, & Peters, 2003). Although the literature has conflicting opinions—both for and against—regarding the use of hybrid records, overall the literature supports the use of EHRs for increased access to previous health histories, to enhance patient safety and improve patient outcomes, to increase access to decision support tools, and to increase the speed and accuracy of order processing. This is a role for the DNP-educated informaticist: to bring the hybrid systems into the future of an all-inclusive EHR.

Theoretical Supports for Nursing Informatics

The nursing informatics specialty covers a wide breadth of clinical care areas but offers the flexibility of pulling from many different theory domains: nursing theories, nursing care models, project management theories, systems theory, behavioral theory, information science, computer science, and education theories. All these theories from within and outside nursing may be applicable to nursing informatics.

One theory that can easily be used to describe change in the clinical setting is Lewin's change theory. Although Lewin's theory has only three steps, it offers the most flexibility. Lewin's theory consists of unfreezing, making changes, and then refreezing. According to Burnes (2004), Kurt Lewin believed that planned change and learning would enable individuals to resolve conflict and understand their world in order to restructure their perceptions. The first stage is unfreezing. This allows people to recognize the need for change from the original process/procedure and move to another by creating the right environment. In informatics, this may occur when frontline staff get involved with redesigning their workflow as technology changes it. Stage 2 involves the actual change to be made. In informatics, Stage 2 might include customization of a computerized documentation system or the implementation of an EHR. Stage 3 is the freezing or refreezing process that allows the new process or procedure to become the new standard and the change to be stabilized and integrated (Boyd, Luetje, & Eckert, 1992). Sometimes there are several iterations of an EHR functionality or a screen display before the final outcome is reached. Lewin's theory is flexible enough to describe these iterations.

Another theory that is applicable to the DNP role and the EHR implementation is Malcolm Knowles' Androgogy theory. This theory is an adult learning/educational theory that concentrates on the art and science of teaching adults. EHR implementation requires working professionals to learn a new workflow. Adult learners can be more self-directed, but there are various learning styles that need to be considered. They are active participants and bring previous life knowledge to build on (Bastable, 2008; Knowles, Holton, & Swanson, 2005).

Future

The future of the DNP-prepared informaticist can only expand. Requirements for data reporting within the healthcare organization, benchmarking, and documentation of quality measures and patient outcomes all continue to increase. Additionally, meaningful use requirements will continue to evolve.

The Office of the National Coordinator for Health Information Technology (ONC) has articulated national goals to be accomplished. Such national goals will secure the place of the doctorally prepared nurse informaticist for the future.

References

Acharya, D., & Shrivastava, A. (2008). *Indigenous herbal medicines: Tribal formulations and traditional herbal practices.* Jaipur, India: Aavishkar.

American Academy of Family Physicians, American Academy of Pediatrics, American College of Physicians, & American Osteopathic Association. (2010). *Joint principles for medical education of physicians as preparation for practice in the patient-centered medical home.* Retrieved from http://www.acponline.org /running_practice/pcmh/understanding/educjoint-principles.pdf

American Academy of Nurse Practitioners. (2015). *American Academy of Nurse Practitioners Certification Program handbook.* Silver Spring, MD: Author.

American Association of Colleges of Nursing. (2006). *The essentials of doctoral education for advanced nursing practice.* Retrieved from http://www.aacn.nche .edu/DNP/pdf/Essentials.pdf

American Holistic Nurses Association (n.d.). *Who we are.* Retrieved from http://www .ahna.org/About-Us

American Holistic Nurses Credentialing Corporation. (2012). *Eligibility criteria for advanced holistic nursing certification.* Retrieved from http://www.ahncc.org

American Holistic Nurses Credentialing Corporation. (2015). *Certification in advanced holistic nursing, AHN-BC and APHN-BC.* Retrieved from http://ahncc.org /certificationprocess.html

American Nurses Association. (2008). *Scope and standards of nursing informatics practice.* Washington, DC: Author.

American Nurses Association. (2013). *Public health nursing: Scope and standards of practice.* Silver Spring, MD: Nursesbook.org

American Nurses Credentialing Center. (2012). *Advanced public health certification requirements.* Retrieved from http://nursing.advanceweb.com/Features /Articles/Public-Health-Portfolio.aspx

American Public Health Association. (1996). *A statement of APHA public health nursing.* Retrieved from http://www.apha.org/membergroups/sections/aphasections /phn/about/defbackground.htm

Association of State and Territorial Directors of Nursing. (2008). *Report on a public health nurse to population ratio.* Washington, DC: Author. http://www .phnurse.org/docs/PHN_to_Population_Ratio_2008.pdf

Barnes, P., Bloom, B., & Nahin, R. (2008). Complementary and alternative medicine use among adults and children. United States, 2007. *CDC National Health Statistics Report #12.* DHHS Publication No. (PHS) 2009–1250.

Baron, R. (2010). Meaningful use of health information technology is managing information. *Journal of the American Medical Association, 304*(1), 89–90.

Bastable, S. (2008). *Nurse as educator* (3rd ed.). Sudbury, MA: Jones and Bartlett.

Bayer, R., Gostin, L., Jennings, S., & Steinbock, B. (2007). *Public health ethics: Theory, policy and practice.* New York, NY: Oxford University Press.

Bersin, J. (2008). *The training measurement book: Best practices, proven methodologies, and practical approaches.* San Francisco, CA: Pfeiffer.

Borycki, E., Lemieux-Charles, L., Nagle, L., & Eysenbach, G. (2009). Evaluating the impact of hybrid electronic-paper environments upon novice nurse information seeking. *Methods of Information in Medicine, 28*(2), 137–143.

Boyd, M., Luetje, V., & Eckert, A. (1992). Creating organizational change in an inpatient long-term care facility. *Psychosocial Rehabilitation Journal, 15*(3), 47–54.

Boyer, E. (1990). *Scholarship reconsidered: Priorities of the professorate.* Princeton, NJ: Carnegie Foundation for the Advancement of Teaching.

Burnes, B. (2004). Kurt Lewin and complexity theories: Back to the future? *Journal of Change Management, 4*(4), 309–325.

Council for Affordable Quality Healthcare. (2015). *Universal provider datasource.* Retrieved from http://www.caqh.org/solutions/caqh-proview

Centers for Disease Control and Prevention. (n.d.). *Local public health system performance assessment.* Washington, DC: Department of Health and Human Services. Retrieved from http://www.cdc.gov/od/ocphp/nphpsp/documents/07_110300%20Local%20Booklet.pdf

Centers for Medicare and Medicaid Services. (2015). *Regulations & guidance.* Retrieved from http://www.cms.gov/Regulations-and-Guidance/Regulations-and-Guidance.html

Cherry, K. (2011). *Lewin's leadership styles.* Retrieved from http://psychology.about.com/od/leadership/a/leadstyles.htm

Chism, L. (2010). *The doctor of nursing practice: A guidebook for role development and professional issues.* Sudbury, MA: Jones and Bartlett.

Commission on Collegiate Nursing Education. (2008). *Criteria for evaluation of nurse practitioner programs.* Retrieved from http://www.aacn.nche.edu/leading-initiatives/education-resources/evalcriteria2008.pdf

Council on Accreditation of Nurse Anesthesia Educational Programs. (2014). *Standards for accreditation of nurse anesthesia programs, practice doctorate.* Park Ridge, IL: Author.

D'Amour, D., Ferrada-Videla, M., San Martin-Rodriguez, L., & Beaulieu, M. D. (2005). The conceptual basis for interprofessional collaboration: Core concepts and theoretical frameworks. *Journal of Interprofessional Care, 19* (Suppl. 1), 116–131.

Dayhoff, N., & Moore, P. (2003). Entrepreneurship: Start-up questions. *Clinical Nurse Specialist, 17,* 86–87.

Dennis, A., & Wixom, B. (2003). *System analysis and design* (2nd ed.). New York, NY: Wiley.

Diers, D. (1995). Clinical scholarship. *Journal of Professional Nursing, 11*(1), 24–30.

Dilts, R., Grinder, J., Delozier, J., & Bandler, R. (1980). *Neuro-linguistic programming. Volume I: The study of the structure of subjective experience.* Cupertino, CA: Meta.

Dimick, C. (2008). Record limbo: Hybrid systems add burden and risk to data reporting. *Journal of AHIMA, 79*(11), 28–32.

Dossey, B., Selanders, L., Beck, D. M., & Attewell, A. (2005). *Florence Nightingale today: Healing, leadership, global action.* Washington, DC: Nursesbooks.org.

Failla, K. (2008). Manager and staff perceptions of the manager's leadership style. *Journal of Nursing Administration, 38*(11), 480–487.

Guyatt, G., & Rennie, D. (2002). *Users' guides to the medical literature: A manual for evidence-based clinical practice.* Chicago, IL: AMA.

Hall, T. (2008). Minimizing hybrid records. Tips for reducing paper documentation as new systems come online. *Journal of AHIMA, 79*(11), 42–45.

Hamilton, W., Round, A., Sharp, D., & Peters, T. (2003, December). The quality of record keeping in primary care: A comparison of computerized paper and hybrid systems. *British Journal of General Practice, 53*(497), 929–933.

Hanson, C., & Bennett, S. (2005). Business planning and reimbursement mechanisms. In A. Hamric, J. Spross, & C. Hanson (Eds.), *Advanced practice nursing: An integrative approach* (4th ed., pp. 543–574). Saunders-Elsevier.

Hasnain-Wynia, R. (2006). Is evidence-based medicine patient-centered and is patient-centered care evidence-based? *Health Services Research, 41*(1), 1–8. Retrieved from http://www.ncbi.nlm.nih.gov/pmc/articles/PMC1681528/

Health Resources and Services Administration. (2010). *HRSA study finds nursing workforce is growing.* Retrieved from http://www.hrsa.gov/about/news/pressreleases/2010/100922nursingworkforce.html

Hyman, D., Gurgevich, E., Alter, T., Ayers, J., Cash, E., Fahnline, D., . . . Wright, H. (2002). Beyond Boyer: The UniSCOPE model of scholarship for the 21st century. *Journal of Higher Education Outreach and Engagement, 7*(1&2), 41–65.

Indiana State Medical Association. (2015). Physician leadership program. Retrieved from http://www.ismanet.org/PLP/

Institute for Healthcare Improvement. (2015). *Triple Aim for populations.* Retrieved from http://www.ihi.org/Topics/TripleAim/Pages/default.aspx

Institute of Medicine. (1988). *The future of public health.* Washington, DC: National Academy Press.

Institute of Medicine. (1999). *To err is human: Building a safer health system.* Washington, DC: National Academy Press.

Institute of Medicine. (2001). *Crossing the quality chasm.* Washington, DC: National Academy Press.

Institute of Medicine. (2003). *Keeping patients safe: Transforming the work environment of nurses.* Washington, DC: National Academies of Medicine.

Institute of Medicine. (2010). *The future of nursing: Leading change, advancing health.* Retrieved from http://www.nap.edu/catalog/12956.html

Jewish Women's Archive. (n.d.). *Lillian Wald, 1867–1940.* Retrieved from http://jwa.org/people/wald-lillian

Keller, L., & Strohschein, S. (2012). Population-based public health nursing practice: The intervention wheel. In M. Stanhope & J. Lancaster (Eds.), *Public health nursing: Population-centered health care in the community* (pp. 186–215). Philadelphia, PA: Elsevier.

Kelly, K. (2010). Is the DNP the answer to the nursing faculty shortage? Not likely! *Nursing Forum, 45*(4), 266–270.

Kirschling, J. (2014). *Reflections on the future of doctoral programs in nursing.* Presented at the AACN Doctoral Education Conference, January 2014. Retrieved from http://www.aacn.nche.edu/dnp-home

Knowles, M., Holton, E., & Swanson, R. (2005). *The adult learner. The definitive classic in adult education and human resource development.* Waltham, MA: Elsevier.

Kotter, J. (1996). *Leading change.* Boston, MA: Harvard Business School Press.

Lemley, B. (2015). *What is integrative medicine?* Retrieved from http://www.drweil.com

Leven, R., Keefe, J., & Marren, J. (2010). Evidence-based practice improvement: Merging 2 paradigms. *Journal of Nursing Care Quality, 25*(2), 117–126.

Lieberman, J. (1993). *Light: Medicine of the future—how we can use it to heal ourselves now.* Santa Fe, NM: Inner Traditions/Bear & Company.

Love, J. (2005). *The visionary entrepreneur.* JLM & Associates, Inc. Retrieved from http://www.advancingwomen.com/entrepreneurialism/35341.php

Luecke, R. (2004). *Managing projects large and small.* Boston, MA: Harvard Business School Press.

Mann, J. D. (2009, January–February). Practicing presence through Breema. *Spirituality and Health,* 1–2.

Melnyk, B., & Fineout-Overholt, E. (2011). *Evidence-based practice in nursing and healthcare: A guide to best practice.* Philadelphia, PA: Lippincott Williams & Wilkins.

Minnesota Department of Health. (2007). *Cornerstones of public health nursing.* Retrieved from http://www.health.state.mn.us/divs/opi/cd/phn/docs/0710phn_cornerstones.pdf

Monsen, K. (2005). Use of the Omaha System in practice. In K. Martin (Ed.), *The Omaha System: A key to practice, documentation, and information management* (pp. 58–83). St. Louis, MO: Elsevier.

National Association of County Health Officials. (1994). *Blueprint for a healthy community: A guide for local health departments.* Washington, DC: Author.

National Center for Complementary and Alternative Medicine. (2007). *What is CAM?* Retrieved from https://nccih.nih.gov/health/integrative-health

National Center for Complementary and Alternative Medicine. (2009). *Homeo-pathy: An introduction.* Retrieved from http://nccam.nih.gov/health/homeopathy

National Center for Health Statistics. (2013). *Health, United States, 2010—with special feature on death and dying.* National Center for Health Statistics. Hyattsville, MD: Centers for Disease Control. Retrieved from http://www.cdc.gov/nchs/data/nvsr/nvsr61/nvsr61_04.pdf

NLN Board of Governors (2002). *Position statement, the preparation of nurse educators.* Retrieved from: http://www.nln.org/docs/default-source/about/archived-position-statements/the-preparation-of-nurse-educators-pdf.pdf?sfvrsn=6

National Nursing Centers Consortium. (2015). *Our mission.* Retrieved from http://www.nncc.us/about-nncc/who-we-are

National Organization of Nurse Practitioner Faculties. (2000). *Faculty practice and promotion and tenure* (NONPF position paper). Washington, DC: Author.

National Organization of Nurse Practitioner Faculties. (2005). *Nurse practitioner faculty practice: An expectation of professionalism* (NONPF position paper). Washington, DC: Author.

New York State Office of the Professions, State Education Department. (n.d.). *License requirements for nurse practitioner.* Retrieved from http://www .op.nysed.gov/prof/nurse/np.htm

Nicholes, R., & Dyer, J. (2012). Is eligibility for tenure possible for the doctor of nursing practice-prepared faculty? *Journal of Professional Nursing, 28*(1), 13–17.

Nightingale, F. (1946). *Notes on nursing: What it is, and what it is not.* Philadelphia, PA: Lippincott.

Nurse practitioners as entrepreneurs: Constrained or liberated? (2008). *Journal of Advanced Practice Nursing.* Retrieved from http://www.asrn.org/journal -advanced-practice-nursing/february-2008.html

Olds, D., Eckenrode, J., Henderson, C., Kitzman, H., Powers, J., Cole, R., . . . Luckey, D. (1997). Long-term effects of home visitation on maternal life course and child abuse and neglect: Fifteen-year follow-up of a randomized trial. *Journal of the American Medical Association, 278*(8), 637–643.

Otto, H. A., & Knight, J. W. (1979). *Dimensions in wholistic healing: New frontiers in the treatment of the whole person.* Chicago, IL: Burnham.

Pelikan, J. (1984). *Scholarship and its survival. Questions on the idea of graduate education. A Carnegie Foundation essay.* Lawrenceville, NJ: Princeton University Press.

Peraino, R. (2011). *Dedicated to change in the delivery of healthcare: Why patient centered care?* Retrieved from http://www.patientcenteredcare.net

Public Health Accreditation Board. (2013). *Standards and measures.* Retrieved from http://www.phaboard.org/wp-content/uploads/SM-Version-1.5-Board -adopted-FINAL-01-24-2014.docx.pdf

Public Health Functions Steering Committee. (1998). *Public health in America.* Retrieved from http://www.health.gov/phfunctions/public.htm

Quad Council of Public Health Nursing Organizations. (2011). *Competencies for public health nursing practice.* Washington, DC: Association of State and Territorial Directors of Nursing. Retrieved from http://www.resourcenter.net /images/ACHNE/Files/QuadCouncilCompetenciesForPublicHealthNurses _Summer2011.pdf

Robert Wood Johnson Foundation. (2011). *APRNs: A "big part of the solution" to the primary care provider shortage.* Retrieved from http://www.rwjf.org/humancapital /product.jsp?id=72775&print=true&referer=http%3A//w

Rollet, J., & Lebo, S. (2007/2008). 2007 salary survey results: A decade of growth. Results of the 2007 national salary and workplace survey of nurse practitioners. *Advance for Nurse Practitioners.* Retrieved from http://nurse-practitioners .advanceweb.com/Article/2007-Salary-Survey-Results-A-Decade-of-Growth-3 .aspx

Rush University. (n.d.). *Doctor of nursing practice degree program of study* (beginning winter 2009 for new matriculants). Retrieved from http://www.rushu .rush.edu

Sackett, D., Straus, S., & Richardson, W. (2000). *Evidence-based medicine: How to practice and teach EBM.* London, England: Livingstone.

Scherger, J. (2010). Meaningful use of HIT saves lives. *Modern Medicine, 87*(9), 8–9.

Shane, S. (2004). *A general theory of entrepreneurship: The individual opportunity nexus.* New Horizons in Entrepreneurship Series. Northampton, MA: Edward Elgar.

Smith, M. (2001). *Kurt Lewin: Groups, experiential learning and action research.* Retrieved from http://infed.org/mobi/kurt-lewin-groups-experiential-learning-and-action-research/

Sperhac, A., & Clinton, P. (2008). Doctorate of nursing practice: Blueprint for excellence. *Journal of Pediatric Health Care, 22*(3), 146–151.

Stanhope, M., & Lancaster, J. (2012). *Public health nursing: Population-centered care in the community.* Philadelphia, PA: Elsevier.

Stefl, M. (2008). Common competencies for all healthcare managers: The healthcare leadership alliance model. *Journal of Health Care Management, 53*(6), 360–373.

Taylor, J. (2006). *A survival guide for project managers* (2nd ed.). New York, NY: American Management Association.

Ten great public health achievements. (2011, May 20). *Morbidity and Mortality Weekly Report, 60*(19), 619–623.

Tracy, M. (2005). Direct clinical practice. In A. Hamric, J. Spross, & C. Hanson (Eds.), *Advanced practice nursing: An integrative approach* (4th ed., pp. 123–158). Saunders-Elsevier.

Trivieri, L., & Anderson, J. W. (2002). *Alternative medicine: The definitive guide.* Berkeley, CA: Celestial Arts.

United Nations. (2002). *End poverty 2015 Millennium Development Goals.* Retrieved from http://www.unmillenniumproject.org

University of Minnesota Integrative Health and Healing DNP Specialty. (n.d.). Retrieved from http://www.nursing.umn.edu/DNP/specialties/integrative-health-and-healing/index.htm

U.S. Department of Health and Human Services. (2008). *Phase I report: Recommendations for the framework and format of Healthy People 2020.* Retrieved from http://www.healthypeople.gov/sites/default/files/PhaseI_0.pdf

U.S. Department of Health and Human Services Health Resources and Services Administration, Bureau of Health Professionals, Division of Nursing. (1984). *Consensus conference on the essentials of public health nursing practice and education.* Rockville, MD: Author.

University of Minnesota, Doctor of Nursing Practice Program. (n.d.). *Integrative health and healing.* Retrieved from http://www.nursing.unm.edu/DNP/ProspectiveStudent/Specialties/Integrative_Health_and_Healing/home.html

Watson, G. (2011). *Definition of entrepreneurship.* Retrieved from http://www.gregwatson.com/entrepreneurship-definition/

Wisconsin Nurses Association. (2015). *APRN Uniformity Act, Summary of Proposed Changes to Statutes.* Retrieved from http://www.wisconsinnurses.org/

Wood, D. (2009). *Why have nurses left the profession?* Retrieved from http://www.nursezone.com/nursing-news-events/more-news/Why-Have-Nurses-Left-the-Profession_29118.aspx

Part III

The Doctor of Nursing Practice Project

Chapter 10

A Template for the DNP Project

Kathryn Waud White and Mary E. Zaccagnini

> *Knowing is not enough; we must apply. Willing is not enough; we must do.*
>
> —Goethe

In 1995, Ernest Boyer delivered a landmark address to the American Association of Colleges of Nursing (AACN). In this widely cited address, he outlined a new paradigm for understanding scholarship in which he detailed the findings of a Carnegie Foundation report, *Scholarship Reconsidered: Priorities of the Professorate* (Boyer, 1990). He outlined the evolution of American academic traditions from colonial times to 21st-century America. Boyer argued that today, the scholarship of discovery is disproportionately valued by academic institutions and that the scholarship of teaching and service is disregarded in many ways (Boyer, 1996). That plays out in the evaluation of professors for academic advancement and creates the curious situation in which it is far better for one's academic career to present a paper at a professional conference than it is to teach a class to undergraduate students and do it well. In his address to the AACN, Boyer proposed a reimagination of scholarship as a concept that has four interdependent aspects: the scholarship of discovery, the scholarship of integration, the scholarship of teaching, and the scholarship of application. He further proposed that each domain should be valued equally (Boyer, 1996).

Expanding on these thoughts and ideas, many nursing scholars and leaders began to believe that the scholarship of integration and application in the field of nursing could be best acknowledged through the development of a practice doctorate for advanced practice nurses (APNs). These practitioners would be prepared at the highest level of clinical practice and scholarship, integrating concepts of leadership and advocacy into the richness of nursing science and theory. The doctor of nursing practice (DNP) course of study for APNs was proposed as the terminal degree for APNs by the AACN in 2004 after a long period of discussion and consensus building (AACN, 2004). The AACN proposed that all advanced practice nursing programs be in the DNP framework by the year 2015. This proposal created an explosion of DNP programs across the country, as illustrated by **Figure 10-1**. The implementation goal of 2015 has not been realized, and thus the master's degree remains the primary educational pathway to advanced practice nursing. The recent RAND report (Auerbach et al., 2014) identified barriers to implementing the DNP that include lack of faculty, costs and budgetary concerns, institutional barriers within large university systems, insufficient clinical sites, and resource challenges associated with overseeing DNP scholarly projects, primarily faculty workload.

The DNP course of study as proposed by the AACN culminates in a scholarly project, as should any doctoral education (AACN, 2006). The

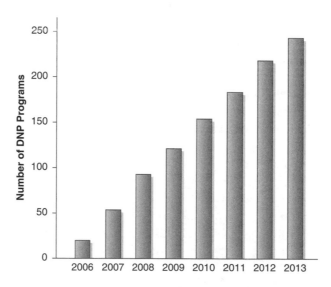

Figure 10-1 Growth of Doctor of Nursing Practice Programs
Modified from Kirschling, J. (2014, January). *Reflections on the Future of Doctoral Programs in Nursing.* PowerPoint presentation at the meeting of the AACN 2014 Doctoral Education Conference, Naples, FL.

nature of the project should be commensurate with the domain of scholarship of the student. For PhD students, the domain of discovery of new knowledge dictates an original research project conducted and evaluated using traditional research methodologies, statistical analysis, and evaluation schemes. The DNP degree focuses on the clinical scholarship of integration and application as elucidated by Boyer in 1996. Therefore, a project intended to discover new knowledge is an inappropriate vehicle for demonstration of the student's scholarship; scholarship for the DNP student is demonstrated through a project that reflects the breadth of the student's education and is a synthesis of the knowledge gained in the course of study (AACN, 2006). It should address a complex practice, process, or systems problem within the student's field of expertise, propose an evidence-based intervention to address that problem for a significant population, use doctoral-level leadership skills to implement and evaluate the efficacy of the intervention, and evaluate the outcomes of the intervention (National Organization of Nurse Practitioner Faculties [NONPF], 2007). The project may take on many forms, but the common element throughout the variety of DNP scholarly projects is the use of evidence to improve practice, processes, or outcomes (AACN, 2006). The DNP student functioning as project leader gains real-world leadership skills conducting the project. The structure and format of the final product will vary with the requirements of the degree-granting institution (AACN, 2006; NONPF, 2007).

Nature of the Project

Although practice doctorate programs are rapidly growing within colleges and schools of nursing, questions remain about the nature of the scholarly project. This is reflected in the many appellations given to this project: leadership project, scholarly project, capstone project, or, from the AACN, simply the DNP final project. Several of the websites of universities offering DNP programs describe the DNP scholarly project in vastly differing ways. Most offer no description of the project but simply give examples of DNP scholarly project titles. There remains ambiguity as to the exact nature of the scholarly project for both prospective students and faculty in schools of nursing.

We can gain insight from other disciplines that have used a project as evidence of scholarship. For example, projects are used in the fields of business and engineering to demonstrate mastery of the subject matter. The use of a capstone project as evidence of scholarship in the engineering field is particularly interesting because there are similarities between nursing and engineering. Both of these fields of study center on the application of evidence-based knowledge to practice problems, and they both integrate knowledge from other fields of scientific study as well as the base field to create interventions. In Ernest Boyer's definition of the scholarship of application, he stated that this type of scholarship moves "from theory to practice and from practice back to theory" (Boyer, 1996). Both engineering and nursing take theories and new knowledge and test them in the gritty world of real life, real people, and real institutions.

Original research, even when illuminating and well executed, may languish for lack of application in the real world. In *Crossing the Quality Chasm* (2001), the Institute of Medicine (IOM) noted that the lag time from discovery of effective treatments to the integration and application of those treatments in clinical settings is 15 to 20 years. The IOM calls for development of an effective infrastructure to support the more rapid application of evidence to patient care. The DNP-educated APN is well positioned and educated to do just that: bring evidence to patient care. This is where the scholarship of integration and application brings life to theory and reality to research in the context of the real world.

In engineering and business, capstone projects are done most frequently at the baccalaureate and master's levels. What distinguishes the doctoral project from the baccalaureate or master's project is the depth of inquiry, the depth of the literature reviewed, the scope of the project, the population served by the project, and the student's use of solid scientific evidence and theory as underpinnings of the project (AACN, 2006). **Table 10-1** outlines Boyer's criteria by which we can evaluate scholarly work in any domain.

To date, no other fields of health care that require a practice doctorate for entry into practice require a capstone project similar to the DNP

Table 10-1 Boyer's Criteria for Evaluation of Scholarship

Are the goals of the project clearly stated?

Are the procedures well defined and appropriate for the project?

Are resources adequate for the stated goals of the project and utilized effectively?

Did the student communicate and collaborate effectively with others?

Are the results of the project significant?

Is there evidence of self-reflection and learning?

Boyer, E. L. (1996). Clinical practice as scholarship. *Holistic Nursing Practice, 10*(3), 1–6. Modified with permission.

scholarly project. In a recent review of accreditation requirements for practice doctorates in 14 healthcare professions, the reviewers found that none of these programs required original research, as would be required in a PhD curriculum. Some accreditation requirements alluded to "opportunities" for research or access to faculty who are conducting research. The only other field of health sciences that requires a clinical project for a practice doctorate is occupational therapy, but this practice doctorate is not required for entry into practice or certification as an occupational therapist. Practice doctorates in health care require a varying amount of exposure to research methodologies and evidence-based practice (Phelps & Gerbasi, 2009).

The DNP curriculum, as outlined by the AACN in 2006, focuses on nursing practice, leadership, collaboration, and integration of science from many fields of study. This curriculum prepares APNs to evaluate evidence for the implementation of best practices and the improvement of patient care. The PhD course of study focuses on vigorous research, generation of new knowledge, and the scholarship of discovery. Therefore, the DNP scholarly project should be the demonstration of the scholarship of integration and application as first discussed by Boyer in 1995. Although the DNP scholarly project is quite different from a PhD thesis (**Table 10-2**), it is a rigorously executed project that is described, and the results documented, in a paper or product of doctoral quality (AACN, 2006).

When evaluating the differences between the PhD thesis and the DNP scholarly project, it is useful to consider the desired outcomes. The PhD-prepared nurse will likely conduct his or her career in the academic or

Table 10-2 Comparison of DNP Practice Project and PhD Research Project

PhD Dissertation	DNP scholarly project
Systematic search for an answer to a research question	Systematic investigation of a practice issue
Outcome is an answer to the research question that is generalizable beyond current study; reproducible	Outcome is a solution to a practice problem that usually involves systems change; may be reproducible in other systems
Not specific to a time or place	Limited to a place and a time
Based in theory and literature	Based in theory and literature
Uses rigorous methodology that is unbiased and can be reproduced	Uses rigorous methods that are appropriate to the scope of the problem

Edwardson, S. (2009, January 14). *MN/DNP colloquium*. Colloquium conducted at the University of Minnesota School of Nursing, Minneapolis, MN. Reprinted with permission.

research setting. The DNP-prepared nurse will almost certainly conduct his or her career in clinical practice. To that end, the emphasis of the PhD thesis is on the rigorous application of standard methodologies and the meticulous evaluation of results using generally accepted scientific analysis techniques that can be reliably reproduced and are generalizable. The DNP scholarly project focuses on a practice problem and the evidence-based solutions for that problem. It is specific to a place or a system and may be applied to other settings, but this is not the goal of the project. Rather, the project focuses on the application of evidence to the problem that was identified. Results may be analyzed using standard statistical methods, but this is not strictly necessary (Edwardson, 2009). Many of the projects will be completed in institutions that utilize various quality management tools and processes for data analysis.

Some important similarities between the PhD thesis and DNP scholarly project emerge as well. Both approaches to problems need to be systematic and rigorous. The literature review should be in depth and rigorous. The PhD dissertation topic is narrow; the investigation is tightly controlled to eliminate extraneous influences. The DNP scholarly project is a real-world project and cannot control those influences. The DNP scholarly project seeks to adapt the research to real situations. Both the PhD thesis and the DNP scholarly project are based in theoretical concepts and literature. The PhD literature review will be focused; the DNP literature review will be broader and have many different points at which a discussion of theory is appropriate. The final product should meet all the academic institution's requirements for scholarly work (AACN, 2006). According to AACN (2015), graduates from both research- and practice-focused doctorates are prepared to generate new knowledge: "Research-focused graduates are prepared to generate knowledge through rigorous research and statistical methodologies that may be broadly applicable or generalizable; practice-focused graduates are prepared to generate new knowledge through innovation of practice change, the translation of evidence, and the implementation of quality improvement processes in specific practice settings, systems, or with specific populations to improve health or health outcomes. New knowledge generated through practice innovation, for example, could be of value to other practice settings. This new knowledge is considered transferrable but is not considered generalizable." The AACN white paper went on to state, "These delineations in knowledge generation are not to be construed as a hierarchical structure of the importance of these two types of knowledge generating methods. The application and translation of evidence into practice is a vital and necessary skill that is currently lacking in the healthcare environment and the nursing profession. The DNP graduate will help to fulfill this need. As a result DNP and PhD graduates will have the opportunity to collaborate and work synergistically to improve health outcomes." What does this mean for the DNP scholarly project? It means that the project needs to be as rigorous, evidence based, and scholarly as a research thesis. The difference is that the DNP project is utilizing the tools of translation science to bring research findings into patient care. The end result is evidence-based quality patient care outcomes or changes in practice.

Because this scholarly project is a synthesis of the student's work in the DNP program, it should be related to the student's advanced practice specialty (NONPF, 2007). The problem to be addressed usually arises from clinical practice issues observed by the student or his or her mentors. The process or practice improvement project is often conducted at the student's clinical practice site. It can also be done in partnership with an agency of the community (e.g., school, health agency, church, nonprofit organization). The leadership of the project is typically handled by the student alone, along with faculty support. The project may be conducted in collaboration with another student if the educational institution permits it. The project should engage a team of professionals to accomplish the change, demonstrating the student's attainment of leadership and collaboration skills (AACN, 2006; NONPF, 2007).

Structure of the Project

A needs assessment and literature review should be conducted to support the need for improvement. The improvement should benefit a significant population instead of a single patient or practitioner (NONPF, 2007). The review of literature for the DNP scholarly project is not done to identify gaps in the body of knowledge, as one would do for the PhD research project. Rather, the DNP scholarly project proposes to fix a gap in a system given the available evidence. The literature review should address the efficacy of the intervention selected for the DNP scholarly project and support the rationale for selection of that specific intervention. It should support the validity and reliability of assessment tools, specifically surveys and data collection methodologies. Scholarly support for the project includes the use of nursing theories and theories from other fields of study to describe the conceptual framework of the project. The student may need to integrate several theories from different fields of study in order to adequately describe this framework.

The implementation of the DNP scholarly project should meet all the ethical standards for conducting any research or quality improvement project. Review by an institutional review board (IRB) is dictated by the nature of the project and the policies of the academic institution and implementation site. As the lines between quality improvement activities and research blur, the tendency for these projects to undergo review by IRBs is stronger than in the past. The expected outcomes of the project should be defined when constructing the project. They should be measurable in the time frame of the project. The elements for the successful implementation of the project should also be sufficiently described to the extent that the project could be implemented at other clinical sites (NONPF, 2007).

Data collection during the project should be rigorous and structured. The tools and methods for data collection should meet accepted standards of practice (NONPF, 2007). They should be defined early in the project for best-practice and best-outcomes evaluation. It is helpful to consult with a statistician early in the project if statistical analysis is anticipated. Data collected can be qualitative or quantitative. Statistical analysis is useful as a measure of change but is not the only measure. The time frame of these projects often does not permit the collection of enough data points to achieve statistical significance. Other measures of change may include graphs, trends, cost analysis, narrative data, and patterns of practice.

The development, implementation, and outcomes of the project should be reviewed by an academic panel or committee per the academic policies of the degree-granting institution and disseminated in a public forum (NONPF, 2007). Modalities for dissemination are diverse and vary from project to project.

Advising the student's DNP scholarly project is different from advising the PhD dissertation and is a highly debated topic in nursing academia. Advising is often quite intense because of the condensed time frame of the project. Instead of one or two PhD advisees, clinical and research faculty in schools of nursing that house advanced practice programs may have 10, 15, or 20 DNP advisees, which increases faculty workload. Clinical faculty who must maintain a clinical practice in order to maintain certification often find workloads unsustainable. Various strategies have been suggested to account for faculty workload, but in this economic climate, it is unlikely that workload accounting practices will be altered to allow for more advising time. Some suggest that the DNP degree will only make the faculty shortage all the more acute in the short run (Fulton & Lyon, 2005). An article by Kelly (2010) suggests that unless faculty salaries improve and workload issues are addressed, the DNP-prepared graduate is no more likely to enter into a faculty role than the PhD graduate.

As nursing progresses toward the goal of educating all APNs in a DNP framework, projects are evolving. The DNP scholarly project parameters, purpose, and process are unclear within academia, employers, professional organizations, and other healthcare professions. It is reminiscent of the Indian fable of the six blind men examining an elephant to ascertain what an elephant is. Each felt a different part and came to different conclusions about what the elephant was because he could not see the whole (www.jainworld.com/literature/story25.htm). In the remainder of this chapter, the authors lay out a schema for the DNP scholarly project. The authors' graphic representation of the process is shown in **Figure 10-2**. This model is one framework for the development, implementation, and evaluation of DNP scholarly projects. This section is primarily written to assist DNP students and faculty and can be used by any practitioner who is developing a new project or program.

The Project

Getting Started

In the authors' experience with baccalaureate-to-DNP students, finding a project idea is often the most difficult part of the project. This is often because they are new to the role and the clinical environment. They may not know the evidence that supports the practice. Clinical guidelines can be found in many sources. A search through clinical guidelines can be utilized to discover gaps in practice that are amenable to a DNP scholarly project. High-quality guidelines and suggested sites for locating guidelines can be found in **Table 10-3**.

The Hexagon Tool (**Figure 10-3**) (Blase, Kiser, & Van Dyke, 2013) can be used as a planning tool to evaluate evidence-based guidelines, programs, and practices during the exploration stage of the DNP scholarly project. Factors that can be evaluated with the Hexagon Tool include:

- Needs (how well the guideline meets the identified needs)
- Fit with initiatives already in place
- Resource availability
- Evidence supporting expected outcomes
- Readiness for replication (exemplars of implementation at other sites)
- Capacity to implement

As the student becomes immersed in the advanced practice specialty and his or her practice area, gaps in practice will become more apparent. Perusing these guidelines during the exploration phase of the DNP scholarly project may help the student identify potential project ideas. The practice guidelines will also provide support for the project during the needs assessment phase of the project.

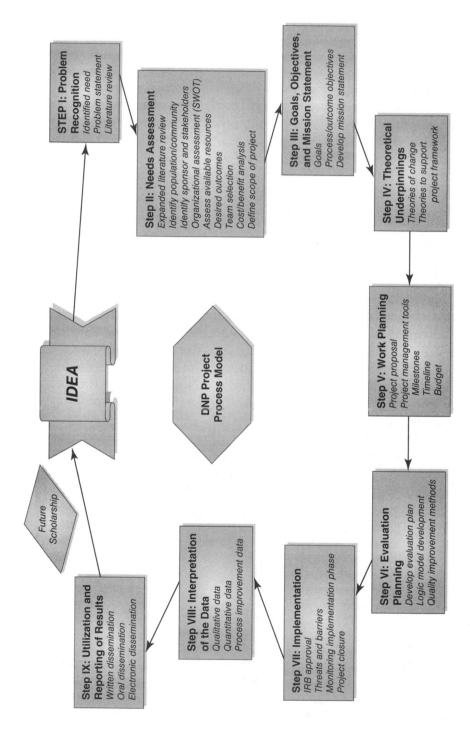

Figure 10-2 DNP Project Process Model

Table 10-3 Sources for DNP Project Ideas

National Implementation Research Network (Hexagon Tool)

Agency for Healthcare Quality and Research

National Guideline Clearinghouse

Joanna Briggs Institute

Virginia Henderson Library

National Academy of Science

Institute of Medicine

Institute for Healthcare Improvement

World Health Organization

Cochrane reviews

Professional guidelines

National Quality Forum

Quality and Safety Education for Nurses (QSEN)

Turning Research Into Practice (TRIP)

Database of Abstracts of Reviews of Effects (DARE)

DynaMed

Evidence Updates

Centre for Evidence-Based Medicine (Oxford University)

Centre for Evidence-Based Medicine (Toronto)

Canadian Medical Association Infobase

Registered Nurses Association of Ontario Best Practices Guidelines

Clinical Key Guidelines

Step I: Problem Recognition

Project ideas typically emanate from a clinical issue or opportunity identified by the nurse who is exercising critical thinking skills. In *Holistic Critical Thinking Rubric*, Facione and Facione (2009) outlined a critical thinker in part as a person who "fair-mindedly follows where evidence and reasons lead." This statement continues to be reaffirmed as a model for assessment of critical thinking in health care.

The problem could be brought forth by an individual, a group, facility administration, regulatory bodies, accreditation organizations, or government agencies. Drivers for the project can be internal or external (**Table 10-4**). The problem must be articulated clearly to the academic advisor or committee working with the student's project. The academic

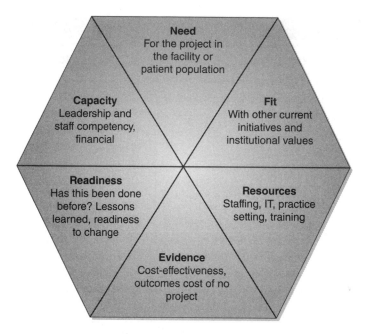

Figure 10-3 The Hexagon Tool: Exploring Context for the DNP Project
Modified with permission from Blase, Kizer, and Van Dyke, 2013.

advisors and student must sufficiently focus the project so that it can be completed within the period defined by the academic institution. The project should be in the student's area of practice scholarship (NONPF, 2007). It also must fit into the mission of the organization in which the project will be developed and implemented and within the constraints of that organization. The next step is to develop a problem statement.

Developing the Problem Statement

A problem statement identifies a situation that requires change and puts it into an organized form. It answers the questions, Why this project? Why now?

Clarity is the key. The following list is a framework for developing a problem statement.

1. Identify the deficits in the current circumstances.
2. Describe the setting of the problem.
3. Define the magnitude of the problem in measurable terms.
4. Characterize the impact of ignoring the problem on the population or organization.
5. Describe where evidence is missing in practice (identifying gaps in practice).
6. Outline evidence-based solutions. (Polit & Beck, 2012; Waddick, 2010)

Table 10-4 Internal and External Drivers for Projects

Internal Drivers	External Drivers
Administration	Public policy
Healthcare professionals	Standards of practice
Budgetary issues	Evidence-based guidelines
Customer needs	Accreditation organizations
Quality improvement programs	Third-party payers
Safety issues	Government regulations
Staffing issues	Mandatory education
Educational requirements	

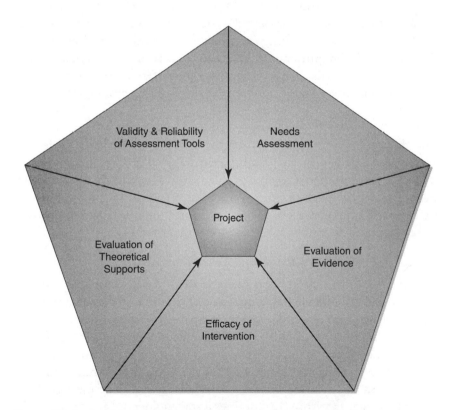

Figure 10-4 Multidimensional Literature Review for the DNP Project

At this juncture, one dimension of the literature review should be done to support the problem statement and should answer the questions posed earlier: Why this project? Why now? The literature review is multidimensional and iterative (see **Figure 10-4**). The purpose of the literature review is to identify gaps between practice and evidence, provide scientific support for the proposed intervention, support the desired goal and outcomes, and identify theoretical supports for the proposed change. The literature review may include scholarly articles, government regulations, national guidelines, clinical care models, regulatory agency policy or guidelines, professional standards and scopes of practice, organizational procedures and policies, certification requirements, reimbursement requirements, and internal institutional data.

Step II: Needs Assessment

Introduction

According to Rouda and Kusy (1995), a needs assessment is the systematic identification of the gap between the current condition and the ideal condition. It involves scanning for problems, upcoming changes in regulations or clinical requirements, business opportunities, and new mandates. A good needs assessment identifies the difference between what is and what should be (Regents of the University of Minnesota, 2015).

Population Identification

A needs assessment is done to gather the information required to develop a plan for the project. That information begins with an assessment of the population affected by the problem. Tools for this assessment may include demographic data from public sources, consultations, surveys, interviews, chart reviews, observations, focus groups, internal organizational data, and external data from government websites.

Identification of Project Sponsor and Key Stakeholders

The next phase of the needs assessment is identification of individuals who have a vested interest in the outcome of the project. Those vital individuals include a project sponsor who can partner with the academic institution to address institutional barriers and help the student navigate the matrix of the project setting. This person could be an administrator in the organization in which the project is being conducted or a similar individual with the authority to facilitate accomplishment of the project goals.

Joanna Briggs Institute (JBI) defines a stakeholder as "any individual, group, or organization having a 'stake' in an issue or its outcome" (JBI, 2013). Stakeholders are key individuals who will be affected one way or another by the project. To identify the stakeholders, consider the individuals who are not only affected by the work but also may have an interest in its outcomes. **Table 10-5** lists examples of potential stake-holders (Mind Tools, 2009). In addition to simply listing stakeholders, it is useful to analyze their roles, interests, and influence over your project. The example that follows (**Figure 10-5**) is a grid developed by Mind Tools for analysis of stakeholder interest and influence.

Table 10-5 Identifying Key Stakeholders	
Internal	**External**
Site administrator	Insurers
Chief financial officer	Regulatory agencies
Medical director	People in the community
Chief nursing officer	Suppliers
Department or program director	Interest groups
Project team members	Families in the community
Nurses	Health advocacy organizations
Ancillary staff	Community health organizations
Patients or residents	Support groups

Modified from Mind Tools. (2009). *The Mind Tools e-book* (6th ed.). Copyright © Mind Tools 1995-2009. All rights reserved. http://depts.clackamas.edu/workBehaviors/documents/MindToolsEbook-Part1.pdf

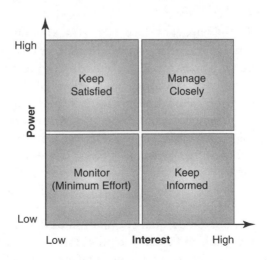

Figure 10-5 Stakeholder Analysis Grid
Cook, Mind Tools eBook, 6e, Figure 1, p. 169. Copyright © Mind Tools 1995-2009. All rights reserved. http://depts.clackamas.edu/workBehaviors/documents/MindToolsEbook-Part1.pdf

Organizational Assessment

The organizational setting and culture should be assessed. This assessment should answer these questions: What are the values of the organization in which the project will be conducted? Are the values of the organization consistent with the values of the project and the project leader? To what extent is the mission of the project consistent with that of the organization in which the project will take place (W. K. Kellogg Foundation, 2004a)? The evaluation of the setting may identify challenges and stumbling blocks for the project. When such stumbling blocks are identified, plans can be made to address them, or the project can be implemented in a different setting. If the values of the project or the project leader are not consistent with those of the organization, the project is likely to fail.

Assessment of Available Resources

A thorough assessment of available resources should be conducted early in the project development and planning. These resources could include, but are not limited to, financial support, personnel, materials for the project, marketing, statistical analysis support, office space and materials, communication costs, consulting costs, grant writing support, travel expenses, survey costs, and copyright costs. The cost of the resources must be thoroughly investigated, understood, and documented before moving on to develop a cost–benefit analysis for the project proposal.

Identification of Desired Outcomes

Outcomes describe the impact of the project. Tracking outcomes involves a concerted effort to identify what impact, benefit, or change resulted from the program. Outcomes can be measured in changes in knowledge (e.g., pre/post-program surveys), attitudes, skills, and behaviors (e.g., reduction in risk behaviors). Outcomes answer the question "What difference did it make?" (Regents of the University of Minnesota, 2015).

Early in the project, the project leader (DNP student) must develop a reasonable estimate of the desired outcomes. These can be defined through the literature review done for the problem statement; alternatively, this may be a point at which the literature review requires expansion to search for predictable outcomes based on other similar projects. In either case, some outcome statements should be developed. The project is developmental, and these outcome statements at this phase of project development are brief and will need refinement before the implementation phase. Nevertheless, the remainder of the project plan cannot proceed without clear outcomes in mind.

In health care, measurement of outcomes is the backbone of assessing the quality of the care delivered. Healthcare providers have a vast array of physiologic measures, patient self-reported functional status, and symptoms that make for rich measurements of outcomes. The difficulty is in attributing any given outcome to the care that preceded the event of physiologic change. Making the connection between any outcome measured and the care that preceded it is further complicated by the variety of care providers a patient may encounter in any one event. An example of this is a surgical patient who receives care from the surgeon; clinic staff; any number of nursing personnel with different educational backgrounds; anesthesia providers; postoperative or home care providers; family caregivers; physical therapists; and others. Attributing outcomes to one provider or another becomes quite complex. Nevertheless, we must strive to demonstrate the efficacy of our interventions. Risk factors and risk stratification can be used to account for factors that impact the outcomes of care, particularly in large populations or an accountable care organization that takes responsibility for care coordination (Agency for Healthcare Research and Quality [AHRQ], 2015, 2015).

SWOT Analysis

A powerful and simple tool for needs assessment is the SWOT analysis. SWOT stands for strengths, weaknesses, opportunities, and threats. It helps the project leader to discern where the strengths of the project lie, make plans to address weaknesses, know where to look for opportunities, and be aware of threats. This is usually a business tool, but it can be adapted to the DNP scholarly project to provide a useful analysis of the project and to generate material for the project leader to consider for solutions and direction for the project. In general, strengths and weaknesses are internal to the organization or project, and opportunities and threats are external; therefore, this matrix is sometimes referred to as the internal/external Matrix Analysis Tool (Mind Tools, 2015b). The analysis is typically summarized in a grid that briefly touches on the important learning in each category (**Figure 10-6**).

The first step in a SWOT analysis is to make a list of each of the categories. When the list is complete, prioritize it to a few strategic items in each category. Use verifiable data whenever possible (e.g., "The project improves compliance with Hgb A1C recommendations from the American Diabetes Association in this clinic population by 20%" rather than "We will improve Hgb A1Cs in our clinic"). Be brutally honest when assessing all categories, seek reliable opinions from outside the organization or unit, and be certain that this analysis is done at a level where it

Strengths	Weaknesses
• What do you (or your organization) do well? • What resources do you have that others may not have available? • What do your customers see as your strengths?	• Where could you improve? • Where do you have poor resources as compared with other similar organizations? • What do your customers see as your weaknesses?
Opportunities	**Threats**
• What social, economic, regulatory, or policy changes are happening that may provide opportunities for growth? • How can you turn strengths or weaknesses into opportunities?	• What are competitors doing that presents a threat to your core business? • Are there impending changes in technology, regulations, policy, or organizational leadership that present threats to your business or project?

Figure 10-6 SWOT Analysis
Modified from SWOT Analysis. Copyright Mind Tools Ltd, 2006-2015. All rights reserved. https://www.mindtools.com/pages/article/newTMC_05.htm

can make a difference. A SWOT analysis on a large organization may not generate enough specific data and ideas to give good direction to the organization or project (Manketelow, 2015). Listed next are some questions to stimulate thoughts about each category.

Strengths are just that. You can contemplate these questions: What does this organization, unit, or project do better than anyone else? What special resources do you have access to that others might not? What advantages do you have? Why do patients choose your organization over other similar organizations?

Weaknesses are areas for improvement. What could you improve about the organizational or unit performance? What do your patients see as your weakest areas? Should you address these areas, or simply avoid them? Do you have the resources to strengthen these areas?

Opportunities often arise from an assessment of strengths and weaknesses. Do your strengths create any opportunities for additional business or a change in direction of the current project? The same is true for weaknesses. Ask yourself if elimination of weaknesses would create additional opportunities or if it would be more cost-effective to let go of a weak area. Scan the environment for changes in regulatory requirements, emerging social phenomena, new technology, new laws, and new markets to identify opportunities.

Threats include obstacles to the project, business, or organization. Identify competitors that you should be concerned about, technological threats to the project, changes in regulatory requirements, impending changes in organizational leadership, and policy changes that may negatively impact your project. At the conclusion of the SWOT analysis, the project leader should have a sense of direction for the project's best chance for success.

Team Selection and Formation

At this point, the DNP student should assemble a team of individuals with the correct skills to conduct the project. There is no defined number or recommended composition for the team. The team membership is dictated by each individual project. These team members may or may not come from the list of stakeholders; however, the project leader is always the team leader.

Team formation is a process well defined in the literature. It proceeds through four phases: forming, storming, norming, and performing. In the forming stage, the people on the team get to know each other and may be hesitant to offer opinions. This is a good time to evaluate individual skills and personalities. The team leader should be directive during this phase. In the storming phase, team members may jockey for position and authority. At this point, some team members may feel overwhelmed by the scope of the project and the tasks necessary to complete the project. Some may be resistant to the project and express doubts about it. At all times, the DNP student should remember that she or he is the project and team leader and is ultimately responsible for the project and that the end product will reflect on her or his scholarship. The project leader should support those team members who feel less secure, work to build positive relationships among team members, and remain positive but firm when the goals of the project or his or her leadership is challenged.

Norming brings the team's strong commitment to the project goals, and as the team socializes more, the members are more agreeable to taking on the tasks of the project and working together as a unit. The leader of the team should facilitate the development of collaboration between team members.

The last stage of team development is performing. In this stage, the team makes rapid progress toward the goals of the project. The team leader may be able to delegate much of the work but remains ultimately responsible for the outcome. The team leader must remain cognizant of the constraints of the team members. In many cases, the members are staff members with other responsibilities. If the project is not dictated by the needs of the institution or community in which it is being conducted, there may be constraints on the time that team members can commit to the project (Eyre, 2015).

Cost–Benefit Analysis

A cost–benefit analysis is a powerful tool to promote the project to sponsors and others with vested interests. The development of this analysis simply adds up the real costs of the project and subtracts them from the benefits gleaned from the project. The point of the analysis is to demonstrate that the benefit of solving the problem is worth the costs (Mind Tools, 2009). For most projects, it is important that both costs and benefits be quantifiable. It is often easy to quantify costs and relatively difficult to measure benefits that are intangible and realized over a period of time. **Table 10-6** provides an example of benefits that are difficult to quantify but useful to name.

Because outcomes can be measured in a number of ways, it is imperative to avoid double counting benefits of the project. An example of double counting benefits follows. Gaining control of Hgb A1C levels in a population will decrease the cost of care through avoidance of long-term complications of diabetes. In addition, it may decrease the number of hypo/hyperglycemic visits to the emergency department. Counting both financial outcomes as a benefit is double counting (San Jose State Department of Economics, n.d.).

In some instances, projects are dictated by regulatory requirements, governing bodies, or organizational administration. In this case, it is still feasible to do a cost–benefit analysis. If the cost–benefit analysis demonstrates more cost than benefit, the analysis will demonstrate how the costs will affect the budget. This does not imply that the project will not be done; often the institution has no choice. For example, regulatory issues may dictate the implementation of the project regardless of the cost. At times the project will proceed simply because it is the right thing to do. Examples of this might be a project that is done to benefit the community served by the organization to improve community relationships or provide service to the community.

There are four additional approaches to analyzing the financial impact of a project or intervention, and each has its own advantages and disadvantages in certain situations (Frick, Cohen, & Stone, 2013).

- Cost-miminization
- Cost-utility
- Cost-consequences
- Cost-effectiveness

For a more detailed analysis of the methods, including how to select the appropriate method for the project and how to decide when to use these methods, see Chapter 2 of *Outcome Assessment in Advanced Practice Nursing* (Kleinpell, 2013).

Table 10-6 Example of a Cost–Benefit Analysis for a DNP Project

Reducing Social Isolation and Loneliness Through the Development of a Computer Resource and Communication Center

Benefit Analysis	Costs of Intervention	Percent of Residents Needing Service (national average)	Number of Nursing Home Residents	Private Room Cost Per Day	Semiprivate Room Cost Per Day	Annual Private Room Cost	Annual Semiprivate Room Cost	Goals/Assumptions	Hours of care will decrease by 5%	Cost of care	PROJECTED annual savings for the sample
Nursing Home Care MPLS Area*			**119**	$228	$191	$83,220	$69,715				
Indirect Expenses											
Room and board (space, lights, heating, Internet, housekeeping)		100%									
Direct Expenses											
Medication management		100%	Possible random sample of personal care	**Calculated hours of care per day/person**	Hours of care per day/sample	Total cost of nursing care*/day/person	Total cost of nursing care*/day/sample	**Goal: Hours of care per day/person with intervention**	Hours of care will decrease by 5%	Cost of care	**PROJECTED annual savings for the sample**
Personal care**		44%	22	**3.07**	68	$51.19	$3,457.37	Maintain - Improve - **Decrease hours of care 3.07**	2.92	$3,288	**$61,658**

(continues)

Table 10-6 Example of a Cost-Benefit Analysis for a DNP Project *(continued)*

Reducing Social Isolation and Loneliness Through the Development of a Computer Resource and Communication Center

Benefit Analysis	Costs of Intervention	Percent of Residents Needing Service (national average)	Number of Nursing Home Residents	Private Room Cost Per Day	Semiprivate Room Cost Per Day	Annual Private Room Cost	Annual Semiprivate Room Cost	Goals/Assumptions
Personal care with one or more ADL**		51% (+ 7% of pc)	25					Maintain - Improve - Decrease
Social and recreational activities**		40%	24					Increase use
Cost of Intervention								
Cognitive Assessment/ Rescreening/ Analysis - Investigator grant funded	$6,750	at 45/hr × 3 hours/ client - if hired outside agency						**Improved mental cognition**
MDS								Improved mental cognition
Mini-Mental Exam								Improved mental cognition
Depression Scale								Improved mental cognition

Facility Costs for Intervention

Space/rental	0	In kind

Equipment for the Intervention | **$8,540**

Computer (includes software)	
Headphones	
Microphone	
Printer/fax	
Equipment already purchased	**$(2,696)**

Remaining Equipment Costs | **$5,844**

Supplies

Paper	$1,000
Toner	$1,500
Ink cartridges	$1,020

Total Annual Supply Costs | **$3,520**

Teaching computer skills to the elderly	$4,320.00	($15/hr 6 hrs/week/ 48 weeks)

(continues)

Table 10-6 Example of a Cost–Benefit Analysis for a DNP Project *(continued)*

Reducing Social Isolation and Loneliness Through the Development of a Computer Resource and Communication Center

Benefit Analysis	Costs of Intervention	Percent of Residents Needing Service (national average)	Number of Nursing Home Residents	Private Room Cost Per Day	Semiprivate Room Cost Per Day	Annual Private Room Cost	Annual Semiprivate Room Cost	Goals/ Assumptions
Staff salary savings attributable to student volunteers	$(11,520.00)			($15/hr 8 hrs/week/ 48 weeks/ 2 students) - not included in calculations				
Total Cost of Intervention	**$13,684**							
PROJECTED Annual Savings (Benefit)	$61,658							
Possible annual cost savings of the intervention	**$47,974.35**							
* The MetLife Market Survey of Nursing Home & Home Care Costs Nursing	Sep-06							

Zaccagnini, M. (2007). *The development of a computer resourced communication center in a long-term care facility* (Unpublished DNP project paper). University of Minnesota, Minneapolis, MN.

Defining the Scope of the Project

Now the scope of the project statement can be written. A well-crafted project scope statement is essential for the project manager to make well-reasoned decisions throughout the life cycle of the project (Bright Hub, 2012). The scope statement will clearly and succinctly state what the project will and will not do (Luecke, 2004). The scope will help to identify potential barriers to the project. The scope statement will bind the agreement between the project leader, the project sponsor, and the organization. A well-thought-out project scope statement will help the project manager identify changes throughout the life of the project and guide modifications to the project to adapt to the changes (Bright Hub, 2012).

Step III: Goals, Objectives, and Mission Statement Development

Goals

The entire topic of goals and objectives is complicated by confusing and overlapping terminology. For the purposes of this chapter, we define goals as broad statements that identify future outcomes, provide overarching direction to the project, and point to the expected outcomes of the project. Goals should be written first. Typically a project has several goals, and each goal will need different objectives to support its achievement. Institutional demands may dictate that the goals of the project be prioritized according to financial savings, safety, or the institutional mission. Simply stated, goals are where you want to be; objectives are how you get there.

Objectives

Objectives are clear, realistic, specific, measurable, and time-limited statements of the actions that, when completed, will move the project toward its goals. In the business literature, the commonly used template for crafting objectives is SMART, which stands for specific, measurable, attainable, realistic, and timely (Lewis, 2007). In the case of the DNP scholarly project, *specific* means being precise. It is not enough to state that you want to improve a process or practice; you must name the who (target population), what (what the project will accomplish), where (project setting), and when (creation of a specific timeline) (Issel, 2013). *Measurable* implies that there are collectible data adequate for measuring change. *Attainable* and *realistic* mean that the scope of the project has been focused so that the project is feasible and meaningful with the resources at hand. Will the project really make a difference, or is it simply an exercise to attain a degree? *Timely* refers to the ability to realistically get the project accomplished in the time allotted by the academic institution. This can be an opportunity to re-check whether the scope of the project is attainable. The objectives should be rigorous but not impossible to achieve (Lewis, 2007).

Although many other types are found in the literature, in this conceptualization of the DNP scholarly project, there are two types of objectives: outcomes objectives and process objectives. *Outcomes objectives* simply address the outcomes of the project as they were defined earlier but state a specific time frame for accomplishment of the desired outcomes. *Process objectives* define the steps needed to accomplish the outcomes objectives. The process objectives are the actions or activities required to implement the project in the time frame stated. Process objectives should be succinct and clear. They function as a real-time check on the progress of the project so that course corrections can be made in a timely manner (Burroughs & Wood, 2000).

Mission Statement

The mission statement is a succinct paragraph that accurately describes why the project is being conducted. The academic institution determines whether a mission statement will be included in the DNP scholarly project. The benefit of a mission statement is that it helps clarify the purpose of the project and the methods of getting the project accomplished. Writing a mission statement is an opportunity for the project leader to take all the information gathered thus far and focus on the problem to be solved, and the methods of solving it, in two or three sentences (Allison & Kaye, 2005). A mission statement can be used to solicit support for the project, and it can be used as an explanatory statement for "elevator conversations," well-rehearsed 30-second conversations that the project leader can turn into an opportunity to inform a person or group of people about the project. A well-crafted mission statement can help keep the project focused throughout the entirety of the project.

To draft a succinct mission statement, the project manager or project team needs to answer three questions: What is the purpose of the project? (The answer should use an infinitive verb and a statement of the problem to be addressed.) What is the population to be addressed in solving the problem? What are the methods to be used in addressing the problem? It is often helpful to engage the project team in developing the mission statement to help clarify the mission to the team itself and cultivate buy-in from the team members and other stakeholders (Allison & Kaye, 2005).

The mission statement for this text is as follows: "This book is intended to serve as a core text for DNP students and faculty to use to achieve mastery of the American Association of Colleges of Nursing essentials as well as a shelf reference for practicing DNPs. The DNP essentials are all covered herein; each essential is covered in adequate detail to frame the foundation of the DNP educational program. This book provides the infrastructure for students, faculty, and practicing DNPs to achieve and sustain the highest level of practice."

Step IV: Theoretical Underpinnings of the Project

Theoretical Underpinnings of Change

The DNP scholarly project leader now has completed the work necessary to begin implementing the project plan. Each project will by definition involve change in a system or practice (NONPF, 2007). Change is notoriously difficult to achieve. The change will be made easier by using a theory to support the change process and building a model of the planned change. Planning expedites change and improves the likelihood of long-term success. Theories of change come from many different fields of study: education, sociology, psychology, organizational psychology, business management, and health care. Expansion of the literature review will assist the project leader in identifying theoretical supports for the project. The DNP scholarly project leader will use the scholarship of integration to select a theory of change that best describes the change that will occur as a result of the project.

Kurt Lewin is noted as the first change theorist. His work had a profound impact on the field of psychology and organizational psychology. His force field analysis is still used to create force field diagrams. He theorized that issues are held in balance by those forces that maintain the current state and those forces that advance change, which he called restraining forces and driving forces, respectively. Until the driving forces exceed the restraining forces, change will not occur. Lewin also created tools to map the driving forces and restraining forces. The resulting force field diagram is a powerful tool to understand the environment in which the project will take place (Thomas, 1985) (**Figure 10-7**).

Kurt Lewin was the first person to develop a model of the change process, and this model is regarded as one of his lifetime achievements. His model of the change process has three stages: unfreezing, movement, and refreezing. Most other theories of change are based in part on Lewin's theory. The first step entails an "unfreezing" of the current status or state. This can be achieved by convincing people to let go of the status quo or old way of doing something. The second step involves movement toward a new state. In this phase, people are persuaded to take a fresh look at problems from a different perspective and move toward a new

Forces for Change in Healthcare Education

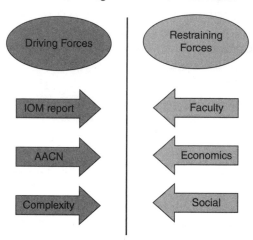

Figure 10-7 Forces for Change in Healthcare Education

paradigm. Movement of the group is supported by respected leaders who understand the need for change. In the third and final step, the change becomes the new norm for the population affected by the change. One mechanism for accomplishing this is to reinforce the new behaviors and institutionalize ("refreeze") them through formal and informal mechanisms. This reinforcement is done to ensure that the change will endure past the project implementation and become incorporated into the organizational culture (Thomas, 1985). There are many other change theorists in addition to Lewin, such as Lippitt, Watson, and Westley; Wheatley; Haverlock; Rogers; Kotter; and Prochaska and DiClemente.

Theory to Support Project Framework

Essential I (scientific underpinnings) of the Essentials of Doctoral Education for Advanced Nursing Practice supports the notion of utilizing theory to create a framework for the project. It states that "the DNP program prepares the graduate to . . . use science-based theories and concepts . . . [and] develop and evaluate new practice approaches based on nursing theories and theories from other disciplines" (AACN, 2006). The theoretical framework helps the project leader to conceptualize the project and supports it throughout the course of the project.

Theoretical frameworks can be constructed using concepts from fields of study other than nursing—for example, Motivational Theory in business, adult education theory, economic theory, social psychology, and theories of medicine. Often theories from different fields will need to be integrated into a theoretical framework that describes the unique project. For example, a framework developed by Dr. Kathleen Casey incorporated a change theory and a nursing theory to support her DNP scholarly project. Casey (2007) used Kotter's theory of change and the American Association of Critical-Care Nurses' synergy theory to create a theoretical framework for her project, "Development of an Innovative Staffing Model: Nurse Practitioner (NP) Hospitalist/Intensivist."

Step V: Work Planning

Project Proposal

Typically, a formal project proposal will be required by the academic institution or the organization where the project will take place. Minimally, the expectation is to develop an executive summary. The amount of detail required varies from institution to institution. Most proposals will include a synopsis of the problem recognition and the problem statement, a summary of the significant findings from the scope of the project and its mission statement, the desired outcomes, the goals and objectives, and, most important, the cost–benefit analysis. It is incumbent on the project leader to check with the organization for the details required for the project proposal.

Templates for project proposals can be found online. We do not support any one software package or website; many good sources exist. One such source for templates is Google drive (The Project Proposal Toolkit, 2015). This website has many other templates (http://project-proposal. casual.pm/). Another reliable website that has templates for project proposals is Mind Tools (http://www.mindtools.com/). If you decide to use additional project proposal software, you must find a package that meets your needs. Many of these software packages include project management tools that will be helpful in the next phase of work planning.

Project Management Tools

Project management is a body of specialized knowledge and skills that equip project managers with skills often developed in parallel with large government projects, beginning with the transcontinental railroad and continuing through the projects of the National Aeronautics and Space Administration (NASA) that eventually landed people on the moon. The common theme is that these projects employed thousands or hundreds of thousands of people who needed to complete highly accurate work on time and within a budget. To manage these requirements, the field of project management was born. Around the turn of the 20th century, Frederick Taylor studied work efficiency in detail and demonstrated that output can be improved by studying the work and breaking it down into small tasks that can be made more efficient. One of Taylor's peers, Henry Gantt, studied the order of tasks, primarily in shipyards during World War I, and crafted the familiar Gantt chart that is used by many to keep projects on task. These skills were applied to the building of the Hoover Dam, thus securing the place of project management in scientific approaches to large projects (Luecke, 2004). Any project developed today is likely to include a Gantt chart, which details the timeline for the project as well as which tasks can be done in parallel and which are sequential. An example of a Gantt chart is shown later in this chapter. Another important tool developed in the 1950s is the Critical Pathway Diagram (CPD), which adds a time and activity dimension to the scheduling of projects, and the PERT chart, which has a more detailed timeline. Activities are described as occurring in parallel or in sequence, and the relationship of activities is described before being incorporated into the timeline. Time estimates in a PERT chart are calculated using the shortest estimated time, the longest estimated time, and average time in this formula:

Shortest time + 4 × average time + longest time/6.

This corrects for overly optimistic time estimates. An example of a PERT chart is in **Figure 10-8**.

Today the field of project management is a distinct field of scholarship and certifications. Using the scholarship of integration (Boyer, 1990), the DNP scholarly project leader can borrow knowledge, skills, and tools from the field of project management that will serve the field of healthcare projects as well as NASA space projects. The point of the activity is to gain benefit from careful work planning and scheduling.

Baker, Baker, and Campbell (2003) defined a project as "a sequence of tasks with a beginning and an end that is bounded by time and resources and that produces a unique product or service" (p. 404). From this definition, the DNP student can discern where project management tools might aid the DNP scholarly project and where the DNP student will need to select different tools. For example, in business, the project is typically assigned to someone who is designated as the team leader. For the DNP scholarly project, considerable time and effort are expended on the needs assessment, which is then used to persuade the leadership of the

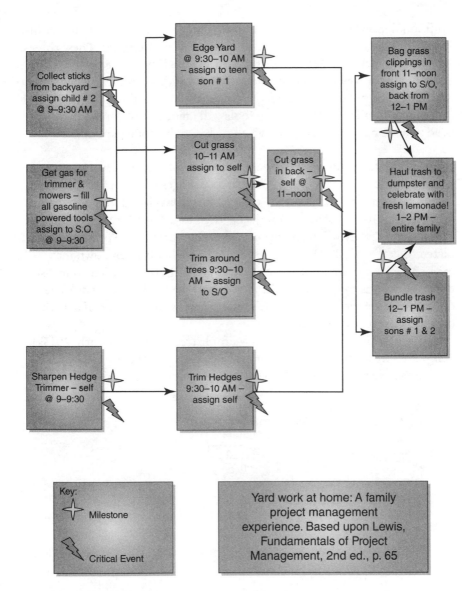

Figure 10-8 PERT Chart: Yard Work at Home
White, 2006.

organization that the project is necessary for improvement of patient or process outcomes.

Defining the scope of the project; identifying key stakeholders; assessing resources, goals, and objectives; and writing a mission statement are project management tools that have already been discussed in this chapter.

Additional tools that can be helpful to the DNP scholarly project leader include work breakdown, timeline tools, and project milestones. These three tools will help the project manager determine the flow of the project, predict when resources are needed, and estimate time to completion, which will in turn help the project leader to estimate whether the project can be done in the allotted time. These tools will identify which project tasks need to be done sequentially and when tasks can be done in parallel.

Work Breakdown and Milestones   Accurate planning of work requires that the work be broken down into small packages that can be easily monitored. Each task of the project is broken down into levels and sublevels or subprojects. Each subproject is then examined for milestones. Milestones identify when an important or large part of the project is completed (Baker et al., 2003). The subproject is further broken down into major activities and then into work packages (**Figure 10-9**). The purpose of this activity is to systematically identify all the work that needs to be done to execute the project. **Table 10-7** identifies the benefits of a work breakdown structure (WBS).

The WBS can be diagrammed as a simple tree diagram (Smith, 2015a). Templates are available online, some at no charge to the user. The work breakdown does not have to be perfect. The amount of detail will vary

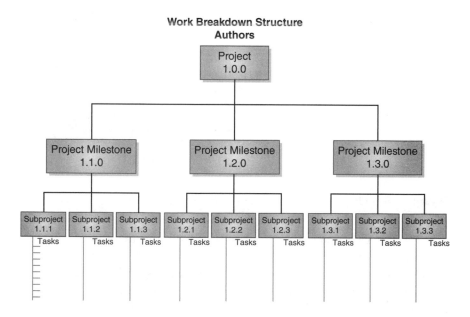

Figure 10-9 Work Breakdown Structure

Table 10-7 Benefits of Work Breakdown Structure

Identifies all the work needed for the project to be completed

Organizes the work in a logical sequence

Predicts when work may be completed

Identifies team members who have the best skills for the tasks

Identifies which resources are needed and when

Helps to prepare the budget

Provides a communication tool for all team members

Keeps team members attuned to the work of all team members

Organizes work tasks with milestones

from project to project and from institution to institution. The project leader will know that the work is broken into small enough tasks when a task can be done by one individual in a defined amount of time, and that task will produce a distinct product.

Once the WBS is completed in sufficient detail, the project leader can begin to estimate the time required to complete the subprojects and tasks. At this time, it is essential to begin to identify whether tasks can be done in parallel or whether they are sequential to other tasks. This can be done by placing the activities into a simple table such as the one in **Table 10-8** (Smith, 2015b). The information in the table can then be placed into a Gantt chart (**Figure 10-10**).

Budget Development   Developing a budget is an important step in project management. Administrators, funding agencies, and project stakeholders will need to know the costs associated with the project to decide whether to proceed with the project. Making a detailed and ac-

Table 10-8 Task Length Table

Task	Estimated Start	Estimated Length to Completion	Sequential or Parallel	Dependent Upon
A	Week 1	Four weeks	Parallel	None
B	Week 1	One week	Parallel	None
C	Week 2	Two weeks	Sequential	Task B
D	Week 5	One day	Sequential	Task A
E	Week 6	One week	Sequential	Task D

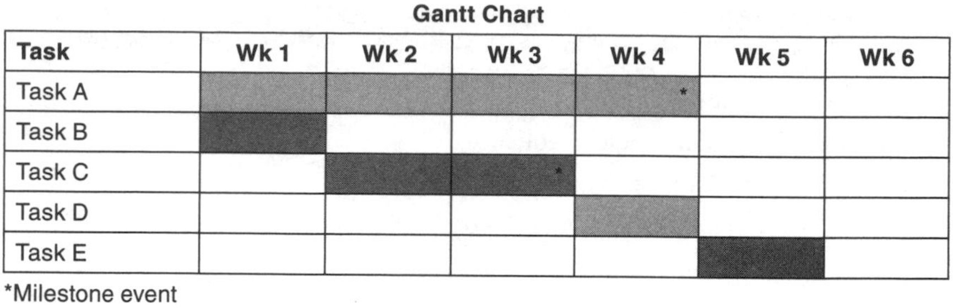

Gantt Chart

Task	Wk 1	Wk 2	Wk 3	Wk 4	Wk 5	Wk 6
Task A				*		
Task B						
Task C			*			
Task D						
Task E						

*Milestone event

Figure 10-10 Gantt Chart

curate budget and staying within the project budget will give the project manager credibility within the organization. One strong source for budget templates and planning tools is the online site of Fiscal Management Associates, LLC (http://fmaonline.net/). Here are a few pitfalls to avoid when developing a budget:

- *Underestimating labor costs.* Even though some of the team members may be salaried by the sponsoring institution, the project manager must include these costs in the project budget. Employee benefits, often estimated as a percentage of employee salary, must also be included in the calculations. They are not free.
- *Neglecting to add in the costs of equipment in use at the institution.* Use of computers, copiers, and other business equipment should be accounted for in the budget.
- *Neglecting to add in the cost of business space.* Estimates for business space can be found from many different sources online for each city or town in the United States.
- Underestimating the costs of external consultants and supplies. Most professionals will provide an hourly estimate for services.
- *Forgetting about travel costs.* Mileage rates for various purposes can be found at IRS.gov if the institution does not have a set rate for mileage.
- *Forgetting to include all the costs for materials.* The team will need supplies such as paper and pencils, pens, printing, and folders. (Luecke, 2004)

Calculating Direct and Indirect Costs   The budget must account for both direct and indirect costs. Direct costs are those that are specifically attributable to the project. This includes items such as labor, materials, supplies, equipment for the project, travel, consultant fees, project training, and marketing. Indirect costs include items that are shared by many different entities in the institution, such as business space, Internet access, information technology services, internal communications such as telephones and pagers, and support staff (Arline, 2015; Luecke, 2004). Indirect costs are often expressed as a percentage of the direct costs. A more experienced colleague or administrator at the project site may be able to assist with the development of the budget.

Templates for Budgeting Most institutions have a template they prefer to use for developing a budget. If the institution does not have a template that it prefers, templates can be found online. Microsoft Excel, Google Docs, and Word also provide templates within the programs. Once the budget is developed and final project approval is obtained, the plan for evaluation can be created.

Step VI: Planning for Evaluation

In today's healthcare environment, funds for projects are limited, and competition for funding is fiercely competitive. To get the best funding for your project, you must have a strong evaluation plan with clearly identified outcomes from the start. It is also an ethical imperative to demonstrate the efficacy of programs and practice changes (W. K. Kellogg Foundation, 2004a). It is no longer acceptable to present materials, give a posttest, and count participants. Evaluation requires a far broader range of data collection involving both quantitative and qualitative data. The focus of evaluation is not simply the DNP scholarly project: these methods should become ingrained into the framework of the professional practice of the DNP.

Unlike research that has a prescribed protocol, evidence-based practice or process improvement programs are applied broadly and thus do not have a defined research question. We are not collecting data to make the project reproducible; we are collecting data to measure change in a population or practice. Although some statistical methods may be useful for evaluation of the DNP scholarly project, many of the methods for evaluation will be different from those of the research project. The purpose of data collection is different as well. Evaluation provides accountability to the stakeholders, demonstrates quality improvement, demonstrates effectiveness in the population involved in the study, and provides clarity of purpose to the program (W. K. Kellogg Foundation, 2004a).

This section presents tools, methods, and resources that can be used for evaluation of the program or project. It is the responsibility of the project leader to select the correct tools and methods for evaluation of the project in a coherent plan for evaluation. This section also presents logic models that will assist in the development of the plan. Like any other skill, development of an evaluation plan requires both tools and practice. As the DNP uses these tools and methods, confidence and competence in project planning, implementation, and evaluation will develop. These are skills that will be necessary past the educational program into DNP practice. They define clinical scholarship.

Finding Tools to Measure Outcomes

The notion of measuring outcomes is not new and is central to demonstrating the efficacy of advanced practice nursing. Measuring outcomes provides evidence for the need for process improvements, and it determines whether the changes made are successful. It has been said that if you don't know where you are going, any route will do, and this is a clear example of that saying. To enter into a project without having clear outcomes to measure is a waste of time and talent, and it may present a hazard to the patients we serve. The ideal measurement tools should be valid and reliable measures that address the domain of health you are seeking to improve. Validity refers to the degree to which an instrument measures the concept it is supposed to measure. Reliability is concerned with the accuracy of the actual measurement tool. Those outcomes tools should also measure compliance with standards, evidence-based guidelines, and recommendations. They should be useful in customizing programs to the individual and they should be easily interpreted and reported to stakeholders (AHRQ, 2015). Here are some questions to answer when selecting outcomes to measure for the DNP scholarly project:

- Does the outcome measure selected answer the question of whether the change proposed actually happened? (Appropriateness)
- Are the outcome measure data easy to collect and report? (Feasibility)
- Does the outcome measure selected produce data that are consistent? (Reliability)
- Does the outcome measure actually measure what it is supposed to measure? (Validity)

- Does the outcome measure identify change over the time frame of the project? (Responsiveness)
- Is the outcome measure acceptable to the patient population? (Acceptability) (Olney & Barnes, 2013)

Sources for reliable tools include the AHRQ, National Guideline Clearinghouse, IOM, and the World Health Organization.

Development of Evaluation Methods

Evaluation should be thoughtfully designed so that it measures the degree to which the outcomes were or were not met. The evaluation design should fit the unique project. The project leader must determine the appropriate methods and types of data to be collected that best demonstrate the outcomes. The evaluation plan can consist of qualitative methods, quantitative methods, or a mix of both. When choosing the methods, there are some indications of whether quantitative or qualitative methods are most appropriate for measurement of your outcomes. If the outcome is to identify how much, how many, how often, or an average response, then the best method is quantitative. If the outcome is to identify what worked, what the numbers mean, how the project was useful, what it meant to the participants, or what factors influenced success or failure, then one should select qualitative methods (Olney & Barnes, 2006, 2013). Qualitative data can provide contextual meaning to the quantitative data in a project that uses both. For example, it is useful to know the number of diabetic patients in a population who develop diabetic retinopathy; it is another thing to understand the impact of blindness in a person's life. Qualitative data provide meaning to the people affected by the project, the stakeholders, the organization, and possibly outside audiences (W. K. Kellogg Foundation, 2004a). Regardless of which approach is used for evaluation, the methods should be chosen before implementation of the project.

Tools for qualitative evaluation may include observations, ethnographic interviews, structured interviews, written questions, and document review. Issues of cultural sensitivity should be kept in mind when developing survey or interview questions. Tools for quantitative data collection include surveys, health factors, laboratory test results, and chart reviews. No matter which methods the project leader selects for evaluation data collection, they should be reliable and valid (Olney & Barnes, 2006, 2013).

Logic Model Development

> *Basically, a logic model is a systematic and visual way to present and share your understanding of the relationships among the resources you have to operate your program, the activities you plan, and the changes or results you hope to achieve.*

> —W. K. Kellogg Foundation (2004b)

The first logic models were developed in the 1970s. *Evaluation: Promise and Performance* by Joseph S. Wholey was the first text to use the term *logic model* (Taylor-Powell & Henert, 2014). Logic models have evolved since the introduction of the Government Results and Performance Act of 1993. This act was intended to improve the effectiveness of federal programs through requirements for strategic planning and program evaluation. It shifted the focus of evaluation onto results and not simply activities. The models identified in this chapter were developed in part in response to this act.

A logic model (**Figure 10-11**) is a picture of how the project developer believes the program will work. It uses a series of diagrams to indicate how parts of the program are linked together or sequenced. There is no one correct way to diagram the logic model. It depends in large part on the purpose of the model. If the diagram is used to describe the entire project plan, it should be detailed. If it is used for communication among team members, it should be less complex. The project developer may need several models for various parts of the project (Taylor-Powell & Henert, 2008). Logic models all have similar components: inputs, outputs, and outcomes (Taylor-Powell & Henert, 2008).

Only the simplest of programs will be adequately described by this model. For example, if you had a headache, it would describe the input as "headache," the output as "take an aspirin," and the outcome as

Simple Logic Model

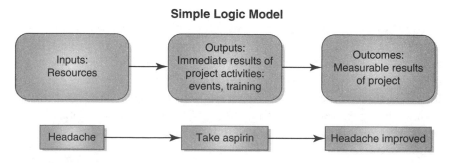

Figure 10-11 Simple Logic Model

"headache is better." This simple model does not identify how projects get from inputs to outputs. No activities are defined in the model. Most programs will require more detail to adequately describe the project.

The logic model template presented in this chapter is an assimilation of several models: the Kellogg Foundation Logic Model, the United Way Program Outcome Model, and the University of Wisconsin Extension Service Logic Model. Resources, templates, designs, and worksheets for development of these models are available online at no charge to the individual. **Figure 10-12** is a template created by the authors.

In the template, inputs are the resources required to implement and evaluate the project. Those resources may include personnel, facilities, equipment, time, and finances. Resources could be constrained by laws, regulations, funding, time, existing culture, and local policy. Constraints can prevent the project from advancing or limit the project in some manner. For example, financial resource allocations may be less than what was originally proposed to support the project. The project leader may either redefine the budget or reexamine the project activities that affect the budget. Activities are what the project does with the resources to achieve the intended outcomes: events, training and education, meetings, development of media and technology, and development of the processes

				Outcomes		
				Short Term	Long Term	Impact
Inputs	Constraints	Activities	Outputs			
Personnel	Budget	Events	Number of participants	Knowledge improvement	Behavior Improvement	Long-term results of the change
Financial	Physical space	Training	Amount of education delivered	Skill improvement	Motivation improvement	
Time	Law, regulations, local policy	Education	Number of hours of service	Improved level of functioning		
Materials	Time frame	Media/ Technology				
Equipment	Existing culture	Meetings				
Facilities		Development of processes				

Figure 10-12 Logic Model Template

necessary to implement the project. Outputs are the immediate results of the project. They could include the number of participants, the number of hours of instruction, the number of meetings, participation rates, and the number of hours of each service provided. Outcomes can be considered at three levels: short-term, long-term, and impact outcomes. In short-term outcomes, the project leader measures the effect of the activities on the knowledge base and skills or level of functioning. The long-term outcomes reflect a change in behavior or motivation. Impact outcomes describe the results of the change on the population served by the project.

Figure 10-13 demonstrates an application of the logic model to a more complex project completed in 2007 as part of the requirements of the

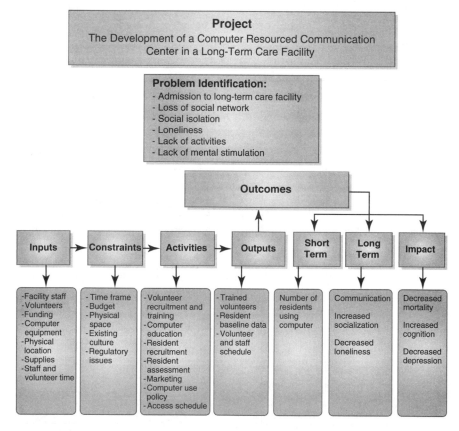

Figure 10-13   The Development of a Computer Resourced Communication Center in a Long-Term Care Facility

Zaccagnini, M. (2007). *The development of a computer resourced communication center in a long-term care facility* (Unpublished DNP project paper). University of Minnesota, Minneapolis, MN.

DNP curriculum at the University of Minnesota School of Nursing. This model describes a DNP scholarly project completed by Mary Zaccagnini, "Development of a Computer Resourced Communication Center in a Long-Term Care Facility." This project addressed the problem of social isolation within a long-term care facility and the resultant problems caused by the isolation. The project leader developed a computer center and trained the staff and volunteers to assist the residents. It demonstrated that the residents who used the computer center experienced an increase in socialization and communication via e-mail and a decrease in loneliness.

> *Thinking about a program in logic model terms prompts the clarity and specificity required for success, and often demanded by funders and your community. Using a simple logic model produces (1) an inventory of what you have and what you need to operate your program; (2) a strong case for how and why your program will produce your desired results; and (3) a method for program management and assessment. (W. K. Kellogg Foundation, 2004a)*

Quality Improvement Methods

After a long Congressional debate, the Affordable Care Act was passed and signed into law in March 2010 (U.S. Department of Health and Human Services, 2011). One major initiative contained in this act was the directive for the Secretary of Health and Human Services to develop a national strategy for quality improvement in health care. The three aims of this national strategy were: to improve the delivery of healthcare services, reduce the cost of quality health care, and improve the health of the U.S. population. The strategy continues to guide the national effort to improve health care for all Americans. As the largest group of healthcare providers, nurses play a pivotal role in quality improvement efforts in implementing these strategies (U.S. Department of Health and Human Services, 2012). The DNP-prepared nurse will have the skill set and an understanding of the various methodologies to develop, lead, implement, and evaluate these quality improvement efforts.

Quality improvement methods have been used in the business world for many years. The earliest quality improvement tools were developed during World War II and continue to be used in healthcare quality improvement today. W. Edwards Demming and Walter Shewhart are considered the founders of quality improvement. Shewhart first developed the PDCA cycle as a methodology for quality improvement. PDCA consists of the following steps:

- Plan:
    - Collect data
    - Analyze data
    - Plan the intervention
- Do:
    - Develop and test potential solutions
- Check:
    - Measure efficacy of solutions
    - Analyze outcomes for needed adjustments to solutions
- Act:
    - Modify the plan as needed

(U.S. Department of Health and Human Services, 2013)

Demming later modified the PDCA model to the PDSA model (plan, do, study, act) in order to refocus the cycle on analysis instead of inspection. Demming's PDSA model is used to this day in healthcare agencies that do *rapid cycle improvement processes* consisting of daily management and continuous development. With this model, small changes are made, evaluated in a very short time, corrected or changed, and reevaluated. **Figure 10-14** demonstrates the iterative nature of the PDSA model. In 1948, the engineers at Carnegie Tech further modified this model with the addition of a first step, "Define the problem" (Brecker, 2001).

Dr. Joseph Juran broadened quality management concepts and focused on the responsibilities of management of the organization. He promoted the concept known as *managing business process quality*, which is a technique for executive cross-functional quality improvement. His

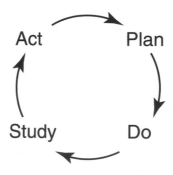

Figure 10-14 PDSA

model, known as the Juran trilogy, is made up of three methods: quality planning, quality control, and quality improvement, which, when complete, will lead to quality leadership. The three methods leading to quality leadership are also known as *total quality management* (TQM) (Ross, 2009). The Juran model gained popularity in business during the 1980s (Juran Institute, 2009).

Another quality improvement method, *value analysis*, also known as value engineering, was developed by Larry Miles, an engineer at General Electric during World War II. The value analysis method focuses on a very structured analysis of materials, processes, and designs by multifunctional teams to seek cost-effective alternatives. The data generated by this very structured methodology laid the groundwork for the *lean* and *six sigma* techniques for quality improvement in health care (Brecker, 2001).

There are many quality models in use in health care. Two focus on patient care: the CARE model and the FADE model. The CARE model is used to support chronic care projects. This CARE model emphasizes the interactions between patients with chronic diseases who take an active role in the management of those diseases, and the providers who have the expertise and resources to aid the patient's self-care. The FADE model is more appropriate for acute care. The four steps of the FADE model are:

- Focus (define which processes are to be improved)
- Analyze (collect and study the data)
- Develop (develop plans for improvement in processes)
- Execute (implement) and evaluate (measure outcomes for success)

The FADE model, like PDSA, is cyclic in nature. Many iterations may be needed until the desired improvement is seen and documented with data (Duke University Department of Community and Family Medicine, 2014; U.S. Department of Health and Human Services, 2011).

In 1986, an engineer at Motorola Corporation, Bill Smith, invented six sigma as a method to count the number of manufacturing defects in semiconductors. He noted that it takes six standard deviations from a normal curve to improve reliability of manufactured parts to compete with the Japanese manufacturers. The goal of the six sigma processes is to reduce errors in manufacturing to 3.4 defects per million, or 99.99966% error free (GE, 2012). These same statistical methods are being applied to healthcare processes in an effort to improve the quality and safety of health care. Six sigma core concepts seek to improve the quality of healthcare process outputs by identifying and removing the causes of errors (defects) and minimizing variability in healthcare practices and processes. Two of the most common methodologies used to achieve six sigma goals are DMAIC (design, measure, analyze, improve, and control) and DMADV (design, measure, analyze, design, and verify). DMAIC is employed when an existing process does not meet customer expectations, and DMADV is used when "developing a new product or service or when a process is optimized but still fails to meet customer expectations" ("DMAIC versus DMADV," 2012). There are many techniques and processes available for quality improvement. This is not intended to be an exhaustive list. PDSA and six sigma are at the core of many of healthcare quality improvement strategies. These quality improvement skills are necessary for the DNP graduate to fulfill as leaders for organizational change and healthcare quality improvement strategies (AACN, 2006, DNP Essential II).

Step VII: Implementation

Institutional Review Board Process

If Steps I through VI went well, the DNP scholarly project is ready to be implemented. Most institutions will require a review from the IRB or human subjects committee. These reviews are a mechanism to ensure that human subjects are protected and have given fully informed consent when required. It also ensures that patient privacy issues are addressed and that the data collected are secure and used correctly. Some projects may require just one review through the academic institution; other projects and settings may require an academic review and a review by the IRB of the institution where the project will be conducted. The timeline and manner in which this review is conducted will be dictated by the institutions that complete the review. Because these reviews can take some time to process, the DNP scholarly project leader must be certain to account for this time in the project timeline. Projects cannot be implemented until the IRB review is completed.

Getting the Project Implemented

The IRB review is a good opportunity to review all the project steps taken thus far. The DNP scholarly project leader should review the goals, objectives, and work plans to be certain that they are appropriate to the problem identified in the needs assessment. The project leader should reflect on her or his own leadership style and the team she or he will be leading. In addition, this is a good time to review the evaluation plan to be certain that it will measure the correct data points to determine whether the project addressed the problem. It is a good idea to plan a formal kickoff event to reenergize the team at this time because enthusiasm can wane over the time it takes to plan the project. The team should select a firm start date for the project and avoid wavering on this date. All of this involves clear and frequent communication. This is a time when every team member should be fully informed and knowledgeable about the project plan.

Threats and Barriers to Project Success

The project leader should think very carefully about threats and barriers to the project. Threats can be divided into those that can be predicted and those that cannot. Foreseeable threats to the project are those threats that the project leader and team members can identify as potential barriers at the beginning of the planning. The threats to the project might include lack of or decreased funding, employee turnover, reduced interest over time, time-frame barriers, and technology challenges. Unforeseen threats are events that just happen and over which the project leader has no control. Events such as a change in institutional leadership, new regulations or policies that affect the project, changes in the economy, business failures, and "acts of God" such as Hurricane Katrina are examples of unforeseen threats (Luecke, 2004).

Although it is impossible to predict unforeseen events, the foreseeable threats and barriers should be addressed with alternative plans for implementation. The project leader should consult with the team to develop different strategies, taking the available resources into consideration. For example, if funding is less than anticipated, the project leader will need to work with the team on a scaled-back plan. Ultimately, if the project is successful, the project can be expanded when additional funding is available (Luecke, 2004).

Monitoring the Implementation Phase

Project implementation is the exercise of leadership and control of the project. This is the time when the DNP has to be the explicit project leader to monitor every step of implementation and measure progress against the goals and objectives, mission statement, evaluation plan, and timeline. This is the time when the project leader must have a clear vision of the project. The leader cannot vacillate about the goals and objectives or the direction of the project. The project leader cannot relinquish the leadership role to another team member or show diminished enthusiasm. Implementation is the time to showcase all the previous work and to turn ideas into reality.

Implementation Science   One consistent finding in healthcare research is the long gap between discovery of new knowledge and implementation of that knowledge in the practice arena. Patients fail to gain benefits from the new knowledge, they are exposed to potential harm, and the healthcare system incurs unnecessary liability and lost opportunity costs (Grimshaw, Eccles, Lavis, Hill, & Squires, 2012). The emerging field of implementation science examines how research is translated from new clinical knowledge into improvements in patient care. Grimshaw et al. (2012) stated that there are two kinds of translational research: the first (T1) is the translation of new knowledge of basic science research into clinical science, and the second (T2) takes new clinical knowledge and implements it in a practice, policy, or process to improve patient care. This field is also known as implementation science. Grimshaw et al. (2012) defined implementation science as "ensuring that stakeholders are aware of and use research findings to inform their health and healthcare decision making." This definition crosses many groups of interest: healthcare providers, policy makers, administrators, regulatory bodies, and patients.

Much of this new science is emerging from Canada, where some translational scientists have created large databases of evidence from systematic reviews. However, housing data in accessible databases does not solve the problem of implementation of new clinical knowledge, nor do continuing education or recertification programs. Scientists at the Knowledge Transfer Study Group of McMaster University in Ontario have proposed a framework for the overall approach to knowledge transfer that could be applied to the DNP scholarly project. The framework centers on the answers to five questions (Lavis, Robertson, Woodside, McLeod, & Abelson, 2003):

- What should be transferred?
- To whom should the knowledge be transferred?
- By whom should the knowledge be transferred?
- How should research knowledge be transferred?
- With what effect should research knowledge be transferred?

Emerging evidence suggests the answers to these questions. In summary:

- The "basic unit" of knowledge transfer should be current systematic reviews or synthesis of current evidence. Only rarely should one study be widely disseminated without the context of other supporting findings.
- Different types of research will have different audiences that may include policy makers, healthcare professionals, administrators, regulatory bodies, industry, research funding agencies, and

researchers. Discerning which of these audiences should be targeted is a key to successful implementation.

- The appropriate person, organization, or body to communicate this knowledge will vary according to the audience but should be trustworthy and credible. Communication of this clinical knowledge will likely need both organizational components (data analysts and training programs) and technological components (accessible databases of systematic reviews).

- Transfer of research knowledge should be planned and take into account barriers to knowledge translation, such as the sheer volume of new science, organizational barriers, structural barriers, peer group barriers, and professional to patient barriers, to name a few. Careful assessment of these barriers will make implementation and permanent practice or policy change more likely.

- Choosing the correct behavioral change strategy is another key to successful implementation. The Cochrane Effective Practice and Organization of Care (EPOC) group has written two overviews of systematic reviews of professional behavior change strategies and their effectiveness in certain situations and for specific audiences. Grimshaw et al. (2012) have summarized this information in an article in *Implementation Science*.

There are other implementation strategies and frameworks in the literature that are variations on change theory. All are relatively recent and thus have not been validated to any great extent. What does this mean for the DNP student trying to implement his or her project? This emerging scientific field has enormous potential to aid the DNP during the implementation phase of any evidence-based change project. The framework for T2 translational science leaves many questions to be answered in the future. Nevertheless, this is a field that bears observation and scanning for new developments that can make implementation of the DNP scholarly project more likely to be successful.

Project Closure

Every project has a beginning and an end. A good project leader plans for project closure. Final details and loose ends must be identified and addressed. Project closure checklists and templates are available online to help the project leader develop the report that will be presented to leadership.

The report should contain several items:

- An objective evaluation of the successes and shortcomings of the project

- Project accomplishments
- Important project data
- Significant project changes that had an impact (positive or negative) on the project
- Issues that need further exploration
- An accounting of the budget and any variances
- Recommendations based on what has been learned in the project

("Project Closure," 2014)

Closure should include a meeting with stakeholders and an acknowledgment that the project is completed, a brief summary of the results, plans for sustaining the changes due to the project, and plans for transfer of leadership to the institution. The project leader should meet with team members, thank them for their contributions, and celebrate the accomplishments of the project team. This is a time for team members to reflect on what went well and what did not go well during the project. Closure promotes sustainability of the project after implementation.

Step VIII: Interpretation of the Data

Quantitative Data

Quantitative data collected in the DNP scholarly project serve a different purpose from those collected for the PhD thesis. They serve to demonstrate the efficacy of the project and are not intended to meet rigorous statistical tests for significance. Nevertheless, funders and other stakeholders will be interested in the project's results, and the correct data must be collected in sufficient amounts to demonstrate the outcomes of the project. Data that describe the outcomes of the project must be collected, organized, and presented to peers, the academic community, and other parties of interest. These data will also help other clinicians with similar issues select an intervention that is likely to address the problems they are experiencing in a similar setting.

Descriptive statistical analysis is the traditional method for bringing meaning to data. This type of statistical analysis describes the population in which data were collected and what was observed in the population. The authors of this chapter recommend engaging a statistician early in project planning if the plan for evaluation includes statistical analysis. Mahn-DiNicola (2014) advised likewise: "The APN may wish to enlist the support and guidance of a statistician or doctorally prepared nurse researcher to insure the end product is methodologically sound and contains the information necessary to convince others" (p. 680). In addition to statisticians, statistical analysis software programs are available. Microsoft Excel has some tools for statistical analysis built into the program.

Even if the project design and sample size do not permit the application of inferential statistical analysis, there are other ways in which the project leader can bring meaning to the data. The project leader can present the findings with other visual tools and techniques, such as charts, graphs, and diagrams. Examples of these visual tools could be run charts that display a change in response over time, pie charts that show relative proportions in relationship to the whole, or flowcharts that diagram processes (Mahn-DiNicola, 2014).

Qualitative Data

The analysis of qualitative data can be daunting because of the sheer volume of records, narratives, and interviews. An organized and logical approach is needed to gain meaning from these kinds of data. The process for analysis of qualitative data includes revisiting the data, placing the data into focus areas, coding the data while looking for themes and patterns, identifying common themes and patterns across data sets, and interpreting the results.

- Step 1 is to review all documents, tapes, videos, surveys, and field notes to get an overall sense of the data. This step will also help the project leader eliminate unnecessary or extraneous information. As this review is under way, the themes or focus areas can be identified.
- Step 2 is sorting the information into the categories and themes identified in Step 1.
- Step 3 is to code the information, naming the themes identified in a systematic manner.
- Step 4 is to look for common threads of meaning or patterns within and across the coded data sets.
- Step 5 is to interpret the data by returning to the outcomes for the project and evaluating whether the qualitative data collected and organized reflect the desired outcomes.

Programs exist to help project leaders assess and interpret qualitative data and can be found readily online. Microsoft Word also has some qualitative analysis tools built into the program (Taylor-Powell & Renner, 2003). Resources for beginners include "Analyzing Qualitative Research" at the University of Wisconsin–Extension website (http://learningstore.uwex.edu/pdf/G3658-12.pdf).

Analyzing Quality Outcomes Data

Analyzing quality outcomes data is considerably different from analysis of carefully controlled research data. Although the data collected certainly may achieve statistical significance, often they do not, and the data cannot be subjected to rigorous statistical methods. Instead, change is demonstrated through the use of pie charts, bar graphs, scattergrams, and other visual methods that show trends and patterns that have clinical significance even if the data are not statistically significant. An adequate selection of these graphic methods of showing trends and clinical change can be found within Microsoft Excel and many other common programs.

Step IX: Utilization and Reporting of Results

Why Disseminate Your Scholarly Outcomes?

There are two purposes for dissemination of the project results: reporting the results of the project to stakeholders and the academic community, and dissemination to other professionals in similar settings. The information and results of the successful DNP scholarly project will have application beyond the immediate practice environment. It is very likely that the problem you identified at the beginning of the project is experienced by others as well. Therefore, it is important to share the findings of the project regardless of whether the project produced the results you expected or different results. There are many venues for dissemination of the project results. The AHRQ dissemination tool can assist authors in deciding where to publish and when they have attained successful dissemination (**Figure 10-15**).

Written Dissemination

Written dissemination is a time-honored method of sharing information. Considerations for selection of the best place to disseminate the information include the targeted audience, the environment in which the project is most likely to be helpful, and the forum in which the project should be published. If the project leader simply wants to communicate the outcomes of the project, an executive summary is a good mechanism for this purpose.

Executive Summary　An executive summary is a document that summarizes the results of the project. It should not exceed 10% of the length of the main report ("How to Write an Executive Summary," 2012). It typically has a problem statement, a short description of the background, a summary of results when applicable, and recommendations. The execu-

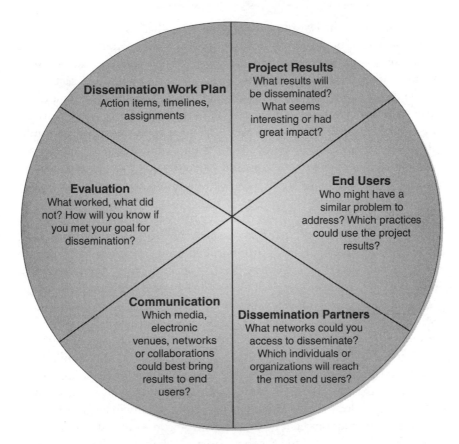

Figure 10-15 AHRQ Dissemination Planning Tool
Data from Dissemination Planning Tool: Exhibit A from Volume 4. October 2014. Agency for Health-care Research and Quality, Rockville, MD. Retrieved from http://www.ahrq.gov/professionals/quality
-patient-safety/patient-safety-resources/resources/advances-in-patient-safety/vol4/planningtool.html

tive summary is used quite differently from an abstract. The executive summary provides the project leader with a chance to present important information to a group that may be able to fully fund a project or continue it past the immediate project. The executive summary must be well written, succinct, smooth, and polished. When creating an executive summary, reread the project paper. Identify and extract the main themes. Create a rough draft from the ideas you have identified as the major points in each category or heading. Reread the summary until you are certain that every word in it is important and clearly communicates the outcomes of the project.

Abstract An abstract is a very short description of the project and significant results. The purpose of the abstract is to give readers a glimpse of the main published work so they can decide whether it contains information they would find interesting or informative. Most journals are very prescriptive about the number of words and characters that may be included in an abstract. Look in the "Information for Authors" section of the journal. Some journals require as few as 200 words, making it difficult to discern which main concepts should go into this type of abstract. The author should keep in mind the purpose of the abstract: What would colleagues find interesting or informative about the project? Focusing on that will help you create a succinct and engaging abstract. Examples of abstracts from colleagues in each role can be found in **Appendix 10-1**.

Peer-Reviewed Journals   If the audience for dissemination of the results of the project is a group of professionals in a similar practice setting, a peer-reviewed journal is an appropriate medium. Thousands of journals are on the market. The project leader must select the most appropriate. For a more general project, select a journal that targets a broad base of professionals, such as the *American Journal of Nursing* or *Advanced Practice Nursing*. A more focused project should be submitted to the appropriate specialty journals. Look at several recent issues of the journal you believe may be the best for publication. Find articles that have similar subject matter to the topic you are presenting and read them to discern the style, format, and themes. Authors can also contact the editor-in-chief with the topic idea to see whether she or he believes it will be appropriate for the audience targeted by the journal. The journal will also note the publication manual used for their journal. That might be American Psychological Association, American Medical Association, Chicago, or Squire Guidelines.

The authors of this chapter suggest the following methodology for writing for publication. Readers may find some of these tips to be helpful.

Set a goal for publication that includes the desired journal, the target publication date, and how the author will manage her or his time for writing.

- Good writing takes time. Set aside regular time when you can write quietly. The most difficult task will be to convey the most important findings in a four- to five-page article. Go through the major sections of your project and select the key highlights of each section to create an outline.
- Keep a folder of articles that you have cited. Make the citations in the text as you write. This is far easier than trying to go back and remember which articles support what sentences.

- Keep the material engaging. This is the author's chance to share important material with other professionals so they can learn about a project that improved a practice or some outcomes.
- Manuscript preparation is crucial to getting the article published. Most journals have information for authors that details how the manuscript must be prepared for that journal's editors to review it. Carefully follow those guidelines when preparing the manuscript. If questions arise, contact the journal's editorial assistant.
- Journals also have specific requirements for the abstract and keywords. Carefully follow the journal's requirements.
- Be meticulous about grammar and style. The editors will not accept an article with multiple grammar or style errors, and such errors diminish the scholarly quality of the work.
- After submission, expect feedback from expert reviewers. The feedback to the author is not intended to make the author feel good; it is intended to make the article stronger and more meaningful to the audience. In general, editors know their business well, and if you incorporate reviewer suggestions into the manuscript, it will be a better article.
- Be patient. This is a process that will take some time.
- Enjoy the results.

Other Professional Publications   Many other types of publications are not peer reviewed but may have a far larger audience. These include non-subscription journals that come in the mail to practitioners, local publications, public media, and newspapers. All of these will be appropriate vehicles for dissemination of your outcomes if the audience is identified correctly. In general, the suggestions for peer-reviewed journals also apply to these types of publications. Reflect the scholarly nature of the project in all forms of communication.

Oral Dissemination

Nurses disseminate much information orally, and clear communication is imperative. Leaving a voicemail message for a patient requires careful thought and consideration of the content and anticipated outcome of the communication. Oral dissemination to professional audiences can be effective as well, and oral communication gives the author the chance to express passion for the topic through voice tones and gestures. Oral dissemination opportunities include poster sessions, presentations, or lectures for professional meetings at the local, state, or national level, and presentations to population-based groups.

Preparing for oral presentations is a bit different from preparing written materials. Nevertheless, the successful presenter must identify the audience before beginning preparation, just as if the materials were being submitted to a peer-reviewed journal. Here are some tips from the chapter authors on preparing oral presentations.

- Understand the setting for your presentation. If you are not familiar with the organization that requested the presentation, learn about the organization by visiting its website or reading the materials published by that organization.
- Contact an organizational officer or member of the board of directors for questions. Know why you were asked to present, what issues may underlie the presentation, the knowledge level of the audience on the topic, the organizational context, the topics of other speakers before or after the presentation, the timing of the presentation, and what is happening before or after the presentation (for example, if there is a business meeting preceding or following the presentation, the audience may be anxious about the impending meeting) (Guffey & Loewy, 2015).
- Review your project for main points and create an outline. Remember that the criteria for citations in oral presentations are the same as for written work. All the points in the presentation will need the same kind of strong support from the relevant literature. Do not use figures or tables unless you get permission from the authors. Cartoons also need permission from the author of the cartoon.
- Recognize that listening is different from reading and that it is difficult for most people to sit and listen for long periods. Thus, it is useful to change the style of presentation by interspersing scientific content with stories or case reports that break up the presentation but still present useful information in a different manner.
- Fill in the outline with the most important findings and results of the project. Be succinct. The rule of thumb is that every presentation should have three parts (Guffey & Loewy, 2015):
  - Tell the audience what you are going to say in the introduction.
  - Tell the audience the information most relevant to the project in the body of the presentation.
  - Recap your presentation in the conclusion.

Presentation Software Packages   Many presentation software packages are on the market. They will assist you in creating slides for your presentation, but the point of the slides is to enhance the oral presentation with a visual component, not to replace the oral materials. The slides should be simple and easy to read to avoid distracting the listeners from the oral materials. Each slide should cover one major point and have no more than seven lines with seven words on a line (Guffey & Loewy, 2015). Remember that many figures and tables are difficult to read when projected, so keep the tables simple and readable, or consider using bar graphs or pie charts instead of tables. Avoid using all caps—IT LOOKS AGGRESSIVE. The font size should be 24 points or larger for best readability (Guffey & Loewy, 2015). The slides should be free of grammatical errors, just as if the presentation were being published (often the presentation slides will be published for the attendees). Plan on no more than one slide per minute of presentation (Guffey & Loewy, 2015).

Tips for presenting to professional audiences include the following (adapted from Guffey & Loewy, 2015):

- Time your presentation carefully and rehearse it meticulously.
- Preparation is the key to a successful presentation. You cannot possibly rehearse too much.
- Learn to speak to the audience, not the slides.
- Check to ensure that all the embedded links work with the equipment at the site before the presentation begins.
- Bring a backup disc with the presentation materials on it.
- Get instruction on how to use the audiovisual equipment prior to the presentation.
- Establish a routine of self-care for the evening before the presentation to get a good night's rest and appear enthusiastic about the materials.
- Avoid drinking caffeinated beverages immediately before the presentation.
- Dress professionally but comfortably.

Electronic Venues for Dissemination

Electronic venues for dissemination are exciting recent phenomena. Our society has quickly incorporated these forms of communication into our culture and language. One astounding example is social networking sites. SixDegrees.com was the first identifiable social network, established in 1997 (Boyd & Ellinson, 2007). Since that time, the use of social networks has exploded and taken off in many different directions from the original intent of connecting friends electronically. As of this writing, there are literally hundreds of social networking sites with different purposes. Many professional organizations maintain a Facebook site, and there are thousands of informal social networking groups of professionals. This is just one example of an electronic dissemination venue.

Table 10-9 Electronic Dissemination Venues

Formal

Peer-reviewed electronic journals

Voice over network (VON) programs

Teleconferencing

Podcasts

Videoconferencing

Organizational/professional websites

Patient education websites

Websites with evidence-based guidelines (National Institutes of Health, Agency for Healthcare Research and Quality)

Informal

Blogs

Professional networks

Social networks

Many more are available to the DNP student or practitioner who wants to disseminate project results to a specific audience. **Table 10-9** lists some of the available venues.

Use caution when publishing to social networks and other electronic media. There is little quality control over content, and most of these types of electronic tools are not peer reviewed. Once an article is published to many of these sites, the author has no control over where it goes or how it is used. Until some of these issues are resolved, be cautious in publishing articles to a website or other electronic medium.

Conclusion

The DNP scholarly project is not simply a requirement for a degree. At its finest, it should reflect a synthesis of all the knowledge and skills gained by the DNP student in the course of studies (AACN, 2006). It should also establish the basis for the student's future scholarly work—the scholarship of integration and application. The state of American health care will benefit enormously from a cadre of expert clinicians who can utilize evidence-based projects and tools to improve the outcomes of care delivered by APNs.

Nevertheless, issues remain with the development and implementation of the project. In 2013, the NONPF wrote a white paper on the titling of the DNP project. This white paper outlined some significant issues and recommended beginning a national dialogue with advanced practice registered nurse stakeholders to

- Delineate and clearly communicate the essence of the DNP project.
- Delineate and clearly communicate acceptable forms of the DNP project, and
- Clarify and unify standards for DNP projects. (NONPF, 2013)

As pointed out in this white paper and through other authors, the curricula and expectations for the DNP project are evolving. As programs transition into the DNP framework, faculty for advising projects is often lacking, and many of the current faculty are either master's-prepared or PhD-prepared and have little experience in the kind of clinical scholarship that is most helpful in advising the project. There is little in the way of resources for faculty to learn about the conduct of the DNP project in the field of the student's scholarship and considerable variation in the curriculum that would guide students through the project. Even the variation in titles for the project leads to dissemination issues given that university libraries cannot archive these projects under a separate category, and this reduces searchability. The call for a national dialogue is timely and can only help to clarify what the DNP project is and what it can achieve for health care.

References

Agency for Healthcare Research and Quality. (2015). *Selecting health outcome measures for clinical quality measurement.* Retrieved from http://www.qualitymeasures.ahrq.gov/tutorial/HealthOutcomeMeasure.aspx

Allison, M., & Kaye, J. (2005). *Strategic planning for nonprofit organizations.* Hoboken, NJ: Wiley.

American Association of Colleges of Nursing. (2004). *AACN position statement on the practice doctorate in nursing.* Washington, DC: Author.

American Association of Colleges of Nursing. (2006). *The essentials of doctoral education for advanced nursing practice.* Washington, DC: Author.

American Association of Colleges of Nursing. (2015). *The Doctor of Nursing Practice: Current Issues and Clarifying Recommendations Report from the Task Force on the Implementation of the DNP.* Washington, DC: Author. Retrieved from http://www.aacn.nche.edu/news/articles/2015/dnp-white-paper

Arline, K. (2015). *Direct costs versus indirect costs: Understanding each.* Retrieved from http://www.businessnewsdaily.com/5498-direct-costs-indirect-costs.html

Auerbach, D., Martsolf, G., Pearson, M., Taylor, E., Zaydman, M., Muchow, A., . . . Dower, C. (2014). *The DNP by 2015: A study of the institutional, political, and professional issues that facilitate or impede establishing a post-baccalaureate doctor of nursing practice program.* Washington, DC: RAND.

Baker, S., Baker, K., & Campbell, G. (2003). *The complete idiot's guide to project management.* Indianapolis, IN: Alpha.

Blase, K., Kiser, L., & Van Dyke, M. (2013). *The Hexagon Tool: Exploring context.* Chapel Hill, NC: National Implementation Research Network, FPG Child Development Institute, University of North Carolina at Chapel Hill.

Boyd, D. M., & Ellison, N. B. (2007). Social network sites: Definition, history, and scholarship. *Journal of Computer-Mediated Communication, 13*(1), article 11. Retrieved from http://jcmc.indiana.edu/vol13/issue1/boyd.ellison.html

Boyer, E. (1990). *Scholarship reconsidered: Priorities of the professoriate.* San Francisco, CA: Jossey-Bass.

Boyer, E. L. (1996). Clinical practice as scholarship. *Holistic Nursing Practice, 10*(3), 1–6.

Brecker Associates, Inc. (2001). *Quality-based problem-solving/process improvement.* Retrieved from http://www.brecker.com/quality.htm

Bright Hub Project Management. (2012). *Examples of project scope statements.* Retrieved from http://www.brighthubpm.com/project-planning/57950-example -and-evaluation-of-project-scope-statements/

Burroughs, C., & Wood, F. (2000). *Measuring the difference: Guide to planning and evaluation of health information outreach.* Seattle, WA: National Network of Libraries of Medicine.

Casey, K. (2007). *Development of an innovative staffing model: Nurse practitioner (NP) hospitalist/intensivist* (Unpublished DNP scholarly project paper). University of Minnesota School of Nursing, Minneapolis.

Duke University Department of Community and Family Medicine. (2014). *Patient safety-quality improvement: What is quality improvement?* Retrieved from http:// patientsafetyed.duhs.duke.edu/module_a/module_overview.html

DMAIC versus DMADV. (2012). *sixsigma.* Retrieved from http://www.sixsigma .com/new-to-six-sigma/design-for-six-sigma-dfss/dmaic-versus-dmadv/

Edwardson, S. (2009, January 14). *MN/DNP colloquium.* Colloquium conducted at the University of Minnesota School of Nursing, Minneapolis.

Eyre, E. (2015). *Forming, storming, norming, and performing: Understanding the stages of team formation.* Retrieved from http://www.mindtools.com/pages /article/newLDR_86.htm

Facione, P., & Facione, N. (2009). *The holistic critical thinking rubric.* Retrieved from http://npiis.hodges.edu/IE/documents/forms/Holistic_Critical_Thinking _Scoring_Rubric.pdf

Frick, K., Cohen, C., & Stone, P. (2013). Analyzing economic outcomes in advanced practice nursing. In R. Kleinpell (Ed.), *Outcome assessment in advanced practice nursing* (3rd ed., pp. 45–73). New York, NY: Springer.

Fulton, J., & Lyon, B. (2005). The need for some sense making: The doctor of nursing practice. *Online Journal of Nursing, 10*(3). Retrieved from http:// nursingworld.org/MainMenuCategories/ANAMarketplace/ANAPeriodicals /OJIN/TableofContents/Volume102005/No3Sept05/tpc28_316027.aspx

GE. (2012). *What is six sigma?* Retrieved from http://www.ge.com/en/company /companyinfo/quality/whatis.htm

Grimshaw, J., Eccles, M., Lavis, J., Hill, S., & Squires, J. (2012). Knowledge translation of research findings. *Implementation Science, 2012*(7), 50. doi:10.1186/1748-5908-7-50. Retrieved from http://www.implementationscience.com/content/7/1/50

Guffey, M., & Loewy, D. (2015). *Business communication: Process and product* (8th ed.). Mason, OH: South-Western.

How to write an executive summary. (2012). *Ehow.com*. Retrieved from http://www.ehow.com/how_16566_write-executive-summary.html

Institute of Medicine. (2001). *Crossing the quality chasm: A new health system for the 21st century*. Washington, DC: National Academies Press.

Issel, L. (2013). *Health program planning and evaluation: A practical, systematic approach for community health* (2nd ed.). Burlington, MA: Jones & Bartlett Learning.

Joanna Briggs Institute. (2013). *A strategy for strengthening the translation of evidence into action across JBI Programs*. Retrieved from http://JoannaBriggs.org

Juran Institutes, Inc. (2009). *Juran Trilogy Model*. Retrieved from http://www.juran.com

Kelly, K. (2010). Is the DNP the answer to the nursing faculty shortage? Not likely! *Nursing Forum, 45*(4), 266–270.

Kleinpell, R. (Ed.). (2013). *Outcome assessment in advanced practice nursing* (3rd ed.). New York, NY: Springer.

Lavis, J., Robertson, D., Woodside, J., McLeod, C., & Abelson, J. (2003). How can research organizations more effectively transfer research knowledge to decision makers? *Milbank Quarterly, 18*(2), 221–248.

Lewis, J. (2007). *Fundamentals of project management* (3rd ed.). New York, NY: American Management Association.

Luecke, R. (2004). *Managing projects large and small*. Boston, MA: Harvard Business School Press.

Mahn-DiNicola, V. A. (2014). Outcomes evaluation and performance improvement: Using data and information technology to improve practice. In A. Hamric, J. Spross, & C. Hanson (Eds.), *Advanced practice nursing: An integrative approach* (5th ed., pp. 645–683). St. Louis, MO: Elsevier Saunders.

Manktelow, J. (2015). *SWOT analysis—understanding strengths, weaknesses, opportunities and threats*. Retrieved from http://www.ventes-marketing.com/References/Marketing%20strategique/SWOT%20Analysis.pdf

Mind Tools. (2009). *The Mind Tools e-book* (6th ed.). London, England: Author.

Mind Tools. (2015a). *Stakeholder analysis, winning support for your projects*. Retrieved from https://www.mindtools.com/pages/article/newPPM_07.htm

Mind Tools. (2015b). SWOT Analysis Discover New Opportunities, Manage and Eliminate Threats. Retrieved from https://www.mindtools.com/pages/article/newTMC_05.htm

National Organization of Nurse Practitioner Faculties. (2007). *NONPF recommended criteria for NP scholarly projects in the practice doctorate program*. Retrieved from http://www.nonpf.org/associations/10789/files/ScholarlyProjectCriteria.pdf

National Organization of Nurse Practitioner Faculties. (2013). *Titling of the doctor of nursing practice project.* Retrieved from http://www.nonpf.org/search/all .asp?bst=titling+of+the+Doctor+of+Nursing+Practice+project

Olney, C., & Barnes, S. (2006). *Including evaluation in outreach project planning.* Seattle, WA: National Network of Libraries of Medicine.

Olney, C., & Barnes, S. (2013). *Collecting and analyzing evaluation data* (2nd ed., booklet 3). Seattle, WA: National Network of Libraries of Medicine.

Phelps, M. R., & Gerbasi, F. (2009). Accreditation requirements for practice doctorates in 14 health care professions. *AANA Journal, 77*(1), 19–26.

Polit, D., & Beck, C. (2012). *Nursing research: Generating and assessing evidence for nursing practice* (9th ed.). Philadelphia, PA: Wolters Kluwer/Lippincott Williams & Wilkins.

Project closure—whether your 1st or 21st project, successful completion involves a few important steps. . . . (2014). *Mastering-Project-Management.com.* Retrieved from http://www.mastering-project-management.com/project-closure.html

The Project Proposal Toolkit. (2015). Retrieved from http://project-proposal .casual.pm/

Regents of the University of Minnesota. (2015). *Conducting a needs assessment.* Retrieved from https://cyfernetsearch.org/

Ross, J. (2009). *Total quality management.* Retrieved from http://totalquality management.wordpress.com/2009/06/07/dr-joseph-juran/

Rouda, R., & Kusy, M. (1995). *Development of human resources part 2: Needs assessment, the first step.* Technical Association of the Pulp and Paper Industry. Retrieved from http://alumnus.caltech.edu/~rouda/T2_NA.html

San Jose State Department of Economics. (n.d.). *An introduction to cost benefit analysis.* Retrieved from http://www.sjsu.edu/faculty/watkins/cba.htm

Smith, C. (2015a). *Stakeholder analysis, winning support for your projects.* Retrieved from http://Mindtools.com/pages/article/newPPM-07htm

Smith, C. (2015b). *Work breakdown structures: Mapping out the work within a project.* Retrieved from http://www.mindtools.com/pages/article/newPPM_91 .htm

Taylor-Power, E., & Henert, E. (2008). *Developing a logic model: Teaching and training guide.* Madison, WI: University of Wisconsin Extension.

Taylor-Powell, E., & Henert, E. (2014). *Developing a logic model: Teaching and training guide.* Retrieved from http://www.uwex.edu/ces/pdande/evaluation/pdf /lmguidecomplete.pdf

Taylor-Powell, E., & Renner, M. (2003). *Analyzing qualitative data.* Madison, WI: Cooperative Extension Publishing.

Thomas, J. (1985). Force field analysis: A new way to evaluate your strategy. *Long Range Planning, 18*(6), 54–59.

U.S. Department of Health and Human Services. (2012). *What's changing and when.* Retrieved from http://www.healthcare.gov/law/timeline/

U.S. Department of Health and Human Services. (2013). *2013 Annual progress report to Congress: National Strategy for Quality Improvement in Health Care.* Retrieved from http://www.AHRQ.gov/workingforquality/reports/annual-reports

U.S. Department of Health and Human Services, Health Resources and Services Administration. (2011). *Quality improvement*. Retrieved from http://www.hrsa .gov/quality/toolbox/methodology/qualityimprovement/

Waddick, P. (2010). *Six sigma DMAIC quick reference: Define phase*. Retrieved from http://www.isixsigma.com/new-to-six-sigma/dmaic/six-sigma-dmaic-quick -reference/

W. K. Kellogg Foundation. (2004a). *Evaluation handbook*. Battle Creek, MI: Author.

W. K. Kellogg Foundation. (2004b). *Logic model development guide*. Battle Creek, MI: Author.

Zaccagnini, M. (2007). *The development of a computer resourced communication center in a long-term care facility* (Unpublished DNP scholarly project paper). University of Minnesota, Minneapolis.

Development of a Computer Assisted Communication Center in a Long-Term Care Facility

Provided by Clinical Nurse Specialist: Mary Zaccagnini

Abstract

There is evidence to support the fact that many residents of long-term care facilities experience loneliness and social isolation. This state is consequently linked to depression, cognitive decline, and an increase in illness and mortality. Conversely, social and cognitive activity is responsible for an improvement in these conditions. This scholarly project will attempt to demonstrate that by using computers to improve socialization and communication, the result in the short term would be a decrease in loneliness and an increase in socialization; a long-term result would be a decrease in loneliness, decrease in depression, and an improvement or stabilization of cognitive status. For purposes of the timeline for this project, the short-term outcomes will be the focus.

The focus of this project was to introduce computer access and education to a sample of 12 residents in a long-term care facility. The participating residents were assessed pre- and postintervention using the University of California, Los Angeles (UCLA) Loneliness Scale, which has been evaluated for validity and reliability. Additionally, the residents were monitored by a sign-in log for the amount of times they used the computer for e-mail or Internet purposes. The established outcomes were to decrease loneliness and isolation and increase socialization through the use of the computer.

The analysis consisted of evaluating the comparison of preintervention scores minus postintervention scores, with a goal of decreasing loneliness, as indicated by a 2-point decrease in score. The goal of computer use was that each resident would access the computer twice during the project. A paired t-test demonstrated a mean decrease in loneliness score of 4.17, with the two-tailed P value equaling 0.0028. Using a one-sample t-test for the mean difference of login revealed an actual mean of 6.33 with a P value equaling 0.0107. These results indicated a statistical significance. Additionally, several anecdotal evaluative statements and observations from participants, staff, and team members provided evidence of clinical significance.

An Electronic Health Record Redesign as a Strategy for Optimal Pediatric Asthma Care Delivery

Provided by Nurse Practitioner: Catherine J. Miller

Abstract

Introduction: The economic impact of poorly controlled asthma is significant and includes unanticipated clinic and emergency department visits, missed days from school/work, and limitations of activities. Asthma action plans (AAPs) are one strategy to improve outcomes. This project explores the feasibility, optimal format, and documented use of an electronic AAP tool within a regional health system's primary care electronic health record (EHR).

Method: Project was directed toward patients 5–17 years of age and diagnosed with mild to moderate persistent asthma who received primary healthcare services within a regional health system. Excluded were patients with severe asthma or with complex or comorbid conditions. The method used a one group prospective pretest/posttest design and qualitative data gained from user feedback regarding the tool's readability, clarity, and likelihood to use.

Results: Redesigned AAPs accessed in an EHR increased provider use from 2% to 54.7%.

Discussion: Improved visibility increases the likelihood the AAP is completed, updated, and shared with families. Findings show promise for the contributions of AAPs toward improved asthma symptom control and self-management.

Key Words: asthma, pediatric, asthma management, action plan, electronic health record

Implementation of Perioperative Blood Glucose Protocol (PBGP) in Diabetic Patients Undergoing Cardiac Surgery

Provided by Certified Registered Nurse Anesthetist:
Dan Lovinaria

Abstract

Hyperglycemia has been associated with increased postsurgical wound infection (SWI), increased hospital length of stay (LOS), and surgical complications, including increased morbidity and decreased long-term survival. The risks are significantly higher for patients undergoing cardiac surgery when blood glucose (BG) is elevated. Perioperative BG control can be difficult during cardiac surgery because of the combination of counterregulatory stress response and cardiopulmonary bypass, which induce profound hyperglycemia, as well as insulin resistance and deficiency. It is well documented that an increased incidence of deep wound infections in diabetic patients undergoing cardiac surgery was reduced by controlling mean perioperative BG levels below 200mg/dL. Recent studies have shown that intensive insulin therapy not only reduced overall in-hospital mortality but also decreased bloodstream infections and intensive care LOS. This doctor of nursing practice scholarly project implemented a perioperative blood glucose protocol (PBGP) in diabetic patients undergoing cardiac surgery. All diabetic patients undergoing cardiac surgery were enrolled in the PBGP. BG therapeutic level is maintained throughout the perioperative and during their LOS. LOS was measured pre- and postimplementation of PBGP program.

Implementation of a Group Prenatal Care Model at an Urban Women's Clinic

Provided by Nurse Midwife: Heather Jelinek

Abstract

Improvements that focus on providing care that is women centered, including more comprehensive health promotion and encouraging greater participation on the part of women and their families, have been recommended in a number of critiques of standard prenatal care. Evidence supports the use of group models of prenatal care that incorporate existing prenatal care standards of ACOG, AAP, and ICSI within the context of a group of 8 to 12 pregnant women and their partners. Group prenatal care has been associated with a reduced rate of preterm birth, a reduced incidence of low-birth-weight infants, and increased satisfaction with prenatal care. The goal of this project was to pilot a group prenatal care program to evaluate its feasibility as an ongoing prenatal care model and also assess whether group care meets the needs of the women and providers at the clinic. Adequate recruitment demonstrated that the benefits and scheduling of group prenatal care appealed to the pregnant population at the clinic. Clinical outcome data for the participants in group prenatal care differed from the average midwifery patient but could not be statistically analyzed because of the small sample size. The women and families who participated in group prenatal care evaluated the program positively on the program evaluation survey. They expressed that experiencing their care with other expectant families enhanced both their feelings of support and their learning of pregnancy-related topics, which mirrored the benefits of group care in the literature. The data from the Patient Participation and Satisfaction Questionnaire (PPSQ) indicated that the participants in group prenatal care were both satisfied with their prenatal care and felt themselves to be actively participating in their care. Shared wisdom was seen as a benefit to patients and providers alike. The successful implementation of this model demonstrated the feasibility of offering a sustainable group prenatal care model at the clinic and may be further generalized to other clinics.

DNP Scholarly Project Process Model

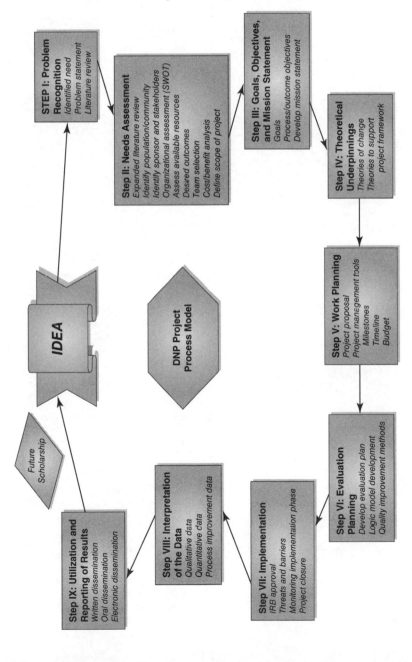

Figure 10-2 DNP Project Process Model

Index

Note: Page numbers followed by *f* or *t* indicate materials in figures or tables, respectively.